MW01248117

HOWEVER LONG
IT TAKES

"We got this, Mom"

Judy Clark

ISBN 979-8-89243-361-7 (paperback)
ISBN 979-8-89243-362-4 (digital)

Christian Faith Publishing
832 Park Avenue
Meadville, PA 16335
www.christianfaithpublishing.com

Printed in the United States of America

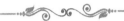

This year I'm going to write a book. Words I genuinely surprised myself by speaking. I feel there's a story within me that needs to be shared. Maybe my adventure can help another gain some understanding in living with and caring for a brain injured loved one. It will also allow my family to relive the last four and a half years shared with my mother following her cerebral bleed and multiple cranial surgeries. These end-of-life years with my mother are truly the most revered years of my entire life. Living my life backward may have increased my depth of compassion in my forty-plus years of nursing.

> Inside each of us is a story.
> My mother's story is one that truly needs to be
>   shared.
> They say a life recorded is twice precious—
> first the experience itself and then the memory
>   of it.

I've recorded very little of my mother's first eighty-eight years, but the last four-plus years are in print. The innocence of her altered brain status is too precious not to be shared. The burden she carried was too heavy to carry alone. The conversations we had are too memorable to forget. The sadness is that she didn't remember it the first time around. Almost everything was happening for the first time in her world. It was hard to imagine starting over with life experiences at the age of eighty-eight.

Where do I start, and how do I start? What should I call my book? Many titles have been used, so how can I pick a title that hasn't been used many times over? How about this? I call my book *243 Postcards*. That wasn't what my story was going to be about, but it may be where the real story started. 243 postcards may hold the secret that bonded me so closely to the woman who gave me life. I wondered if she ever knew just what each postcard meant to a daughter away from home at school. In hindsight, I honestly think she did. How do I know this, for we never really discussed the postcards? Because she didn't stop sending them. Even on days she didn't have much to say, she would write anyway. She would write to tell me that she didn't have much to say—but I still received a postcard from those days also. Somedays she used pencil, somedays a pen, but they came a few every week.

I went into nursing school right after graduation. It was a hospital school of nursing, so it was quite a challenge to me. We stayed in the residence, with classes in the afternoon, and working on the nursing units in the mornings. We were "away from home" and monitored by a "housemother" who walked the halls of the residence and enforced the rules. We were to be in the residence by 8 pm, and no guests were to go beyond the large guest and living room on the first floor. It was a different time than the coed dorms and college life of today. Mail was received in a small wooden box in the housemother's office. Several times a week, there would be my solitary postcard sitting in the little box. I seldom received any other mail, but I did not need any other mail. I had a mother that wrote a postcard about the life on the farm several times a week. I do not think she knew that I kept every single one. I spent eleven weeks living away from home at a psychiatric institution, and I received twenty-one postcards there. I had a thirteen-week affiliation at a children's hospital, and she sent twenty-four of them there. While I spent four weeks at a rehabilitation facility, eight postcards found their way to me there also. I don't think she knew how many she wrote. I wish we had discussed the bond that was built from the loyal mailings of those postcards. I still have every card she sent me.

I love you, Mom. You believed in me.

My parents had encouraged and allowed me to apply into a nursing school, back when times were different. I finished thirty-six months of hospital-based nurses training, without a student loan. My nursing education was entirely paid for by my dad. I graduated and passed my state boards without owing a cent. I was so blessed.

My nursing class met for a fiftieth class reunion this year. I couldn't attend as I was with Mom here in Florida. They sent me a pamphlet they created about everyone in the class. As I read about the girls, I looked over at my Mom. I then realized I had no one to talk to about the updated stories. She was the only one who knew the girls I went to school with. She went through every week with me. She had met all the girls I lived with during those three years. I read the pamphlet and couldn't tell her about anyone in it. I couldn't even read her the story on me. My story had a picture of me with Mom, stating that I had been her caretaker for several years.

My youngest son, Brian, had told her that I was a nurse many times. She responded that she had a daughter that was a nurse. Brian made it possible to take care of my mother, his grandmother, at home for the rest of her life. I think it would have been too overwhelming if I didn't have him available—any hour of the night or day. We never challenged or confronted her with reality. We climbed into her world and made ourselves comfortable. She was content with our presence in her world, more than she was in ours. She knew I was always familiar and wanted me in her vision. Bri was my relief pitcher and her knight in neon work shirts. This seemed to be as close to acknowledgement as we would get, and we accepted that. She couldn't remember, and she would say "I should know, but I don't." It's okay, Mom. We know. We will remember for you.

I have three younger sisters, and my dad had previously purchased a farm from his uncle's estate sale. Although he never considered himself a gambling man, or a risk taker, I must disagree. After all, this man bought a farm with a wife and 4 daughters. He always told everyone that "the boys will come later," and they did.

He qualified for exemption from the draft. He signed up feeling it was his patriotic duty. He served two years, with one year in Europe. He told me the transportation to his military assignment in

Europe took thirteen days—by boat. He also added he was physically sick most of the trip. I guess his first ocean trip was not fun.

During his military service he was quite homesick. After all, here's a farm boy far from home with strangers in a foreign country. He started to play volleyball with a team on the military base. This kept him physically toned but mostly it kept his mind off being homesick.

He was a highly intelligent man. He would help me with Algebra homework by checking my answer with math. It did not look anything like my Algebra problem, but he always come up with the right answer without ever learning Algebra. He had failed two grades in school. I don't know what the problem was in school because I've never met another man with his level of common sense.

He had strong morals and intense convictions. He was opinionated. Oh, was he ever opinionated—but he earned that privilege. He was devoted to his family. He worked hard, extremely hard, his entire life. Even on the day that he bought the farm of his dreams at a public auction, he left for work to report for the evening shift at the Steel Mill. He was always working while we were growing up.

My father was the dominant person in our family and in my life.

He didn't tell me how to live. He lived and let me watch him do it.

He loved his grandchildren. He always took time for them. He inquired about their life, their jobs, and their activities. He showed he cared. He didn't tell any of us he loved us…it seemed he didn't have to. Every action, every example, every lesson from this man left each daughter, every grandchild with the knowledge that they were dearly loved. He was respected. He was revered. He was a provider that loved our mother. He took care of her, provided for her later years, and sheltered her from big decisions, bill paying, and financial obligations. This was wonderful. It was the way of his era. The thing it didn't do was inform our mother how to do this for herself, with his demise. After my father died, we discovered my mother had never balanced her checkbook. She felt there was always enough money deposited to cover what she withdrew or spent. I guess we weren't aware of how she did things until her health changed. She got by, so no problem was ever noticed. My younger sister, Jane, would soon be challenged.

A year or so after my father died, Mother heard that her grandson Mark had been looking to buy a farm, or more property. Mom presented him with the option to buy the family farm instead. We knew the farm was more than she could handle, and the two sets of stairs in the house were an issue as Mom aged. They were steep and short. I can assure you they would never have met the specifications put on construction in our era.

Her grandson loved the prospect of buying the family farm. She loved the thought that the farm our father loved would remain in the family. Mark grew up next to the farm and was always walking the short distance up to the farmhouse with his twin brother Matt. I can remember my mother telling me that they could stay "seventeen minutes." Somedays they could stay "fourteen minutes," always limitations put on their visit time by their mother, my sister Jane.

When asked where she would live if she sold the farm, she said she could go into the "Highrise or something." Rather than have her in a Senior Highrise, her family members encouraged her to set a trailer up on the farm. Several of her grandsons, their friends, and other family members decided to start the set up for her upcoming mobile home. My sister Jane took her shopping for her next "home" and she found one that suited her basic requests. Some changes had to be made, but the order was placed. The boys started preparing for her new home's arrival. The sight was chosen with sewer connection, water, electric, and propane tanks for heating and cooking. It would be positioned on the field located between the farmhouse and my sister Jane's house. The fact that it was during the winter in Pennsylvania, did not affect the family's preparation efforts. It was made more difficult with frozen ground, winter wind chills, and frigid hands during their work outside. The new home was delivered and the set up was initiated and completed. The family had built a wooden deck on the front and the back, giving her two porches to sit outside with her two beloved dogs. Our mother had packed what she wanted to move into her new home. A lot of extra belongings were put in a garage sale managed by my sisters.

To love is to place our happiness in the happiness of another.

This left her begin a brand-new chapter in her life. A clothes washer and dryer located on the main floor, right outside her bedroom. She no longer had to go down steep basement steps to wash and dry clothes. She no longer had to mount a long set of steep steps to go upstairs to her bedroom or bathroom, for now everything was on one level. She had picked a layout with a kitchen that opened into a large living area. She knew her home would be busy with family. Soon afterward, she purchased a car port, that kept her car out of the winter weather. It was set up right off the back-porch steps. Home was just as she wanted it, and she was so very content. She had moved into her new home in the spring.

The most important thing a father can do for his children is to love their mother. My father had that covered.

I now live five states away from my mother. I had just been back "home" and spent about six weeks with my mother in her mobile home. It was located on the farm where she and my dad had lived. The farm was still in the family and my mom's location was bordered on one side by her daughter Jane's home, and her grandson Mark and his family in the farmhouse on the other. It was summer. I had flown up to Pennsylvania to attend my niece, Sara's wedding. During my stay, I felt there was something different going on with my mother. It was difficult to figure out exactly what because it wasn't consistent. The changes in my mom's memory were quite notable. She had given up her volunteer work at Meals on Wheels and more recently quit the church bowling league that she had bowled on for many years. She said her balance had become too wobbly. In just this one half of a year, she had a bad fall on the ice in front of her back-porch steps. We figured she must have hit her head, or at least had a terrible jolt to her head from her fall. She did admit to having a lot of muscle discomfort from the twist of her fall. She had to be helped up and into the house by her granddaughter, Theresa. Her eyeglasses were badly bent and had to be adjusted by the eye doctor's office. My mother did not complain. She never wined. She didn't want to bother anyone, even if she needed help.

Just a few weeks later, she was driving her car and was almost home. She made a left-hand turn; unaware she was turning in front of an oncoming car. She was broadsided by this car, which was coming in the opposite direction. The hit was to the passenger door area. My mother didn't show any signs of injury or pain at the time. She also declined being checked out at the hospital. One of her grandsons had just happened at the accident sight and gave her a ride home, while another family member took care of giving the police report and having the car towed home. The police then came to the house to take her statement. The other car and its occupants had left. In the end, her car was totaled. Again, she didn't complain of any physical problems, so there were no red flags to draw attention to her condition.

In hindsight, we wonder if her head may have hit hard against the driver's door window. This would put the trauma to the left side of her head.

As we look back, it seemed that these two accidents may have been the cause of the changes in our mother's mental status. She had been started on a blood thinner many years earlier for a blood clot. A blood clot had affected her one eye and took half of the vision in that eye. She said it felt like her upper eye lid was only halfway open.

My nieces wedding was the last big social event my mother dressed and attended before all our lives changed. She was seated up front at the wedding of her granddaughter Sara to her fiancé Ty. She was escorted by the usher to her seat, and I was asked to please sit with her. The wedding was performed by a dear friend Carol. My sisters and I had "adopted" her as our fifth sister. Carol performed the most personal wedding ceremony that I ever witnessed.

At the reception, Mom stayed seated at the table with family, keeping conversation within a small group. In a different day or year, this lady would have been busy making sure everyone was comfortable and checking to see what needed done. She was comfortable in the kitchen and out of the limelight. I'm sure she would have been working with the servers of the food, but not this time. Not at this family event. Not this year. Not ever again.

No one realizes how beautiful it is to travel until they come home and can rest their head on the pillow next to their mother.

SOMETHING WAS CHANGING

Sara's wedding was the last event my mother could remember from the whole month of August. I had been staying with her for six weeks in her home in Pennsylvania. I had noticed a change in her ability to perform simple tasks that she has been doing for the better part of her eighty-eight years. She didn't want to make decisions and even had problems making simple choices like what food she was hungry for or what she wanted to wear that day. This was not the mother I remembered.

We had noticed signs of confusion and forgetfulness which had become more apparent during the previous year. She had trouble with names. She knew she was forgetful. She also knew that she was getting "wobbly," as she described it. She had already decided not to rejoin the church bowling league which she had been a member for many years. It was a group of older ladies, members of her church, who seldom broke one hundred with their scores. Mother did have an exceptional game at one time, where she threw five strikes in a row. She loved to talk about that game. The family always listened in wonderment, while wondering just how that game happened.

She used to bowl on an evening bowling team, but the last few years she had transferred to an afternoon team. She said she had become uncomfortable with driving after dark. I wonder if it had to do with the darkness, or did some confusion and disorientation increase in the evening hours? This group of women didn't bowl in any competition, they just had fun.

They always went out to eat after they had played. Later I learned she always ordered a BLT. I think she was unsure of the

1

menu, as I look back. When we dined out, she always had me order for her. She loved trying different foods, but she would never order it herself. She would get confused with too many choices. The BLT was a safe win, so she didn't need to fix something that worked. No one considered this an issue. They just thought she really like the bacon-lettuce-tomato sandwich. It wasn't something that was broken. It wasn't something that anyone questioned. I think this special lady had found a way to handle the subtle mental changes that she knew was occurring during her daily life. Changes were occurring, but my mother had developed a defense mechanism that shielded the changes. She covered her situation well.

She had volunteered at Meals on Wheels for many years. She would drive into town early in the morning when it was still dark. She was a "helper" with the meal preparation. One morning she drove into town but couldn't open the door of the building where the meals were prepared. It was either locked or difficult to open, and she was of the era that didn't use a cell phone. We had tried many times to get her to carry a cell phone in her purse, so she could contact someone if she needed to. She just couldn't seem to retain the directions to use it. So she sat out front of the building in her car. Pounding on the door went unnoticed. She sat for over an hour waiting for someone else to arrive and enter. This never happened so she then decided to drive home. What she didn't know was they had missed her and tried calling several numbers to see why she hadn't reported to help or reported off. She was driving home when her son-in-law, Dave, passed her. He was coming to find her. She was worked up, and so were the people who thought something had happened. I'm sure the anxiety she experienced this day was a determining factor in her decision to resign from working.

Right after my arrival in late June she showed me bruising along the entire left side of her body. She swore me to secrecy, promising not to tell my three sisters. If you are reading this Sisters, please respect her wishes and maintain my secret. She apparently got up to go to the bathroom during the night. She somehow bumped into the door to her bedroom and slid down the wall. Her total left hip and thigh were black and blue, along with her inner legs. She said her lower leg had hurt, but it was getting a little better. She hesitated to tell me but felt maybe she should. I sensed she knew I would see the bruising anyway. Half of her body was purple or yellow, it would be impossible to not notice. Maybe she had other falls and felt someone should know, this time.

She is very content in her mobile home…and seemed quite comfortable. She lives with her two beloved dogs, Mickie and Annie. She hasn't been driving as she did. Family have been taking her shopping. She does drive about half mile to the church where she has been so active.

Since she had been on medication that thinned her blood for many years, skin tears would bleed quickly, and she did bruise easily. Otherwise, her physical health seemed good. She stayed active and loved mowing her own yard with her riding mower. She wore her pink Pirate Baseball hat each time, along with her oversize sunglasses. When summer came, she planted flowers and set out lawn decor that she had used at the farmhouse.

Do what you can, with what you have, where you are.

LIFE STARTS SPINNING
OFF BALANCE

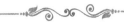

I t is a warm summer. One evening I killed seventeen flies within five minutes on her ceiling. She kept saying she couldn't see them. She lets her doors open for the dogs, and all the flies come in.

I soaked her feet and cut her toenails. She says she wants a home permanent to curl her hair before I return to my own home. She likes having her hair done.

She watches TV but falls asleep while sitting up. She watches a Pirates Baseball game but admits she doesn't know who won or what the score was. So often she asks me, "What am I trying to say?" And so I complete it for her. I thought maybe I could get her to come back down to my home in Florida with me, but she said, "Someday, just not yet." She said she wants to come down later. I'm looking to return to my home toward the end of August.

I'm reminded of my visit with her just last summer. We took several different weekends and traveled to family campsites. We found our way to the Rattay camp named "Thumbs Up." We had spent the day along the river and enjoying family comrade.

On another weekend we went to the Geltz Camp, named "Our Place," which is deep in the mountains.

One more weekend we traveled to see a good friend, Ms. Doris, and visit a campground where my son, Brian, was staying while he worked in the Pittsburgh area. We had a really good time together that summer, as we always do. Mom did mention that we didn't have to do that again for a while. It was a good driving distance compared to her few mile trips to town.

Sometimes happiness comes when we least expect it and in the most surprising ways. Keep your eyes open for the surprise.

When I was planning for my trip back to Florida that previous summer, she timidly asked me if there was room on my plane for "one more." Her question stopped me in my tracks. I told her there is always room for one more. She asked me how I knew that without checking? When I asked her if she wanted to come to Florida with me, she said she did. I planned for her two dogs to be kenneled in the neighborhood boarding facility and changed flights to put us both on the same flight at the same time. She flew down with me and we totally enjoyed time together. She was very content in the warm climate and we kept quite busy.

Her return flight back to her home that summer was traumatic for her. Even though I had her listed to need assistance boarding and exiting the plane, she later told me she worried the whole time in the air. What if there is no one to pick me up? What if I get lost at the airport? She told me she just fretted being by herself for the entire flight. I was at the gate on this end and watched as the stewardess came and put her on the plane first. She took her from my side, and they walked down the ramp together. When she arrived in Pittsburgh, her son-in-law Ken was waiting at the end of the ramp at her gate also. She said she was so happy to see him. He was in a place that wouldn't miss her.

I didn't think it would be that scary for her. I then decided I would never put her on a flight by herself again. I will have someone fly with her if the situation arises again—or I will fly with her myself. Never did I think my mother would have been so frightened to be alone. Ken and I had you covered, dear Mother, even if you didn't know it. You were safe, we knew exactly where you were while you were in the air, and on both ends of your trip.

The lady I took on those road trips was nothing like the lady we are with now. I stand in awe at what a difference a year has made.

Things are never quite like we expect them to be. Keep your eyes open for the bend in the road but remember-it's just a bend.

RESISTANCE TO LEAVE

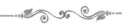

My flight back to my own home five states away was nearing. I was having problems packing, as I felt there was something changing in my mother's world. Her comments made it even more difficult to make plans to leave. She kept telling me that I could stay as long as I wanted. She would justify her request by telling me it gave her someone to talk to. I felt "pulled" in two directions.

We consulted her doctor. Her doctor ordered blood and urine tests, but they came back within normal range. All vital signs were within normal range. We couldn't obtain the urine specimen, so Jane was to try and obtain one from her and take it to the lab. This would rule out a urinary tract infection, which often causes confusion and behavior changes in the elderly.

Her health seemed good. I had found some partially burnt tea towels and a few burnt potholders in a box in her utility room. This gave me great concern. My mother has a gas stove in her home. The knobs are in the front, at waist height. I talked with my sisters and discussed the dangers that an open flame has apparently caused. My sister Jane is going to purchase an electric stove and have the one with the open flame removed. We felt we were extremely lucky thus far, but we weren't going to push the envelope. She would change the stoves out as soon as she finds an electric one to purchase.

I packed one morning and was taken to the airport. It was on a Wednesday, the end of August. Within hours I was back in my own home in Florida, but my concerns were still within the confines of my mother in her home. After I had left, Mom showed my sister Jane an onion on the kitchen counter. She told her that was what she had for lunch. She was only partially dressed at the time. She could not figure out how to put on her bra. Two of my sisters, Jane and Jody, decided she needed to be seen by her family doctor. They took her to the office and from there she was sent to the local hospital for a scan of her head.

The scan was positive for a cerebral bleed, and the blood was putting pressure on her brain. She was transferred to another hospital that very evening. This second hospital had a neurosurgeon on staff. My sisters found their way to that hospital later that night, but not without problems. Neither like to drive after dark, and then to find the hospital while trying to absorb the traumatic news they had just received about their mother left emotions high. They waited at the second hospital until my mother was admitted, then drove back home with heavy hearts.

I received the phone call about her condition Friday, which was one and half days since I had left. I didn't know how acute or active this bleed was and questioned if she would still be alive when I see her again. I was back on a plane the next day to be with her and my sisters. I arrived at the airport and was taken directly to the hospital by my sister Jody and her husband Ken. Since I travel with two small dogs, Ken stayed outside in the parking area with my travel companions which allowed me to enter the hospital. Our mother was being assessed for probable cranial surgery. The decision for surgery would have to be made by her 4 daughters, since she was not able to decide for herself. Did this all happen only two days after I had spent six or seven weeks with this lady? In just two days, our worlds were changed.

The axis of our world was in a hospital bed, no longer in control of her life.

How Our Lives Were Changing

This was our eighty-eight-year-old mother. Grandmother to fourteen children. She was also a great-grandmother to many and so loved by them all. We grew up a very close family. Just as we did, these kids loved spending time with this lady. Her cookie jar was always full. Her door was always open to their visits. She colored with them, put puzzles together, played jacks and pick up sticks, and took a great interest in their activities. She had big family meals on every holiday, and Christmas was an event she planned for all year long. This same lady had quite a following of kids she grand-mothered at the local elementary school, where she was the solitary cafeteria worker and food server for many years. Having worked in the small school during many of her own grandchildren's time there, she was called "Mawmaw" in the school. The children have since grown up, but the memory of "Mawmaw" during their school years has not been forgotten. My sisters and I have special stories relayed to us about moments that were very important to small children away from their own homes during school hours. Her daily presence in the elementary cafeteria was comforting to kids in the whole township. She took special time with anyone who needed her attention. Since her own grandchildren call her "Mawmaw," she became "Mawmaw" to a township of children. What a legacy she has as the "lunch lady."

To the world you are a mother. To our family, you are the world.

We don't know if we will still have this same lady. We don't know if we will have our same mother. We don't know if she will know us and be able to live alone, as she had been. So many unknowns. But there was also some "knowns."

8

The surgeon and his staff felt she was physically strong enough for surgery and relieving the pressure on her brain may allow a few more years in her life. We don't know what the quality of those years may be. These decisions do not come with any guarantee. The outcome is optimistic, but the team would not really know what they might find until they surgically enter her head. Four sisters felt our mother would want the chance to live longer. She loved life. She lived for her family and we loved having her in our lives. Maybe we were selfish, but we wanted to keep her longer. We didn't know what was ahead for her. We didn't know what was ahead for us. We didn't know what was ahead—period. If we don't opt for surgery, her outlook is dire, unstable, but obvious. We don't know what the Master's Plan is, but we felt our mother would make the choice to try. Consents were signed. Surgery was scheduled. The entire left side of her head was shaved in preparation for the operation.

Sometimes life hands you a situation when all you can do is put one foot in front of the other and live moment to moment. We have arrived at one of these situations.

The Surgery Date Was Set

Surgery was scheduled for Labor Day. This lady has four daughters, and three sons-in-law. We were all there waiting for her to return to us after surgery was finished. We were told it went well. We were told the blood clot was large and had been there quite a while. Apparently, it would bleed, then clot. Later it would bleed again, and clot. There were layers involved in the pressure being put on her brain. We were told she tolerated the surgery well. She was alert and talkative as soon as she came out of the anesthesia. We were all in awe. In checking her identity and neurological status, the staff of the hospital would ask her what her name was. They would then ask her when her birthday was. She would recite her birthdate, accurately every time. This proof of identity and neuro checks went on with every staff member who came into the unit to give her care. All at once, in her total state of innocence, she commented loudly, "If they can't remember my birthday, they need to write it down." Without letting her know how much her response entertained us, we could only smile out loud.

It's almost scary what and how much a beautiful smile can hide.
The world always looks brighter from behind a smile.

The first few post-op days was so encouraging, but then one day things changed. She was having trouble with her speech. She was seeing things in her room, things that the rest of us didn't see. She has a large U-shaped incision on the left side of her head with forty-nine staples. The skull bone had been lifted out for surgery, then replaced and held with 4 metal plates and screws.

Apparently, she was experiencing a form of seizure activity. We are told this is common when the brain is traumatized, as hers was.

Her brain was stressed for an unknown length of time with the pressure of the ever-increasing blood clot. To correct this condition, she had to be put under heavy anesthesia.

Next was the trauma to her brain during surgery to remove the clotted blood. She was started on a low dose of antiseizure medication and we waited to see how this would affect the desired outcome following the surgery. Whatever the end results are, whoever we are left with, she is our mother and we will take her home and love her as before.

She has a beloved canine companion. Her name is Mickie, and she has extremely limited vision, and our mother and Mickie are devoted to each other. When we return home from the hospital visits, driving my mother's car, Mickie keeps circling the car. She patiently waits for Mom to get out of the car and give her the beloved greeting she is used to. But Mother is in ICU in the hospital, so she doesn't get out of the car. Even after we lock the car for the night, Mickie waits for a door to open and our mother to get out and walk into the house. How do you explain to a heartbroken dog, where the lady of her life is? She didn't say goodbye. She just left for an appointment one day and didn't come back home. It makes we wonder how many pets are left in this situation with broken hearts, maybe thinking they did something wrong and were abandoned? How many wait and wait—for their loved ones to return for them?

I make it a point to talk to Mom's dog, and even more amazing, she is listening.

Along with this entire family and our mother, Mickie is also very traumatized. Mickie doesn't want to eat. After the first week, she is showing signs of failing to thrive. I sat down on the floor and talked with Mom's beloved canine companion. I promised her that we would bring Mom back home to her. I told her she had to eat so she would be at home waiting when Mom is discharged. I told her Mom would need her very much, along with her other dog Annie. I told her Mom has a long row of recovery to hoe, and Mom will need her help. I patiently explained to Mickie that she had to eat and stay healthy, for our mother would really need to see her when she comes home. Mickie rallied and started eating again. Her dog's hearts were breaking, for they didn't understand what happened to their beloved companion. She would take them in her car and drive to the Dairy Queen in the summer, purchase vanilla soft freeze ice cream, and bring it home. They would all have a dish together. It seemed that this lady lived to love her two dogs. She would buy many bags of certain dog treats. She chopped lunch meat up finely and mixed it into their dry dog food. She would not eat in front of them without giving them treats to eat also. They were always sitting next to her or lying at her feet. She talked to them all the time. One day she left with her daughters and didn't return. I can still see her giving them treats before she eats, then shake her finger and say "that's all, there isn't any more, that's it." I also remember that it wasn't true, there was always more, and those dogs both knew it. All they had to do was sit and look at Mom with their sad-eyed-dog stare.

Home from the Hospital

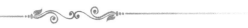

When we brought our mother home from the hospital two weeks later, her beloved canine companions, Mickie and Annie, were waiting for her.

In her first week, she has been admitted to home health services by a visit from the Admissions Nurse, then an RN came and drew blood and did an assessment, the Physical therapist came, the Occupational Therapist came, the Speech Therapist came, then the Physical therapist and RN made second visits—all within six days.

She is scheduled for a CT scan of her head in one week and to be seen by the Surgeon on the same day. She is then to be seen by her family doctor. Our mother has a healing incision on the left side of her head. She is not happy with all the therapists coming into her home, not a bit happy.

If you want to see a rainbow, you must put up with some rain. Mom is not pleased with "the rain"—she tenses up whenever one of the medical staff enter her home.

At Home for One Week

It is eighteen days since her cranial surgery and six days since we brought her home from the hospital. Our lady requires nonstop attention. With her altered thought processes, our mother does not realize that she has four daughters. Sister Jody is having problems dealing with the change she sees in her mother. Jo can admit she isn't handling it well. She offers to prepare food, wash dishes, or get us anything we need, but says she doesn't know how to deal with this other mother. She has difficulty trying to carry on a conversation with this newest version of our mother. Our first mother was so easy to talk to. Conversation flowed like sunshine and covered many topics, people, food, handicrafts, and stories of her great-grandchildren. This second mother needs conversation to be directed. She cannot answer questions, and there is no recognition of who she is talking to. There are no questions referencing children or grandchildren because if you don't have daughters, you just don't have offspring from non-existent kids. This is so difficult for most to accept. They were so important to their grandmother, and she showed such interest in all their lives. Now they have another grandmother that honestly has no idea who they are.

I understand the difficulty my sister is having. Caregivers come with all different abilities. Some can carry out the personal care, cleansing, feeding, and rehabilitation needed to support life. Some can acknowledge the lack of familiarity and accept the loss of abilities. Others reinforce the caregiver, providing the necessary materials or food needed to carry through all the days and nights. They entertain the caregiver with outside crafts or activities or just simply visit as company and offer good conversation. It takes many pulling together to enable all aspects of care needed when you keep a brain injured loved one in the home.

A bundle of sticks is always stronger than a single twig.

Some people sustain a head injury from a car accident and seem "just fine" right after the accident. They can adamantly state there is nothing wrong with them, then suddenly, they're having problems. Within a short period of time, they begin to get more and more confused. In a closed head injury, pressure builds up and damages' brain tissue. They wonder why they're doing some silly things. Why did they put their shoes in the refrigerator? Why did they put the milk in the closet? They have odd events, but they keep rationalizing them away.

The strongest souls have emerged out of suffering. These strong characters are seared with scars.

If you hand Mom a get-well card and it has been opened, she doesn't always know to take it out of the envelope. She reads the envelope and holds it. Today she said she was reading the card. When I ask her to read it to me, she didn't stay anything. I looked and she had it upside down. She is such a sweetheart. I ask her last night what inning the seventh inning stretch occurs in the baseball game. She thought awhile, then said, "I don't know." When I ask her how many innings the pirate game had, she answered with a question, "Seven?" Just then she looked at the game on the TV and said, "that guy is really running." She knows she can't converse as others, so she interjects the subject that is in front of her during the moment. I let it work. We take her subject and let it lead the conversation.

She doesn't like the therapy people coming in. She becomes quite anxious as she waits for them to arrive. Speech Therapy is coming in tomorrow.

I have her appointment set for October 1 to get her staples out. There are forty-nine staples in her scalp. We must get a CT scan of her head before the appointment. I have no doubt that all her tests are going to be great. She is using the inspirator that they gave her in the hospital. We've already been able to move the marker up, as she has improved. It used to provoke a coughing spell but now it doesn't.

I'm sure the fluid must be gone from her lungs. Yes, I'm an optimist. I don't know any other way.

Sometimes, you must bow your head, say a prayer, and weather the storm.

She is talking much more and recalling some things. She still doesn't remember where the bathroom or her bedroom is, as far as which direction to walk toward. She doesn't want anyone coming into her space. She won't sit outside on the porches when there is anyone around. She is so very content right here in her house beside me. I've been trying to get her to lay in her bed but she doesn't want to. She laid in her bed about seven minutes and had already stood up and had her walker. This is good but she won't call me for assistance. She just gets up and she is so off-balance. No matter how many times I ask her to call me when she's done in the bathroom or laying down, she won't. She gets up and says, "I didn't know where you were." She isn't dizzy, so she isn't aware that her balance has been affected. When she does start to lean toward a fall, she has no reaction to try and catch herself, or protect her head or body in a fall. I thought about a helmet during her ambulation. A section of bone was removed from her skull and replaced at the end of the surgery. This makes her head so vulnerable to injury should she fall. She sleeps in the recliner in the living room and the dogs and I sleep on the sofa. We have an empty bed on both ends of the mobile home. The empty beds remain empty all night long.

She is physically doing so very well and eating and cooperating. She is trying so hard. She will eat something every time I give it to her. Liquids is a little harder, for she won't drink unless it's put in her hand and told to drink it. She still doesn't initiate anything on her own. We are keeping her mind busy and causing her to think and try. Jody is bringing in food. Jane will do any shopping. They are here during most of their free time. My youngest sister, Jeani, makes stops on some evenings. She said she was coming out and bringing hoagies the other night. I had to explain to her how little mom is eating and how we are trying to get protein in her. One of her diagnosis was "malnutrition." We have a computer disc of her CT scan from the hospital when they found the hematoma, but I don't know how to open it. I guess all my years of working with the visiting nurses and all the years with gerontology was bringing me to this situation. Amazing how life works, isn't it? Or maybe I should give due credit to the Master's Plan. It is only opened and laid before us with his own timing. Has his plan now surfaced?

Jody brought over some old jeans and material and I told Mom we would start working on some Christmas stuff. She likes that. She just sits and watches me do things. When I sit on the sofa, she wants to sit there with me. I opened the laptop tonight and she watched it with me.

I know where I need to be, and I just can't be anywhere else. Mom is asleep on the recliner. I'm going to have to log onto my household bills and see where I am with that. I just haven't taken time for anything concerning myself or my life in another state since I climbed inside my mother's altered life. Certainly, since Labor Day this year, my priorities have changed.

This is a voyage we are on. It is a time of new discovery. We must see it through new eyes.

It's late September. This mother has been home eleven days. It's been twenty-three days since her surgery. I can't believe how little free time I have. Mom's appointment went well. Office staff took the staples from her head wound and she had another CT scan of her head. Apparently, nothing has changed since her last scan. She has a small amount of blood still in the cranial area, but the surgeon says he is watching it. He said it hasn't changed. She returns the end of October for another scan and appointment. She was weary with the travel today and the waiting for all involved. I decreased the RN visits and discharged the occupational therapy. I'm holding onto the speech and physical therapists. Mom isn't happy with any of them. She has developed an attachment to me. She is sleeping on the sofa now. When I go to bed, I wake her and toilet her, then she sleeps in her double bed and the dogs and I sleep on the twin mattress on the floor next to her. Often, she sits up in bed during the night and I hear her fret a little.

I say, "Mom, I'm right here."

She says, "Okay," and lies back down.

Her memory is attempting to return, but she apparently doesn't remember anything shortly after the wedding on August 2. She remembers nothing of the entire hospital stay or the day or so after we brought her home. She's using a walker, and the therapist is working with her with a cane, but she's not ready for the cane yet. Speech therapy is interesting as to what she can answer and what she can't. The puzzle sheets and questionnaire sheets all have different purposes in regaining her ability to find and use words. My thanks to Janice, the speech therapist, for working so well with my mother. We work with the work sheets when she is able.

What a trip you have taken us on Mother. You are driving our family caravan down an unknown road. We are traveling to an unknown destination. We may not know where we are going, but I can assure you, dear lady, that we are all on board.

I have her eating about every two or so hours. She is gaining strength and energy but the frequent eating sure isn't helping me at all. She weighed 142 before the hospital stay and 130 when she came home. Therapies will be in tomorrow, then Friday she has an appointment with her family doctor. We also have the appointment with the cardiologist coming up, along with the neurologist. Mom is trying to understand what happened to her. She is really working hard at sorting it out.

God made the world round so we would never be able to see too far down the road. Thank you for your foresight God.

Just managing "today" is enough for now.

Move on to the end of September. It's twenty-eight days post op, and sixteen days at home with our revised edition of our mother. I am in contact with her 24-7. Just as I start to see some improvement, she does something out of the perimeters of "normalcy." She put the large spoon from the gravy into the cottage cheese container and then into her mouth. Just as I think she has the direction within her house worked out, she heads in the wrong direction to go to the bathroom. She wants to do more—but walking from the table to the sofa tires her. She is tired of doing nothing, but she still can't work through simple things yet. I brought out the old maid card game and she finally was able to lay down pairs. We played Connect 4, but she couldn't get the concept of getting 4 in a row. She was upset when the checker would go the whole way to the bottom, instead of stopping somewhere in the middle, apparently where she wanted it to stop. She couldn't stop me from getting 4 in a row nor could she figure out how to get her 3 in a row. This game goes back on the shelf for a while, as it causes frustration and anxiety. We worked on "find a word" but altered the rules to just "find a letter," and she did get that. I tried some simple words with "find a word" and she did find them—with some help.

She shows absolutely no interest in the TV shows that she used to watch. She looks at the Pirate baseball game but doesn't really pay attention. Later in the afternoon, she becomes a little worse. In nursing homes, they call it "sun downing." As later afternoon occurs in her day, confusion seems to occur. I understand this is a time of day when she needs to go home, as the sun goes down. "Going home" is somewhere that we can't seem to find. In her confusion it is more of a comfortable safe place in her mind, than an actual physical place. This allows us to provide her this place, without leaving the area where we both reside. She will try to explain something to me that I can't make sense of. Last night she was trying to ask me how to "mark something on the wrong side—so we will know what it is—then when we sell it—like this blanket—but mark it so no one can see it." I ask her if she wanted to sell the blanket. She said "no—but I want to know how to do it—how to mark it on the inside." I couldn't figure it out—and she just got more frustrated.

Her speech has improved, and sister Jane is certainly her best cheerleader. When our mother has a good day, a good therapy, a good visit, or even a good minute, Jane has called it a "woo-hoo" event. Mom has started to refer to Jane as "woo-hoo." When Jane is walking up to Mom's mobile home, I will say, "Here comes woo-hoo." She knows exactly who I mean. Some people get a name, maybe not the one they were used to, but they get a name. I haven't received one yet, but I must remind myself that she does have a "brain injury." She has developed an "attachment" to me and if she can't see me, she gets up to find me. Her gait and balance are altered. She uses a walker with wheels but will tend to "drift" to the side. She is such a "fall risk" that I keep her within reach so I can catch her. She will sit up in bed at night and I can hear her.

I say, "Mom, we are all right here with you."

She says, "Oh, good, thank you, okay." She then lies back down. She knows her mind is affected so she doesn't want to be left alone. She still has a degree of confusion.

Referring to the brain, it is beyond my understanding as to how it functions. It is amazing. Different parts of the brain have different functions. The brain also has the ability to compensate for damaged sections and attempts to pick up the missing functions. It appears to function normally, then it "takes a turn and goes down a side street." Hopefully, as the seizures are controlled and the brain settles, it will all come back. She has no idea how to play solitaire which she did all the time when alone. She just sits and watches me and tries to help. She wants to do more but says "not now" to all my ideas. I cut her hair real short so it would be more even. It is growing back in on the operative side, but still long in length on the opposite side. It really looks cute, but it is nothing like the way she used to see her hair. I put mousse in it, and it kind of stands up on end. She turned down great-granddaughter Sophie's request to have a picture taken with her. She kept saying, "Not now." My guess is she wants to wait until she is pleased with her hairdo.

I witnessed her struggle and I feel so bad for her. I keep drawing pictures of what was wrong with her head and how her brain must heal. She remembers nothing of her hospital stay and most of the month before. Of course, she doesn't understand how she lost all that time without any memory. She won't go back to bed. She lies on the sofa until I go to bed. I then wake her and take her back to bed with me and the dogs.

The other night, she said, "When do you go to bed?"

I said, "Later than you, but I always take you back with me. I never leave you in another room."

She said, "Oh, thank you. I wasn't sure. I'm so glad."

Family does appreciate what I am doing, and they don't hesitate to ask how they can help. Sisters Jane and Jody often send in our lunches or suppers and come over often. From the farmhouse, granddaughter Jamey, who is married to Mark, sent down our supper another day. Jane gets anything we need from town and Jamey often calls me to see if I need anything brought home when she's in town. Jody brings over all kinds of supplies to keep me busy with sewing. She's always bringing over some homemade sweets or desserts.

Light is the task when many share the toil.

I worked with the speech therapist, Janice, when I was employed with the VNA, so she is quite familiar to me. She helps me with therapy sheets to work with our mother when she isn't visiting our home. I know this therapy is very important. Helping our mother with her speech is just one area of her work. She also works with reading comprehension and writing skills. I understand she also works to teach memory strategies. The work sheets she has our mother working with, in what I call her "homework" works toward these goals.

Grandson Lee was given a wheelchair for scrap. He just had it at his house and the kids played with it. He took it to work and welded it and fixed it. It works well for Mom when we leave the house for an appointment.

We are at the end of September. We are now twenty-nine days post op, and seventeen blessed days home with our recovering mother.

Another day of moving from the sofa to the chair to the kitchen to the chair and back to the sofa. We were up about 7:00 AM, so it's been a long day. Mom is constantly getting up and wanting to move. I don't think she is aware of the short periods of time she stays in one place. She is restless, but without any destination or plan. She was able to dress herself after morning care until she got to her pajama top. She couldn't figure out how to get her arms into the top. Later she had her fleece jacket off, and when she tried to put it back on, she had one arm down into the pocket. She wants to do more. She feels useless. She wants to help me do things, but she tires after walking from one place to another.

We sat on the front porch for a while this afternoon. She had on her jacket, her hat, and I took the heated blanket out with us.

She soon asked, "Aren't your legs cold? Where are your shoes?"

I said "Mom, are you ready to go in?"

She said, "Whenever you are," so we came in.

I heard what she wasn't saying.

Her endurance for activity has increased. I can see it, and the physical therapist comments on it. In her world, she only knows what she could do before her hospital stay. She still has trouble grasping the concept of the miracle of her surgery, so she doesn't see the miracle of her slow progress.

Her incision looks good. I had been using Vaseline on the incisional line. I cut her hair very short, so it didn't have the "Mohawk" appearance. I put a little coloring on the new growth to even it out. She saw it for the first time this morning and thought she looked awful. She thought the same thing when her hair was long on top and the sides and shaved on the entire left side of her head. I thought she looked beautiful, as did her other three daughters. Her one granddaughter, Heather, who is my youngest and only daughter, thought she looked beautiful as she had seen her own son, Gage, with the same type of incisional ink. Not only once, but twice, after tumor removal from his brain at a young age.

Sister Jean came out after supper. Mom barely ate. She said she didn't want any coleslaw for breakfast. I told her it was supper, not breakfast. I told her she would get a nutritional milkshake later. I took the dogs outside and Mom kept trying to see out the kitchen window. She said to Jean that she didn't like to let the dogs out before the kids get on the school bus.

I said, "Mom look at the clock and tell me what time it is?"

She looked and said, "Oh, it's 6:00."

I said, "It's six in the evening, Mom. The kids are already home from school and had supper."

We are going to increase her half antidepressant to a whole one tonight. She seems to have slipped into a lower mood than she was. I'm going to be a professional on depression in this lifetime.

If I'm dealing with Mom, I don't get to the phone. I also keep the volume on mine turned down real low because I can see where the noises from texts and phone calls bothers her. Even the dogs barking bothers her, and they never seemed to upset her before. Even the therapist noticed a more negative attitude today. I told her that was so far away from my mom's personality that it is very much a problem.

Oh, my dear mother. These are mountains that you are carrying. I honestly believe you were only supposed to climb them, not carry them.

Take my hand, Mom—together we got this.

I'm going to let Mom lay down on the sofa. She won't go to bed until I do, and she's asleep around eight every night. We have come to an agreement that she will sleep on the sofa and then I wake her when I go to bed and take her with me. I don't let the dogs get in bed with her, so they sleep on the floor area with me. I put a pillow down and tap on it for Mickie, and she comes over and lies down. Annie goes under the bed for most of the night.

Moving on to the beginning of October. We have been home for eighteen days now. Surgery of this beautiful lady was exactly one month ago.

I think Mom is just "getting through" the days. She doesn't show any emotion. She shows no enthusiasm. She's not interested in any activity, not even the Pirates baseball games. She still loses her way to the bathroom and heads the other way. She's laying on the sofa right now. She had been asleep, then woke up and didn't know what she was supposed to do. She just seems to do what I say—even when it comes to going to the bathroom. As soon as it starts to get dark, she wants the doors all locked and the blinds pulled. Speech therapy worked with her today. She left sheets of different topics to work with her. She won't be back for the week, so I teased Mom that she had "homework." She can only work with things for about half hour, and then she is weary.

She isn't pleased with the therapists coming into her home. Jane has tomorrow off. She wants to know if I want to get out for a while. I may take her up on it. Mom's lack of energy and inactivity can pull another's energy and initiative down. I want to stay positive in my interactions with this marvelous lady. I may need a day to recharge.

She seems withdrawn and depressed. She doesn't care to have any visitors. I am tiring, as my laptop just fell off my lap. I must have nodded off. I'm signing off, closing my laptop, and taking this lady and four dogs back to bed. Tomorrow is a brand-new day.

Sometimes we need someone to simply be there. Not to fix anything, or to do anything, but just to let us feel that we are cared for and supported.

Hello to another day. It's Thursday, and already two days into October. I got up with the dogs and toileted them all outside. I then helped my mother into the bathroom, then breakfast. She's using the walker and needs clues every time she goes into the bathroom. The walker is too wide for the doorway, so she must turn it sideways and walk in that way. There is a white sticker in the center of the handle of the walker, so I've showed Mom how to aim the white sticker to the doorway and pivot in. She does it well, except sometimes she forgets to put herself in the realm of the walker and then she ends up trying to push the walker from the side. She still needs very frequent verbal cues. She will stand up, and then ask which way she is going. She will stand and ask me where I want her to be. She pays no attention to the TV, and often closes her eyes and loses attention during visitors' conversation. She has no hunger or thirst, so that is a constant push.

Today I skipped her water pill and encouraged liquids. I thought maybe her energy and enthusiasm was compromised by some dehydration. It's the first time she has held the left side of her head and told me it hurt. There is some swelling on the left side today, so I pointed it out to Jo and Jane. We will watch. I gave her a Tylenol, and she fell asleep for several hours. That was truly a change, as I can never get her to even nap. When she woke it was late afternoon. Jane and I spent hours getting her to realize that it was "night." She kept wondering when the kids school bus would come. Then when Jane told her she would be getting her nighttime snack soon, she said "Jane, I just got up." I'm guessing, and it's just a guess, she didn't get a "Woo hoo" this time from Jane.

She has some new exercises from the therapist today—standing at the sink and working on her balance. She walks her with a cane, but she's a bit wobbly. Mom relies heavily on the walker. Jane and Jody stayed with her while I ran up to Walmart for a few hours. I bought some food and some sewing stuff. Joanne Fabrics is leaving lower Burrell and moving to the Mills shopping Mall. I am truly affected with their decision. I tease Mom a lot and joke with her. Some days it becomes easier because she smiles. Some days it's a lot of work. I keep telling my sisters not to give her the option of saying "no." They will ask her if she wants something to eat, or does she want something to drink. I know that answer is always "not now." I just sit it in front of her.

She hates getting a shower. I must remember that there was no shower at the farmhouse she lived in for so many years. Showers were not a daily ritual in her life. She told me it was so cold, and then she makes a shivering noise. I've told her if she drinks enough water, I won't have to rely on the shower to get water into her. Sometimes she gets my sarcasm if I keep it simple enough. Today I kept a tally and got one and a half quarts of water into her, and that was counting all the liquids (including coffee) from the waking moment to bedtime. It requires constantly pushing her. She doesn't want to do the exercises or do the speech papers and a lot of the time she just closes her eyes and shuts out the world. Hopefully the antidepressant will kick in.

She still isn't happy that therapies are coming into her home. I discharged the RN and occupational therapist, but we need the other two therapies—despite Mom's resistance.

I have sewing and craft stuff all over Mom's house again. I keep myself busy with sewing purses for the great-granddaughters, and now I'm making something in the bag-type for granddaughters. Mom has no interest. Jody comes over and spends time with me, but she tells me she still isn't handling Mom's status well. She wants her other mother back. Jean hasn't grabbed the reality of this lady's brain damage. She comes and visits, shows mother many pictures on her phone. Mother looks at all the pictures, nodding as she does. She has no questions about any of the pictures. She has no knowledge of who these pictures are. Jean gives names and descriptions, and mother just nods. Jean is encouraged by Mom's response to her pictures, not realizing that the response is automatic on my mother's part. Our mother has found a way to cover up her memory problem, enjoying the interaction and attention, not wanting to be excluded. It hasn't been all that long since she had surgery and yet her brain is fast forwarding defense mechanisms. These shield my mother from any embarrassment of being found out.

A creative mess is better than tidy idleness.

Jean calls and asks if I need anything. Jane comes up almost every day, does the grocery needs, works three days a week and sees the reality close hand. She keeps telling Mom that she needs her and wants to be with her. Mom seems to feel useless and thinks she should be doing something but doesn't have the energy. We need to realize that trying to talk, trying to remember and relearn, trying to think of what she wants to say truly takes a whole lot of work. It doesn't come as naturally as it used to. I keep telling Mom we all four met and discussed whether to put her through this surgery. I told her we wouldn't have consented if we hadn't expected a good outcome. I think sometimes she thinks there is more to it and just doesn't think it's worth the effort. She is better certain times of the day, rather than others. When she gets tired, everything goes downhill.

Granddaughter Angie-on-the-hill (I call her that because she lives up on the hill, across the road from the farm), who is married to Matt, came down today and told me I did a really good job on Mom's haircut. And that came from a beautician. Jamey brought down four pizza burgers for Mom's and my supper. I truly have a good family. I've told Mom that not only were all four of her daughters at the hospital the entire day of her surgery, but so were her three sons-in-law. She was amazed. Oddly enough, she seems to remember the sons-in-law, and still doesn't remember the daughters. Dave, married to Jane, is the son-in-law that mows her lawn. Mike, married to Jeani, is the one that took her and some other people (one being her daughter Jean) to the pirate baseball game, and Ken, married to Jody, is the son-in-law that picked her up at the airport. We know she refers to someone that lives on the corner of the yard that does her banking. This would be sister Jane. Mom hasn't put together the "banking lady" Jane and the Jane that lives in the house on the corner as the same person. In fact, she tells us "Dave lives in that house." We tell her Jane lives in part of the house, and we leave it at that.

Now just what Judy, Jane, Jody, or Jean brings to her mind in a memory, we have yet to find out. She is such a sweet lady to have to relearn so much. She's trying to write again. I can't imagine not being where I am. She is nonstop observation. I never want her to fall on my shift.

Tomorrow will be a brand-new day. We are ready. We will do it together. Bring it!

Already we are into the first week of October. Twenty-four days of recovering at home.

Mom is carrying on conversations much better now, and naming people. She is often initiating conversations which didn't happen at all previously. The great-grandkids that she has seen are flattered that she sometimes calls them by name. As we all look back, she had some tough days even before her hospital admission. Most often she has received prompting in what name to use. Physical therapy has started walking her with a cane, so we are to increase her endurance for walking, either with the walker or the cane. I've been sewing some Christmas gifts for her to give to the many girls in the family. She watches.

Tonight she said, "I'm going to bed and you go ahead and do what you're doing."

I said, "Are you going back to your bed?"

She kept walking toward the sofa and said, "No, I'm going to sleep right there until you go to bed." My dear mother has developed quite an attachment to me. She also remembered what our bedtime routine is every evening. This is a "woo-hoo." Where are you, sister Jane?

God does promise a safe landing, but not always a safe passage.

My sisters tease her that I am bossy, and she agrees and makes funny noises to imitate me. I try to keep it fun and humorous. We try joking and teasing with her—when it is appropriate. The physical therapist is young, has a one-year old boy and comes in bubbly and raving about the day, among other things. She is just a little hard to take and I chalk that up to "inexperience" and youth. An older person who is struggling with depression and relearning all the simple things that came easy before her surgery only becomes defensive and barely tolerant of what the therapist requires. I requested her to cut our visits down to one weekly but continue to guide us as to what to do. It is easy to compare yourself to those in your immediate environment. I think my mother is working hard to accept her own present appearance and limitations, acknowledging that she is advancing toward end of life. The therapist's excitable personality appears to be too much of a stimulant to this patient, our mother. She keeps asking Mom if she would like to see the mental health nurse. She informs her she may want to talk through some problems with the mental health therapist that she can't talk over with her family. That suggestion just makes my mother tighten up even more. She doesn't want her here, let alone inviting another service in. Mom has problems with simple conversation. The suggestion to "talk over her problems" with another stranger when this dear lady doesn't know what "her problems" even are, truly upset her.

I understand the therapist's suggestion. I understand that the offer for "someone that's not family" would give a more objective point of view. I can understand this. But it is not me that the mental health nurse is offered. I watch as the young therapist attempts to explain to my mother how this other stranger may be helpful. I wonder if she is even watching my mother's face? She has already overloaded her with conversation. Too much information put in multiple sentences has already left my mother far behind. She is now only hearing the end of her speech. My mother's defense has kicked in. She declines. She doesn't understand so she makes no changes.

This brings to mind one other time when I had taken my mother to the bank. She had social security direct deposit, so at least once a month she withdrew cash from her account. She did not have a charge card. She did not have a debit card. She paid with cash.

The teller said, "Mrs. Clark, have you considered our suggestion to make some changes to your account?"

She immediately responded, "No, I'm not making any changes."

I stopped my mother for a minute and inquired as to what the teller was asking. It seems she had been suggesting making a change in my mother's savings account into another type plan that would make more interest. She told me she could make more interest, and offered it to my mother every time she came in. I made an appointment for my sister and I, along with my mother, to meet with the bank staff. This was something that my mother declined, rather that deal with any change that she didn't understand.

The speech therapist is older and works for the VNA that I worked for many years ago. Her experience is so appreciated after the "rainbows and care bears" physical therapist.

Today Mom walked for the therapist and after she left, I walked her to the kitchen table for lunch. She couldn't hold her spoon properly, and then spilled her protein drink all over the table. I just downplayed it and cleaned it up. I now realize she does best with the little green coffee cup that she always uses, for the other ones have skinnier handles and they roll in her right hand. She had 4 club crackers with chicken salad on, and some cottage cheese and peaches. She was trying to pick her crackers up with her fork, using the spoon in her left hand to help slide the cracker onto the fork. Of course, that cracker fell on her clothes. She worked with the fork and spoon until she ate the crackers and salad. Her speech and attempts at conversation were not making sense, so I brought her in and had her lay down on the sofa. I put a blanket over the window above the sofa, and then pushed the recliner up against the sofa, and sat down. I sat there until she fell asleep.

I sat and embroidered, and when she would start to get up, I said, "Mom, I'm right here, go back to sleep."

She said, "Oh, okay," and she did.

I must lay or sit right beside her when she naps, or she won't stay. I realize she has no concept of what time of the day it is.

We will keep pushing forward, chipping away at the negative feelings and helping the brain to heal from the damage the blood clot did. She is the dearest patient I have ever had, and I attempt to payback for the sixty-seven years she invested in me. My sisters are grateful that we have found a way to keep her at home. I was the obvious choice as caregiver. I have no spouse, no dependent family members living with me, and possibly forty-four years of nursing experience in my back pocket. My itinerary put me at the front of the line of applicants. In Florida, I live within walking distance of my son Brian, who is single. I see that most were unable to handle her in their home, or even in mother's home. Jane and Jean still work outside the home, and Jody is busy raising two of her granddaughters. I am where I am meant to be.

God has placed you where you're at in this very moment for a reason. Remember that and trust He is working everything out. I must let go—and let life happen

The second week of October puts us at twenty-eight days, four full weeks working at recovery at home. Has it really been just four weeks? Has it not been a long four weeks? It went fast, but it went slow. How is that possible? These questions come from myself, who is standing outside and looking into my mother's world. Just how it looks for my mother through her compromised vision, through her compromised mental state, through her confusion as to who she is, where she is, and why. Dear Mother, my heart aches for you. Take my hand, together we got this.

"It's a wonderful day in the neighborhood." That's what I tell Mom every morning as she has breakfast sitting at the kitchen table and gazing out at the fields. Pittsburgh's Mr. Rodgers has left us with some special sayings and many happy memories.

I decided to send out a little group email as an update on this amazing eighty-eight-year young lady. You will see that emails are mixed in with the story I'm writing. You will see how some of the story was recorded during life with my mother, while other memories are recorded after her departure. I've never written a book, so bear with me. I have many years of nursing in my pocket, so I'm not afraid to lead in that field.

She is now sporting a hairstyle like Kolt and Nickolas, two of her great-grandsons. She says it looks good on them, says it looks terrible on her.

I asked Mom whose birthday it was this morning, since it was October 11.

She thought long and hard, and then said, "I think it's Kens."

I told her she was right, and she won a dish of frosted flakes with half banana and protein powder sprinkled on. A few minutes later I said something to her, and then ask, "Now what do I win?"

She told me I won a cup of coffee. Ken is one of her sons-in-law. She not only remembered his name, she remembered his birthday.

I'm still not called by name, and without causing stress in her day, I'm pretty darn sure she has no idea when my birthday is, even though she was there. She was right up front, sort of the VIP involved in my entrance into this world.

The ability for her to give comebacks to some statements is wonderful news. She is sitting and carrying on conversations with family. This afternoon we watched a little dune buggy in the field up above the road. It was left sitting there all alone. After I pointed it out to my mother, she often walked with her walker over to the window or door and checked to see if it was still there. I informed her that someone just drove the dune buggy up the hill with a little white dog bouncing along beside them.

She said, "It must be Jackson driving it." (Jackson is another of her great-grandsons that live within walking distance of Mom's home. I have been informed it was probably the puppy Jagger running with him.) I was amazed that she just came up with Jackson's name. She was correct.

Sophie and Sam, grand twins of Janes, came up to see Mom this evening. Mother carried on a conversation with Sam telling him the whole story of the dune buggy happenings of the afternoon. She told him about the buggy, the driver, and also how the dog was running alongside. This was so amazing. Her memory is improving, and her conversation skills are improving. She is like an unopened package at times. You can guess what might be inside, but there is no way to know until the contents are revealed. She is remembering the names of some of the family.

Every day may not be perfect, Mother, but there are perfect moments in every day.

One day she walked over to the dog's water dish and checked to see if there was water in it. Such a wonderful landmark in her recovery. She checked for water in the dog dish. The next day she walked to the flowers and tree that was in the living room and reached over to check and see if they needed water. She washed dishes several times, which helped her to maintain her balance while standing at the counter.

She had homemade worksheets that Speech Therapy had left to help her improve the function of her brain. On this day she did two and a half sheets without stopping to rest. I could see her tire while doing the worksheets. It was more of a strain on her mentally, with her attempts at thinking, than any physical workout.

Mother is paying attention to her environment, walking with her walker on her own, asking if we should do some more of "that lady's papers"? My mother is telling my three sisters that I am "bossy" and "strict" and I talk a lot. I may be just that, but she is the best patient I have ever worked so closely with. I can take the criticism, as my sisters have always taunted me for "pulling rank" with my parents, as I was the oldest. I'm sure I committed the crime, but I thought I did it so discreetly.

Another day she was trying to figure out how to flush the commode. Somedays she goes to the bathroom, other days she doesn't know if she was going in—or coming out. She knows the commode flushes, but she doesn't know when to flush it. We take for granted so many things that my mother has brought into the light.

We did not have a professional recreational therapist come into the home. When I define that therapy, they help people reduce depression, stress, and anxiety; recover basic physical and mental abilities, build confidence and socialize effectively. I find they help people to reclaim the enjoyable parts of their life. I think we have been wearing that hat for quite a while now in my mother's daily activities.

She took a nap from about two till four thirty one afternoon. She woke up and we walked to the kitchen. She looked at the clock for a while, and then said, "I don't know how you people live like this?" I asked what she meant. She said, "I'm getting up of at four thirty in the morning, and now you tell me we are going to eat." I take the hit graciously and smile to myself. Is this a sampling of what our future holds with this awesome lady? It is what it is, and I will take it in love.

Family is not an important thing. It's everything.

God blesses us with not only a beautiful matriarch, but a large family to surround her with. If I have been too busy to thank you for this blessing, God, please know how grateful we all are.

I tried to reorient her to the time, but it wasn't happening easily. When I showed her supper she said, "we are having this for breakfast? I suppose I could learn to live like this, but I don't know why you don't turn the clocks back?" I explained that we would, in November. She then asks me "how many people do that? How many people turn their clocks back?" I didn't have any more answers, I got nothing.

It's like I stopped thinking and forgot to start again.

Sometimes a person needs to stop thinking too much. I must accept that I don't know the answers, and that is okay. I must trust the answer will come when I least expect it.

Time flies when we are having fun. We are at twenty-nine days here at home. It is only one day since Ken's birthday. Why did I think time was flying? So much happens in some time periods, while other periods of time slide by without notice.

It's Sunday. This evening Mom walked over to the kitchen sink with her walker. She picked up her green cup, which I had washed and turned upside down on the rack. She fiddled with it for a few seconds until I finally ask what she was doing. She said she wanted to get a drink of water. I watched for a few more long seconds, as she tried and tried to find the opening on the bottom of the coffee cup. I showed her that she had to turn the cup over, then showed her how to get a drink from the faucet. She thanked me. This is another first—she went to the sink on her own. And to make it even more wonderful—she went to get a drink of water. This is a "woo-hoo" Jane.

She is trying to do her worksheets and often does well. She can lose her focus very easily if the area she is working with is not blocked off with some colored paper. She may drift back to the former category, or if a word on the sheet addresses something different—she may just drift off in that direction. She tries so hard and that's heartbreaking to watch. Her struggle with the simplest instructions makes me realize just how far we have to go.

Tonight, I ask her if she had any more questions about how her brain is and if she understood why she must relearn and retrain in so many areas. I ask her if things "come back" when she comes upon them or is it like it is totally new again. She said it doesn't "come

33

back," it's just new. She asks me what happened to her brain to make it like it is. I again explained the blood clot, and how it put pressure on her brain. How the skull bones wouldn't move, and as the clot got bigger, it pushed on the brain. She wanted to know if it was all blamed on the blood thinner medicine. I explained that is why she had the slow bleeding area on the left side of her head. I explained, again, that it was all removed but it had leaned on the brain for a while. The brain had to heal and rebuild from the area that was damaged from the pressure. She asks me why there was not even a small drop of blood that we could see. I told her it was all contained inside her head and couldn't be seen from the outside.

She just nodded and said, "Oh."

When her granddaughter Jen, Jane's daughter, and Jen's son Sam stopped in to deliver our supper, we were working on worksheets. She tried to cover them up, but Jen showed interest. She told her a little about what she was doing and then she told Sam, "I have to learn to write all over again, Sammy."

When I showed sister Jean the papers the other night, I asked Mom to show her how she works with the papers.

She said, "So you can see how stupid I am?"

I realized then that this is a fragile area to her right now. If she hasn't yet figured out what happened to her, how would she understand why she doesn't remember the things she is relearning.

I've been letting her fix her own supper plate, which is working out. Some funny things occur but it's a learning process. Gravy was put across her buttered dinner roll. Cottage cheese went on her vegetables. The gravy spoon went from the gravy dish right into the cottage cheese container, then directly into her mouth. From there her cottage cheese covered spoon went into her coffee. Life is truly like that assorted box of chocolates addressed in the *Forrest Gump* movie.

Mom had her left hand lying on her lap, as she was trying to use her fork to pick up food off her plate. She couldn't get the right move involved. She then laid down the fork and picked up the spoon and tried scooping up the food, but she just ended up chasing it around her plate. I asked her where her other hand was. She held it up and waved her fingers and said, "Here it is," then put it back on her lap. She resumed her struggle with the food.

I said, "If you let your left hand help, you will be able to get the food you want up to your mouth to eat."

She studied my face until she understood what I said. She then said, "Oh, okay." She was able to finish her meal with the spoon in her left hand and the fork in her right. She was able to analyze verbal words of explanation to relate it to physically carrying it out. Let's put another notch in that belt of accomplishments. I can hear Jane give her another "Woo-hoo."

I have noticed that she isn't doing well at problem solving. If her walker gets hung up in the doorway, she keeps trying to push it through. She doesn't seem to be able to come back at a problem from a different angle. When she spilled her iced tea across the table and onto her lap, she just sat there and used her napkin to wipe up the table. She left an ice cube lay on her lap until I reached over and moved it off.

She is watching the dogs more and asking me if "they are all in." She is telling them to be quiet and calling them to her when they start their incessant barking. Previously if I gave Mom three treats to give to the dogs, one dog could end up with all three treats, and it didn't occur to her that something was not right. Now she pays attention as to who got one and who didn't.

It is very interesting to be continually with Mom and see just what she really isn't aware of. She hasn't figured out how to flush the commode yet, but she knows it flushes. I tell her repeatedly, which way to turn when she gets up from the sofa to go to the bathroom. She always turns the wrong way, even to where she moves the chair blocking the way into the extra bedroom. I said to her, "you are always trying to go into my bedroom to pee, do you know that?"

She said, "Then why don't you let me do it, and get it over with?"

Again, I got nothing. That comeback is so refreshing coming from Mom's healing brain. Her sense of humor is so vitally and miraculously saved. Unless maybe she is not using sarcasm. Maybe it wasn't a "comeback." Maybe it wasn't her sense of humor, but rather an actual statement questioning my redirection of her need to use the bathroom?

Maybe we are not here to see each other—but instead to see each other through...

We discuss the rules of Catechism, the women of the church group she belongs to, the family and different things going on with them currently. She can add to any conversation, but the simple functions of daily activities of living are lost. Go figure, just how that mysterious brain works.

She remembers she saves her change all year long to wrap and then use the money for Christmas.

Woo-Hoo's Birthday

The Geltz group was celebrating Jane's birthday today. I mentioned signing a card and sending it down. Later she told me, "I don't give cards any more to the adults. I used to, but there got to be too many. I give the kids a card if I attend their party only. It's too easy to forget one now, because there are so many." Sometimes she recalls things so easily, but other activities must be relearned.

How amazing the brain is? How complex it is. How much we take it for granted. One of the best well-used sayings is, "You don't know how much you miss something, until you don't have it." The brain would fit in that analogy.

Don't Reorient, Just Rejoin

I tried to reorient her to time, but it wasn't happening easily. When I showed her our supper, she said "We are having this for breakfast? I suppose I could learn to live like this, but I don't know why you don't turn the clocks back?" It seems that Mom feels the reason she is unable to tell time is due to daylight savings time. You may be right, Mother. No argument coming from me. If that explanation works for you, I am delighted to join you.

I explained, once again, that we would turn the clocks back in November. Then she asked me how many people turn their clocks back? I didn't have any more answers, at least not on this day. As I would soon learn, there would be many times that her questions would leave me with no answers. I have never been known as "being speechless," but my mother has found a way.

Some things just fill your heart without trying.

Mother, the innocence of your questions continues to fill my heart.

Her youngest daughter, Jean, came to visit one evening. When she left, Mom walked her to the door and then told her to call when she got home. We watched as her car went up the driveway, and then Mom walked over to the sofa and tried to pick up one of the speakers to my laptop. Mom then reached to pick up the TV remote. I watched quietly for a few moments before I asked, "What are you doing?"

She was trying to find the phone so we would be able to answer it when her daughter called. She inquired as to what she was supposed to do now. I picked up the landline phone and I showed her how to push the talk button after it rings and then to say "hello." She returned the demonstration, and then sat on the sofa looking at the handset. She kept saying, "Come on, Jeani, call!" Finally, the phone rang, and she pushed the button and answered the phone.

Mom, you make my world more beautiful.

Mother admits she never knows what time it is. She is working at relearning how to tell time. She can read the digital clocks but has some problems with the numbered ones. It is better on some days. I'm keeping a rolling record of her condition and behavior. It shows me just how important every little thing is and what it means. "Relearned" or "remembered" information from her former independent life is gradually returning. One might not even notice these clues, but they are there. I could do a happy dance if I knew how to do one. I'll have to watch Dave on QVC shopping channel and imitate his dance. He does it so well when things are going well on his show.

Mom is doing better at fixing her own dinner plate. She is helping put the lids on containers. Some versions are her own inventions, but I don't step on any of her efforts. The other day she took the napkins and folded them nicely, then placed them right into my large glass of iced tea. We both sat their quietly—I wanted to wait and see her next action. There wasn't one. She had folded the napkins so nicely—and then put them directly in to a full glass of iced tea. In this new world she resides in—she was not aware that anything was wrong.

The cream of enjoyment in this life is always the impromptu. As I sit with a glass of iced tea soaked folded napkins, I must smile mother, you have truly mastered the art of impromptu.

She knows she makes mistakes, and sometimes we address them, laugh, and move on. She does better with her little green coffee cup, as the other cups seem to twirl on her fingers and spill.

Somedays she tried to eat her crackers with spread, by sliding them onto her fork with the spoon. Now that's not a simple task. If you think it is, just try it.

Somedays the spoon ends upside down and won't hold the food from her bowl to her mouth. No matter how long I watch, she doesn't figure out how to correct the problem. It is easy to see that problem solving has been replaced with multiple attempts to do a task over and over again—exactly the same way, making no changes, but expecting different results.

Somedays she drops her fork, and then continues to try to eat with an imaginary fork in her hand, wondering why she couldn't get it to work. It's okay, Mother, my imaginary fork never works either, so you are not alone.

Sometimes you can't explain what you see in a person. It's just the way they take you to a place where no one else can. I find your world a most interesting place my dear mother. As I am only a visitor, I don't have enough imagination to know what residency in your world is like. I just visit when you can't find your way into my world.

She shivers and shakes with her morning care, so I put the little space heater in the bathroom, throw her clean clothes in the dryer, and then put warm clothes back on her. She loved the warmth.

What do we live for, if not to make life less difficult for each other?

She is starting to question things, and even inquire more detail on things. These are big landmarks for her. She is now on medication for depression. Previously she appeared to only be going through the motions, following commands, asking me what I wanted her to do and where I wanted her to go. She was needing verbal clues, not wanting to make choices on her own. She needs a lot of verbal clues for a lot of activities, but overall, she seems to be healing well. She still hasn't grasped the concept that she isn't "doing nothing." She doesn't understand her brain is healing and needs rest to function properly. She does best in the morning, or after a nap. Her productivity declines quickly when she is tired.

It is important to know that the head-injured person may have a fatigue problem, meaning they get tired very quickly. They may have only three or four good hours in the day before they are wiped out. They may fall asleep easily, or maybe not be able to concentrate. Evenings are often tough on a head-injured person. Visits should be scaled down and shorter in length. It's quite a balancing act to determine how much a person needs socializing and just how much they can deal with.

Some days her right hand uses utensils for eating properly, other days not so well. On those days we have many spills to wipe up. She has speech and physical therapy coming into her home and she is ambulating with a walker, but her gait is often unsteady.

Some days she can carry on a good short conversation, and other days the words cannot be found. Often, she knows what she wants to say, but the words are scrambled and slurred.

The game of life is not so much in holding a good hand...
As playing a poor hand well.

She is very content to be in her safe zone, here at her home. She isn't very receptive to outside visitors or company currently, since she is very aware of her issues. She looks in the mirror and isn't happy with the way she looks, as she has always taken pride in her appearance. She has a large incisional line on the left side of her head, which has healed well. Her hair is now starting to grow in nicely, but she isn't able to see herself in that light. How do you accept the difference in your appearance, if you don't know how or why it has changed?

Since Mom has some rough days as far as her speech and often her inability to perform routine actions, we tend to protect her from the public. We find ourselves guarding her dignity. We know the impression she had with people her entire life. She is not able to maintain that image, as she is not entirely in control of her actions, behaviors, speech or even her appearance.

There may be days that I cannot help you, but never a day that I will not try.

She has several follow-up appointments in the next few weeks, and is still having some medication changes, therefore we don't know how close we will get-as far as the lady we knew. She is followed by the cardiologist, the neurosurgeon, the neurologist, and her family doctor. Some days she does well with worksheets from the speech therapist, other days we slide them to the back burner. Some days we follow through with the exercises set up for her, other days we just get through the day as best we can.

Sometimes your heart needs more time to accept what your mind already knows.

Mom has a lot to relearn. She is learning to write and works daily on remembering the months of the year, along with other information that she has known most of her life. She is amazing, because she is realizing now just how much she must do to "catch up," as she calls it.

As a few more week pass, Mom is not retaining the daily routine activities that we do every day. She still doesn't know which way to turn to go to her bathroom. She will not go to her bed until I go back to her bedroom. I have left her sleep on the sofa until I go to bed. Her doctor has increased her antiseizure medication, and she is now on an antidepressant. She smiles and laughs more now. Antiseizure medication calms the brain down a little bit, decreasing the odds of having a seizure. I must remember that other brain activities are also calmed down. Some seizure medications tend to produce fatigue in people. All seizure medications have an influence on your thinking to one degree or another. So now we add medication side effects to the daily challenges.

I put little colored lights on the tree that is in her house. I have the kitchen window where she sits all the time decorated with Halloween window stickies. We ordered new carpeting for her home, that should be installed next week. The original carpeting has stretched and has many loose areas where it rolls, presenting an accident waiting to happen. I have a lot of work to do, for Mom has stuff under the beds and layered everywhere in boxes or bags. Most will need to be moved to the canvas garage so the carpet layers can work. Mom truly has fifteen pounds of stuff in a five-pound bag. I now know where I acquired those genes. Mom is totally unable to help in this situation.

I have had her cutting out pictures from old Christmas cards and pasting them onto name tags for Christmas. This activity now presents itself with sacrificial lambs. The T-Rex is missing his head. The kitten is missing her ears. Santa is also missing his head. Loved as she is, I see no family member that will critique the tag on their Christmas gift, regardless of their missing body parts.

It's the things that you do that say all there is to be said.

Two Months Post Op

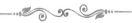

It is now two months since her day of surgery. Speech therapy is coming to the house, as is physical therapy, often on the same day. The physical therapist knows she is back to back with speech but tells me "it's my call whether she comes or not at this time, but otherwise, she has a full schedule." So I have the choice, do I let her come when Mom is tired, or do I have her remove her from her very busy schedule? I just love the inexperienced comments from the younger generation of the health care field workers. I miss the older tempered home care workers that knew they were there to work for the patient, with the patient, and it was all about the patient. This therapist knows that my mother will be tired from working with just one therapist a day, but her schedule is more important than my mother's ability to get the most from her visit.

I don't think this therapist has ever worked with a person from the older generation with a brain injury. They haven't learned that they can't be treated as you would a twenty-two-year-old with a sprained ankle. Of course, this is just my opinion resulting from my observation.

Mom was seen by the neurological team. The doctor feels she is right where he expects her to be currently, not further ahead, but also no further behind. He knows we "lost" about two weeks progression with her backslide following seizure activity. There have been no further episodes since her antiseizure medication was increased, but she didn't just bounce back either. Apparently, my mother was not on a therapeutic dose of antiseizure medication from the beginning.

On our way home from her appointment, we stopped and ate out. We chose a table in the back of the restaurant, where it was very private. This has been her best week yet. This lady truly likes eating out and it's such a pleasure to see her enjoying something.

There ain't much fun in medicine, but there is a heck of a lot of medicine in fun. Today we had some fun.

Relearning What Can't
Be Remembered

S he is questioning how to turn on a light in a room, how to turn on or off the porch light, and how and if she should flush the toilet. She has picked up the remote to the TV and turned it on. Now she is trying to discover how to work a few of the buttons, sometimes successfully. She hasn't mastered holding down the volume button continually, either up or down. We have experienced some exceptionally "loud" days where she says, "I messed it up" and hands it to me.

It's not what I say, but the tone of my voice that's important.

She makes me smile. Her job is to cover the dishes or put the lids on the containers after a meal. Sometimes they are partially on, sometimes it gets more interesting. She couldn't figure out which cover went on the mashed potato bowl, so I told her it was just covered with tin foil and then handed her the piece of foil to recover the dish. I put a few more things away, as my sister Jane was washing the dishes. Mom then handed me the tinfoil with the spoon from the mashed potato bowl wrapped nicely inside. I have always used and encouraged humor, rather than frustration, to meet the challenges of life. I shared this with my sister Jane, completely in front of our mother. As we laughed, "with her," she said, "I never used to do things like that." It's hard to see that your mother must relearn everything, when she is the one who taught you everything to begin with.

Sometimes you will never know the value of a moment until it becomes a memory.

She then dried all the dishes, standing for an extended period at the sink without holding on. This was one of her balance exercises, but with a purpose, letting her feel useful. Her conversation ability is improving greatly, as is her memory recall of things both from the past and recently. She listened intently as her daughter Jody told her of the people that she saw at the election house the day before, and it often had her thinking of someone in the past. She worked with recall until she was able to bring it forward and offer some information to the story. You can see her mind working hard to remember something, often seeking cues from one of us.

Jane came up this evening and Mom stood at the counter and talked with her for the longest period. She can carry on a conversation with one person so well now, and it's amazing. More than one person talking at once can get her confused, and she then loses her focus in what's being said. She tends to put pieces of several conversations or something being heard from the TV together into a mismatched thought. I have discovered that some of the shows on TV become the "news" or "weather" in her world. If we watch *Ice Road Truckers*, she awaits the snow arrival out our windows.

She still doesn't know which way the bathroom is in her home. She tried to tell Jane there was one on both sides of the mobile home. That would explain why she stood up and ask me which restroom is up and functioning now? She is still working out the sleeping situation in her home. She has told Jane that she sleeps on the sofa, and then "they carry me back to bed." She still doesn't go to her bedroom alone, not for a nap or not at nighttime. She is going to the bathroom without assistance now, after she gets directed in the right way.

She removes her glasses and her slippers, positions her pillows on the sofa, and settles in for the night. I turn the volume low on the TV and try to do some quiet activity until later in the evening, as she starts preparing for sleep around eight or nine, at the latest. The evenings are quite long for her right now, so I may move supper to later, so there is less hours of evening. She wants the window blinds closed and the doors locked as soon as dusk settles, and then she watches the clock. I don't know why she watches the clock, that I haven't figured out.

The home has a well and we were discussing a diminished water supply to the home one evening when my mom reminded me that "this never happened before." She feels I am doing too much washing and drying, referring to laundry. I wonder "why" I would have more laundry than she has had in the past? I will not remind her of the many iced tea and coffee spills, various mishaps while trying to use the spoon or fork upside down or using her shirt sleeves or shoulder to wipe off her mouth. Could these actions possibly cause more laundry? Dear Mother, life as we both knew it, has changed. That goes for both of our lives, mother, but I am fine with that.

How cool it is that the same God who created mountains and oceans and galaxies looked at our mother and thought the world needed one of her too.

Mom had her appointment with the neurological team on Tuesday. She was very pleased with "Dr. Mike." This visit she listened intently as Dr. Mike had told her not to waste good energy on what she doesn't remember about being in the hospital, but instead focus on moving forward. We also had him reinforce the fact that she does need to rest during the day. He explained that the brain doesn't show pain or swelling or redness, as an extremity would do to tell us it needs to be rested. The brain may show other symptoms as slurring of speech or more difficulty walking or doing simple tasks or maybe increased agitation or frustration, meaning it is tired.

When she gets tired, she must learn to rest, not to quit.

I gave Mom three choices for supper this night. It took her most of the day before she was able to pick one. I told her I was getting her back into the activities of daily living. She informed me that it's my turn to choose the next time. She doesn't understand that even that comment, shows the progress that she is making.

Then we shake up the box and shuffle the cards. We know we will have to be ready for the challenges ahead. Every day is unique—no two are alike.

With Brave Wings she flies, even though she is not sure of the direction.

She still hasn't figured out how to flush the commode, but she knows it flushes. She doesn't remember that she is to flush it when she has used the toilet, and always comes out to the living room and asks what she is to do now. I always have an answer for that question. Do I get a "woo-hoo" too, Jane?

The problem with a head-injured person is often with short-term memory. They may have problems with long sentences. They have problems relating to more than one person at a time. Their long-term memory tends to be good. That is the information that we recall after a day, weeks, months or years. With a head injury, short-term memory isn't working, so information has a hard time getting to long-term memory. Since little events of the day are forgotten, time seems to fly by for a person with a brain injury. I had never looked at the content of her days in that way. My eyes are opened with so many aspects of my mother's condition.

She talks easily when we discuss life in Rimersburg, the town where both of her parents came from. She likes to talk about her sister Franny but does refer to her as "my daughter" at times. The life she has given four daughters has disappeared. She does delight in the presence of small children, babies, and toddlers. She expresses concern that a toddler could fall and get hurt. She frets that we are handling a baby too much and we need to let him go. Now these protective thoughts are real to her. She protected us intensely when we were small. Some of her feelings are easily dealt with and we can then move forward. Some I don't quite understand. Therefore, I don't know the best way to deal with them. It is then that I find it best to change the topic. I use the three *R*s at this time for it always brings a smile to her face. Rimersburg, Roller Skating, and Rumble Seats are her favorite subjects for conversation. You could say her needs of "readin', 'ritin', and 'rithmatic" have been replaced.

Her parents are both from the small town of Rimersburg. Her father came to the town she grew up in to work at the steel mill. They didn't own a car; he rode the trolley to work. My mother's grandfather or Uncle would drive down from Rimersburg on holidays or special events. They would take the family in their car to Rimersburg. Mother and one of her siblings would ride in the Rumble Seat with her father, while the younger kids rode up front with her mother. This memory was so vivid to her. I can understand how she held onto it. We have so many constraints, put on a child traveling in a car these days. Can you just imagine a few children riding in a rumble seat these days?

The roller-skating rink was the "hangout" in her teen years. She loved roller skating and she was good at it. We would marvel at our mother skating backward. We were not coordinated like she was. Skating wasn't easy to us. It was hard work.

After high school, Mom went to work in the Working Man's Store, across the street from the hardware store. They put a pair of roller skates in the window one day. She went into the hardware store, and the skates were her size. She had them hold them until she got her pay. She has them to this day. When she looks at these skates now, it seems all the memories they hold come alive in her world. We have sat the skates on the kitchen table and just watched her face. She lets herself travel back to a time that causes her face to glow with a soft smile and no spoken words.

RETEACHING, BUT NOT RETAINING

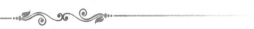

Again, I needed to explain to her what happened to her head. She wanted to know why her brain is like it is. It is about two months since her surgery. She told me she told her nephew that she had to learn to write all over again. I don't correct her. I'm seeing that her daughters tend to be referred to as her sisters. That would truly make her grandson, her nephew in her world.

She's doing better with her worksheets if she has rested. When she gets tired, everything gets mixed up. Watching her work her brain to get the proper answer is something that shows how tired she is. Her brain just isn't running on all cylinders. At least not yet.

She is trying very hard, but still seems to be having some seizure-type activity of the brain, that alters her progress. It has been that way since the surgery was over. The first week she sailed through, we were all in awe. Then one Sunday, she had issues that scared us. Apparently, the brain was adjusting, and she developed "stroke" type symptoms, affecting her right side and speech. She was started on antiseizure medication at this time. The dose was low because staff felt it was making her too sleepy. Since she had been home, I realize just how tired she is and how much rest she needs. I tell her we are giving her brain a rest, so it can heal. At the same time, she has had some returning issues with the use of her right hand and her ability to talk. Since her brain was injured on the left side, her right side is affected with the injury. Right-handed people have the ability to understand and express language from the left temporal lobe of the brain. We think and express in terms of language. This makes the left temporal lobe critical for day-today functioning. Sadly, this is where our mother's brain injury is located.

I had made a phone call to the neurologist, asking if a probable increase in the dose was needed.

She feels "useless," so we ask her to dry dishes, unwrap candy, make choices, or sort buttons for a craft, when needed. Jody was making some little acorn candies with her, so her job was to unwrap the candy kisses.

I'm so grateful Jody didn't give me that job, as those chocolate kisses would be so tempting.

We have tried to get her to color coloring pages or cutting some cards, but it doesn't come easily at this time. I read her some of the newspaper to help her keep up on present issues. She followed the sale and auction of Laurel Point Elementary School, because of her many years working there in the cafeteria. During hunting season, she asks daily about hunting successes of her hunting family. We go through some of her former crafts in an effort to stimulate her memory. Sadly, she admires the beautiful projects without knowing that it was she that had done them. I see that her sewing and crocheting projects will never see completion and I find that so sad.

She chooses to stay in warm knee socks and her flannel pj's, so we have bought her a new pair and a colored jersey to wear under them. She keeps the top of the pj's open, like a jacket, so the colored shirts are a pretty accent. She likes the home quite warm, so I am usually in bare feet and shorts. I still warm her clothes in the dryer during her morning care and run the little space heater in the bathroom while she gets bathed. I have started warming her bed blanket before tucking her into bed. Watching her face with the warmth of the blanket is precious.

It breaks my heart when she asks me "just what happened to my brain," and "why is it taking so long to get back to being right?" Now that requires an answer that I haven't discovered yet. I openly give her a hug and just simply say, "We got this, Mom, together we got this." If there is a better answer, I am open to suggestions. Reassuring my mother, she is not in this alone has become my priority.

To love a person is to see all their magic…and to remind them of it…when they have forgotten. I remember, Mom, and I will remind you!

You were full of magic and you displayed it wherever you went. The world loved you. Your family loved you.

The world and your family still love you.

Sometimes my mother knows I am someone staying with her, and sometimes she knows I am one of her four daughters. Up until recently, she couldn't understand how she had four daughters and doesn't remember anything about them. She will tell me "I know I have four daughters, because you told me I do. How can I have four babies and not remember them?" I so wish I could climb into her brain and help her sort through her tangled mind and put things back where they used to be. The sad result of not knowing you have daughters, eliminates the knowledge of any grandchildren or great-grandchildren that those daughters would have produced.

To be able to look back upon one's past life with satisfaction and love is to live twice. Our mother is shortchanged in this department, and it is so sad to watch her try to locate the missing pieces of her life.

Sister Jane sat with our mother while I ran to a store. When I got home, she told Jane if she would have had a rope tied to me, she would have pulled me in. She's dependent. That's a whole new adjective for her to wear. I know it's because she has so many missing places in her memory and her inability to do things herself.

It is a curious thing in human experiences to live through a period of stress and sorrow with another person. I find it creates a bond which nothing seems able to break.

I make sure I call everyone by name when they stop to see her, and always tell her who is on the phone when they call. This informs her of the caller's name but doesn't identify their relationship to my mother. She lives in a mobile home on the farm that we grew up on. Mom insists it had three bathrooms, and we must have had them taken out. She still doesn't know which way to turn to go to the bathroom. She only has two choices, left or right. She never picks the right direction. She then gets upset because she knows she did it wrong. She just looks at me with confusion.

So what if you turn the wrong way, Mom? You now look at me and say nothing. I look back at you and say nothing. This is something that happens so often, that a hand gesture of the direction you need to go in is adequate and understood. The unspoken communication is remarkable mother. It is a step forward in the world of communication. We are communicating mother, without any words.

She has tried to put her jeans on over her pj's, and somehow didn't know she had to take off her pj's first. Some things she does or says makes us laugh or smile. It must be so tough to live inside her head now. She will be eighty-nine and she is fighting to relearn and retrain and remember...all over again. She can remember some things so well that we are amazed, and then she will turn around and throw us a curve ball by asking me which dogs are hers, and how many does she have?

She was letting the dogs in from outside and trying to count them. She has two and I have two. She kept counting the dogs and getting five, then she asks me how many more were outside.

I look at her in love and say, "Mom, we only have four. Stop letting dogs in when you get to four. The other ones must not be ours."

She says, "But I already have 5."

I just calmly say, "No, Mom, we only have four. They just aren't staying still for you to count, so you are counting someone twice."

My oldest son, Brent, was here one evening. I told Mom to tell him what the doctor did to her head.

She said, "Brent, they opened up my head and took all the old wood out."

We laughed together and I reassured Mom I was never laughing at her, but I was laughing with her. She has a good sense of humor. I thank God that she has a sense of humor, for some days that's solely how we get through.

Attitude defies limitation and exceeds expectations.

Waking up to the beginning of November.

We have been working closely together now for fifty days at home.

I had no idea what turn my life was about to take or the terrible turn my mother's life took. I think she is doing better. Her antidepressant pill has really kicked in. Her antiseizure medicine has been increased. She hasn't had any of those spells where her words were nonsensical, and her speech was garbled. Her right hand still doesn't work as well as it had. We see the neurologist on Tuesday morning so it will be interesting to see what he says or does. She has regained some sense of humor and sarcasm, even in the altered mental state she is in. She has absolutely no balance without her walker, yet she forgets and walks away from it. She took a real fall in the kitchen the day the carpet layers came back, but she apparently didn't hurt anything. When she goes to fall, she doesn't even attempt to catch or protect herself. The entire left side of her head appears healed, but it is still quite sensitive to the touch, telling me it is not yet finished healing. She is no longer on any blood thinners, so one point in our favor.

I did get out for about four hours today. Jody came and sat with her. I went to Joann Fabrics and the dollar store. I am making two of my grandchildren, Jeffrey and Samantha, an advent calendar line. These are my oldest son Brent's two children. I have made fifty little or big bags, clipped them to a long piece of rope with a clip clothes pin and numbered them from November 30 through December 24. They will both have their own line. I have been putting little gifts in them for all those days. Jane has picked up most of the things for me in her travels and shopping trips. I think this is the second time I have gone somewhere without Mom. I sure don't know what long range plans are in my future. I only know where I am now. I won't be leaving here anytime soon. My mother still doesn't know which way the bathroom is. She often gets confused as to where she is going and for what.

I've been bringing stuff in from the garage where we took everything to get the rug replaced. It was trailer carpet and it had so many rolls and tripping bumps in it, it wasn't safe.

Mother has got to the point where she will carry on a conversation with someone. Previously she would answer with general answers, but not initiate any conversation. I read the newspaper to her. We get it on the internet. I show her patterns online and we go over things she has done. We talk about what she might be able to do in the future. We talk and talk all day. We talk and talk—somedays I am almost hoarse by evening. If I don't, she will sit and all at once her head will drop, and she shuts out the world. She is showing more interest and trying to figure things out. What a state of mind she must be dealing with. Sometimes she will be trying to tell me something then throw her hands up in frustration when she can't find the words. We welcome and count fifty-four days at home attempting to regain ground lost.

Speech therapy is coming around nine thirty, physical therapy around eleven. The physical therapist knows she is back-to-back with speech again but tells me she has a full schedule on Friday.

I speak to several of my mother's grand and great-granddaughters. Jen, Angie Jo, Sadie Jane, and Jul, as you are active in the medical field, hear what I am trying to say. Hear these words from your grandmother's life experience. Keep the focus on your patient, not on the convenience of a schedule. Don't let schedules rule over what is best for the patient. Patients need recovery time. You may be able to take care of numerous patients, one right after the other. On the other side of the coin, it doesn't work that way for the patient. My mother was exhausted after time with one therapist. The second therapy that followed was often a lost cause, wasted time for my mother, but the therapist could document the visit and insurance will make the payment. Win for some—but not a win for the key player.

Her conversation ability is improving greatly, as is her memory recall of things of the far past. Not so well with the near past.

She has no more medical appointments until after Christmas. Then she has a script for blood work before seeing her family doctor. No appointment has been made, as we can schedule it according to the weather.

My little Chihuahua Ricky has been on the sofa with me since I got up. It is 5:10 AM, and Mom just got up and went to the bathroom on her own. One of her dogs, Annie, came out and relieved herself on the canine training papers. The newest rescue we have, Joie, just came out and peed on the papers. They have all returned to bed. The domestic canine system we are living in is up and functioning well. It's a wonderful day in the neighborhood.

Fast-forward to day 61—that we have been working rehab at home.

I'm watching a Hallmark Christmas Show. Mom is sleeping on the sofa. She will be there until I wake her up and walk her to bed. Her balance is unstable, so she needs the walker. When we leave the house, we use the wheelchair because the walker would be too much if we have a good distance to walk. She still won't go into her bedroom until I do. She has developed quite a dependency. I never thought my mother would require a caregiver 24-7. I never thought she would have to relearn all the basic needs for daily living.

Today we were in the kitchen for most of the day. My sisters stop in often. I had Mom mix the ingredients, all three of them, for a Hawaiian cake. She mixed hard. She used her right hand, until she asks Jean to finish stirring it. Her right hand doesn't have the fine motor movements that it used to have. It makes writing an extremely hard task, usually ineligible. We are working on answering the phone but haven't even touched on her calling out.

Anxiety happens when you think you must figure everything out at once. You're stronger than you think. Take a deep breath. You got this. We got this. Together, we got this.

Tomorrow I'm going to watch her brown ground turkey, then add crushed tomatoes and mixed vegetables. It's called turkey chili.

Days have been tough. It takes so much longer to help Mom read a recipe over and over and over, and then help her put them together. She is so proud when it is completed. Tonight, she told Jane, in an excited voice, the few ingredients it took, how it was mixed, and then in the dish. She has determined that "the next time" she will let it brown "just a little more." She has been feeling so useless. Just recently we discovered her contentment in the kitchen. I've been going through her cupboards and arranging them better, so she can see what she has. Jane did some shopping after I had made a rather long list of foods she needed in her kitchen. We are going to work with simple recipes, so we have a rather safe chance of it turning out well. It's hard to see my Mom struggle so much with things that she did so well before the accident.

We let some of the therapies go yesterday. Mom would get so anxious when she knew one of them was coming. I will work more with the work sheets and exercises throughout the day. Mom was to walk for five minutes nonstop to build up her endurance. Today she walked for over fifteen minutes through the house. She questioned how long people usually must have a walker. I had to explain to her—again—that "balance" is one of the things affected with the left side of her brain.

I just walked Mom to the bathroom. She still wants to go the wrong way in her house to the bathroom. I'm where I need to be right now.

The cerebral bleed didn't happen all at once. It was going on slowly for months before her admission to the hospital. We can see that now. We thought Mom had some progressive dementia, but it seems it was the cerebral bleed causing pressure. Fortunately, the surgery went well. If she hadn't had the problem with the seizure activity, I don't think her recovery would be so intense.

Don't be afraid to take a big step if one is indicated.
You can't cross a chasm in two small jumps.

We celebrated Thanksgiving with Ken delivering our Thanksgiving breakfast to our kitchen table. He took time and sat with us while we ate. He cooks for his family every year, choosing breakfast over the big afternoon meal because the big meal used to be at our mother's home. This has been the year of changes. The lady that had the change, isn't aware of exactly what happened. Her health causes ripples in our lives that I watch go into high tide some days and low tide on others. There are days the ripples seem to turn into tsunamis.

LETTER TO SANTA

Dear Santa Clause,

It's getting close to Christmas, and I'm not sure you have been able to keep track of me recently. I thought I should send you a letter, letting you know that I have been good this year, at least most of the year. For sure, the last ¾ of the year. I have been working with my mother's rehabilitation 24-7. I seldom leave her home and have left my house in Florida empty for quite some time now. I am trying to help her regain her independent living status. At the present time, we have not reached that goal. I don't know how long it will be before—or even if—we can attain that. I start to think of long-term plans, and then I stop. I just keep working from where she is. Some days we move ahead. Some days we just try to regain ground we have already covered. I just wanted to let you know that I am at my mother's house for Christmas this year. I guess you could say, "I'm home for Christmas." So, Santa, please update my whereabouts on your navigation system, so you don't forget me.

Thanking you in advance.

Judy

CARD SHOWER

We are having a birthday card shower for Mom, since she doesn't attend any social outings yet. So far, she has received forty. She tells us that there must be someone with a big mouth telling people about her birthday. We have assured her that there are 4 daughters with big mouths, and they love her dearly.

Take time to laugh. It nourishes the heart and makes music for the soul.

For a fleeting moment, I sit and wonder what my own future holds. Then I see the struggle that lays before my mother, who will be eighty-nine next week, and my world and future look just fine.

Each day comes bearing its own gifts. Just untie the ribbons.

It's not easy getting her interested in doing anything. I'm trying to get her back to knotting a quilt, but every time she sits down to work on it, it's like starting all over. I spend more time teaching and reviewing things for her, over and over. When she walks away from knotting the quilt, I must reteach her to get her started again. I keep hoping the repetition will start to jolt her memory. I thread her needles, then untangle her thread, then she asks me, "Where was I?" and I help her find her focus again. This is something that she could do in her sleep before. Surely something will return to her memory, or at least she will remember it from the repetition.

We have found that she must take a nap in the afternoon. When she gets tired, her speech becomes garbled and the words she chooses to use are wrong. Up until a few days ago, she would only nap on the sofa while I sat or laid in the recliner by the sofa. She would often look to see if I was there. She would go to sleep on the sofa at night and tell me to take her to bed when I go. She tells me she can't find her pattern or scissors or thimble. Trying to help her find an interest and to help her with her boredom, takes about twenty-five times longer to accomplish than it would normally. She still has some residual weakness in her right hand, and her gait tends to be a bit wobbly, especially when she is tired.

She was a lady that was shy and modest, and always stayed in the background. She is a lady that's not quite the same lady that I have known all my life. She still cannot grasp how to use the microwave, or even what it is. She reheats her coffee in that same little handle-less pan on the stove. If that's not a word, maybe it is an unhandled pan. I don't know how far we will get, or how close I will come to find the lady we had before, but I keep looking for her. God blessed us with the best mother in the world, so we are taking the kind of care of her that we learned when she gave it to us. I have been sewing, along with direct care of our mother. She watches whatever I am doing. Sometimes she pulls up a kitchen chair so she can get closer. This lady knows she can't function like she used to, but she sure does cover well when other people talk with her. The sad part is she can only keep up the facade for a very short time, and then she has run out of generalized conversation. It's sad to watch her ability to converse end abruptly.

We had a piece of pizza for lunch the other day, and a small dish for our peaches and cottage cheese. I noticed Mom didn't have any cottage cheese on her peaches, so I slid the container over to her so she could put some on her peaches. She spooned the cottage cheese onto her pizza. That night I made French toast with eggs and sausage. Some evenings we have breakfast for supper. When she was finishing her plate, she took her spoon and ate all the syrup that was there. Sister Jane sent supper up to us on Sunday. She sent some pizza burgers and other dishes. Mom spooned some coleslaw right onto her pizza burger. She seems to have lost so many things within her precious head and it breaks my heart. We keep it light and use humor to get through our days. Mom told some people that came to visit that she feels like she is such a burden to her girls. She then told them that she may go to Florida for a while to give them a break? I looked at her and said, "Hey, Mom, I'm taking you with me. We will still be together." But since I'm usually not a daughter, her heart is in the right place. She wants to give her daughters a break. I commend her for her comment, and I smile at the thoughtfulness behind it.

Nothing is quite as funny as the unintended humor of reality.

I'm not sure she always knows who I am, but she knows she can't stay by herself yet. She's trying hard to show us she can, but there just isn't enough of regained memory. She can talk about distant times when she was a young girl or a young single woman without a problem. I would tease her that she loved to talk about the "three *R*s." These would be roller skating, Rimersburg, and rumble seats. Now the three *R*s seem to be remembering, relearning, and retraining. "Readin', 'ritin', and 'rithmatic" are things of the past. Sadness occurs with the lack of memory of her children and their offspring. In this mother's life, we don't exist. This lady tires easily and then just sits and watches what I'm doing. When I talk on the phone, she quietly listens the whole time. I find this is not always a good idea, as she hears only one side of the conversation. There have been times she has asked me if I was talking about her. It is then that I try to remember what she would have heard, as she apparently puts her own thought into the conversation that was unheard in the phone call.

She can't initiate any activity on her own. If I lay down, she is uncomfortable, and if I fall asleep, she appears to become frightened. She just wanders about. I am not used to seeing my mom like this. I am so grateful to have her, but I miss the mother that I knew before.

Many family members call. My mother only hears one side of phone calls. I can watch her, and she knows we are talking about her, but she doesn't hear the whole conversation. I have decided to keep family informed with emails. I hope it is as effective. I won't "forget" to tell everyone the same thing, so all will share her progress. These I can create after "my roommate" falls asleep on the sofa. They can also be passed onto other family members that love this lady. This way she doesn't hear one side of a conversation—and take it the wrong way.

We have been home ninety-three days. What a ninety plus three days it has been.

Mom is working hard to regain her memory and level of function. Just when I think we have taken a step forward; I get a reality check.

Last night we left the dogs out when Jane left to go home. When the dogs all came in, my mother kept counting them. She kept counting to five.

I said, "Mom, if you left five dogs in, we might be in trouble."

She said, "Well, did they all come in, or are there some still outside?" She counted them again and kept coming up with five.

Finally, I said, "Mom, we only have four dogs, and they are all in." I again remind her to stop leaving dogs in our house, when she gets to four.

She then got up and walked into the spare bedroom to go to the restroom. For some reason, she felt there was three bathrooms in her house, and she has asked us who took them out. Things are not consistent in her world. Even repetition after repetition doesn't hold an even course. Some things come back to her in the strangest way, then the next time she gets blindsided. Even doing things in the kitchen is a challenge. We are working with simple recipes thus far. She can reheat her coffee in the little pan on the stove. It's a little round pan without a handle. She sets the table and gets out condiments. Condiments can be an interesting assortment of bottles she finds in the refrigerator. Often, she adds something she sees in the room to the assortment. When she gets tired, her memory and word finding suffers.

At least she is going back to her own bed at night. This has just started this past week. She still naps on the sofa after lunch every day and I must lay on the recliner so she will sleep. Otherwise, she keeps getting up. It appears she will never regain the concept of time.

I watch my mother, who will be eighty-nine next week. I look at the struggle she has in front of her. In comparison, my world looks fine.

If she only knew how much those little moments with her mattered to me.

Her birthday card shower was a success. As they came, I hung them on the wall so she would be able to see them all the time. Anything out of sight—didn't exist. Ironically, she received eighty-nine birthday cards. How does that number of cards appear on her eighty-ninth birthday?

We celebrated my mom's birthday and Christmas differently this year. We had a very large cake and ice cream. The door was open to all, and they came at somewhat different times, not to overwhelm our matriarch. This was a difficult task as we have always wanted to be together at the same time. I guess we didn't want to miss anything. Mom does love parties and all the attention was on her. She did not feel shut out by her limitations.

Even my computer wasn't behaving until this last week and it still doesn't have all my programs on it. I'm thinking I may need to bring my mother and her dogs to Florida. I just don't see how she can be left alone for an extended period. Two sisters still work, and Jody now has a difficult health diagnosis, along with raising two of her granddaughters. I am the only one without a real agenda.

Not all storms come to disrupt your life. Some come to clear your path.

So I have not had much exercise. I've been fixing breakfast, lunch, supper, and snacks. I'm writing up grocery lists, carrying for four dogs, trying to find some sewing or cooking that Mom can do and yet be in her sight 24-7. She tires easily and then just sits and watches what I'm doing. When I talk on the phone, she quietly listens the whole time. She just can't initiate any activity on her own. I've been fighting a head and chest cold, so I took some cold medicine and laid down in the recliner this morning. She just wandered about. She looks at the newspaper but doesn't really read anything. I never thought I would see my mom like this. I am so grateful to have her, but I miss my other mom. I am with my mother 24-7, yet I miss my mom so bad.

We don't look back. We don't rethink. We don't redo. We are not going backward.

I tell this lady that a brand-new day is ordered for tomorrow. No matter what today was like, no matter what frustrations we handled this day, we have tomorrow to start all over. We do not carry over the problems of today into the fresh beginning of tomorrow. It has become our motto. We got this, Mom.

Just when I was getting used to yesterday, along came today.

Now we have expanded our horizon. We have gone from a brand-new day to it's a brand-new year. The holidays have passed. My mother is now eighty-nine years young. The old year has exited, and a new year has landed on our doorstep. My youngest son has celebrated another birthday. Welcome January.

Mom woke up with a headache again today. I gave her a cold pill and helped her go back to bed after two cups of coffee and breakfast. When she got up the second time she felt better.

I took my mother and I to the eye clinic for exams yesterday. My left eye needs a big correction in the lens so that must be why my eyes feel dry and tired. Mom's eyesight didn't change at all with her brain injury. I sat in the room with her, and I still don't know how the technician knew what she needed.

I'm trying to encourage her memory of things that she used to do. I get so weary preparing 3 meals a day plus snacks for her. I hoped that she would have started initiating some tasks by now. I watched her go through everything in the freezer a few days ago. I had hoped she would suggest or try to prepare something, but absolutely nothing. The only thing she will do without instruction is put some coffee in her little pot and heat it up on the stove. She can't seem to remember how to work the microwave. She refers to it as "that heating up thing." She can't remember her white dog's name. She still continually goes to the spare bedroom when looking to go to the restroom or to her bedroom.

She still tries to delay our trip to Florida. She tells Jane she has a lot to do before we can go. I surely would love to know what she plans on doing before leaving. I was so hoping that some daily tasks, especially some things in the kitchen or preparing some food or having some ideas of what she would like to eat would return. I feel like I always must address or encourage or ask her to do some things. When she walks into the kitchen, she will say, "What can I do?"

I say, "Whatever you want to do or fix."

It never goes anywhere. I guess I should be grateful that she does bath herself and helps to put her clothes on. She constantly fuses or pets or talks to the dogs. She gives them treats every time she thinks of it. Sometimes she will have four dogs around her at the table, and as she hands down each bite, I watch the same dog get all the treats. She talks to the dogs and gets upset when I scold or reprimand one of them. She will tell me, "Don't yell at them." I know she is more comfortable talking to them. When talking to or with the dogs, she doesn't seem to have any problems with word finding or speech. They never ask her any questions, so she never has to search for an answer. She is in total control of what she says, and what she feels their responses are. It's such a win/win situation for her. No wonder she enjoys them so much. I offer more of a challenge. Plus, as she tells everyone, I am bossy.

I'm getting new glasses, then I am going to make plans to start the trip south. A friend gave me a number for a pet friendly hotel about halfway there. Dave, Jane's husband, is going to get the car inspected and check it out before we leave. There are some visitors that Mom seems to be relaxed around, and then there are others that she gets edgy and irritated.

The world changes so fast that you couldn't stay wrong all the time if you tried.

FLORIDA, HERE WE COME

I have been packing for her. We are working with some material and she is trying hard at knotting a quilt. It tires her so much. She lies down on her bed several times daily and then sleeps about ten or twelve hours at night. She's doing so well, but she has lost so much. She is little-to-no help in the kitchen, and she did so much with meal planning, preparation, and serving it all of her life. I am sitting out her breakfast, cooking lunch and supper, and then giving her bedtime snacks. She sets the table, and it is quite interesting at times. For lunch, she set the table for three. When I ask her if we had company for lunch and asked if there was somebody here that I couldn't see, she looked around the living room. I told her I had enough food so she could invite them. She apparently didn't have anyone in mind. For supper, there was six forks and six knives on the table. Every day dawns a new experience.

She still thinks the bathroom and her bedroom is on the wrong end of the mobile home. She still goes to the doorway and looks in, and then shakes her head and goes the other way.

My sisters and I met with the attorney and straightened out Mom's power of attorney and updated her will. She signed her own name in all the right places. A few months ago, that couldn't have happened.

I am with Mom constantly. Even if I want to go somewhere and leave one of my sisters with her, she says I leave her with a "babysitter." God has truly blessed her present state of mind, as she doesn't know how much she has lost. In her previous mind state, she would be so upset knowing how much she depends on others for everything.

The heart has reasons that reason does not understand.

PREPARATION FOR TRAVEL

I am trying to gather all the pieces required to take my post-surgical mother to my home in Florida. Her large cranial incision appears to be healed. Her medication seems to have been regulated to control symptoms. She is doing well with basic activities of daily living, if she is directed to the right room and given some basic cues. I am the only daughter without a spouse, retired, living alone, and without a personal agenda.

I've been with my mother for over four months since her initial day of surgery. I was with her two months before her hospitalization. I've started the plans to take her and her two dogs to my home in Florida. I would like to make this move before the really cold weather hits Pennsylvania. I'm getting copies of her medical records, either to hand carry to physicians or be sent. I can have the physician's referrals as needed. She has a mail order prescription plan, so I've called to have them sent to my address. Now to do this, they need her permission to allow me to change the mailing address where her drugs will be sent. The man on the other end of the phone was saying too much. He didn't keep it simple, and her face showed it. I had to take the phone and explain to Mom what he wanted from her, then explain to the man on the other end what I was doing, and then give her the phone back. He needed her to give permission for me to speak in her behalf. It sounds simple, doesn't it? The man on the other end was saying too much too quickly and talking too long. She then falls behind. Just as she does when there is too much company in the room with her, and too many conversations going on at once. She just sat there for a bit, and then said, "I am lost, I don't know what's going on."

Again, I explained to the man on the other end of the line that he needs to ask one simple question slowly. He needs to then wait for her answer and say no more. We finally accomplished this mission, but not without issues. I am wondering if this man on the phone will change his phone habits when dealing with elderly? Even before her surgery, she did not reorder her medication via her mail order script pharmacy. She would call her doctor's office and ask them to reorder what she needed. Apparently, some confusion has been going on for longer than we knew.

I had spent months thinking over this trip. I had planned on driving her car with our now five dogs. When I first came up to stay with my mother, I had two dogs and she had two. My niece, Angie Jo, was concerned with a little Yorkie in her neighborhood that ran the streets. He was no longer wanted by the owners, so they left him run the neighborhood. It is soon to be winter, and he is a small dog. She brought him out to meet us one night, and we were smitten. Now our canine family has increased to five. We have now rescued a small five-pound Yorkie. He is a little boy that runs every chance he gets. That's all he has known, because the owners would let him outside and just let him go. He would surely freeze to death, if not hit on the roads before. So before our trip, we have a new little boy that doesn't know he has new owners or even where his home is. He doesn't even know his name, or the fact that we are keeping him and loving him. Why not add another new adventure into the challenge of our already complicated, combined lives?

I had been planning a thousand-mile trip, alone with my mother and five dogs in a car. I totally thought out every action, all toilet stops, every needed dog walk or gas fill up. I imagined what this trip with five dogs and a totally dependent mother could possibly be like. I thought through every circumstance. Toileting my mother and myself while five dogs were left alone in the car. Walking dogs while my mother was left in the car. Wondering what would happen when I tried and needed to take a power nap. I also wondered what would happen if my mother "sun downed" and didn't know who I was or what we were doing. I may get arrested for elderly-napping or worse, elder-abuse. Take a minute and imagine an elderly woman with an apparent injury to her head yelling "help me" to strangers, while five dogs are going haywire in a small automobile packed for a long drive. To complicate the situation, the automobile is registered to the elderly woman. The driver is then handcuffed and put into the back seat of a patrol car.

You would still hear me yelling "I got this" as they dragged me away. I can hear my mother saying to the officer, "Who is that doing all the yelling?"

I can get her medications filled for three months. I have had her eyes examined. I'm exploring AAA. I need to take out one of those programs for a few months anyway. I will pick one and get it started. That way, if we have problems on the trip, at least there won't be a weary ole lady helping an older woman walk along the road with five dogs on leashes. I'm sure we would be on the eleven o'clock news that night. I'm kinda going with the time that my glasses are done to plan on leaving. I'm thinking about Sirius radio, to be able to maintain pleasant music and not static during our two-day adventure. I did call it an adventure, as I'm trying not to look at it as a disaster. Time will tell.

None of my premonitions or impending results were positive. My mother was dragging her feet about leaving her house, so that didn't help. My son, who lives in Florida, was anxiously awaiting our arrival. All of my attempts at working out a plan, did not take into consideration an engine problem, a flat tire, a missing dog, a sick passenger, or if something would happen to me and I had a car full of dogs and a frightened, dependent mother. Every action that I thought through seemed to swirl downward into a grand fiasco. And that is just taking into consideration those within the confines of the car. What would happen if someone decided to rob us or attack us, or strangely enough, steal the car?

A task ahead of us is never as great as the power behind us. Are you there, God?

One night, while talking with his grandmother on the phone, my son offered to fly up to Pittsburgh and drive the car down. My mother jumped at this suggestion. I called him on this. He said he could fly up on the weekend, and we could leave from the airport.

He could rest up on the remaining weekend day so he would be fit and rested for work on Monday. If those requests could be met, he could make it happen. I went to the computer and reserved a one-way ticket for the following Saturday. This would answer the prayer that I hadn't even sent yet. I hadn't formed the words of a prayer yet, because I didn't know what request would work best for the trip. After Bri's phone call, I could just picture God quietly shaking his head as he observed all my planning. That would be a silent action that my dad would have done also…just stand and shake his head.

God already has the master plan in front of him and I'm sure he figured he would be so busy watching my mother and I with five dogs on that two-plus day trip he wouldn't get around to watching the rest of the world. I can see he already knew he would be putting Brian in our car, and just wanted to see what my plans looked like. I've proved God does have a sense of humor and just gives us time to realize he's waiting and watching patiently. God truly hears our unspoken needs, because I was so busy trying to make a plan—when it was already sketched in the master's workbook.

The car has been inspected and my brother in law had four new tires put on it, new brakes and routers, and new fluids in the car. It is now road ready for the long trip. It is filled up with gas. I have spent the entire week attempting to pack for my mother and my trip. My son Bri is to arrive at the airport at 10:50 AM. I had packed everything that we could take in the car. I had bathed and trimmed all the dogs attached to our lives, which would now be five. I had packed for my mother and attempted to take as much other stuff as possible for our car trip.

We had a lot of company, frequent visitors and phone calls, as my mother is so loved. Spending 24-7 with my mom, I understood why they wanted to see her before we left.

Funny, Mom has been counting five dogs since her hospitalization, In her altered mental state and innocence, was she aware of the chance that we would be rescuing a fifth dog? I feel there are no coincidences—things happen for a reason and as the master has them planned. I also feel that God gives insight or visions to some people at times. It may be brain injured or compromised adults and children. As I learn later during my time with my mother, those that have passed before her often quietly visit her. This didn't scare her, no one talked, they just made their presence known—but only to her.

I limited the dog's food and water the evening before we were to leave and had them outside several times, in hopes they would relieve themselves before our departure. My mother does not totally understand the whole plan.

Change the way you look at things and the things you look at change.
Bri's flight is to arrive at ten fifty this morning.

I put Mom and the dogs in the car and left from her home. We went up the driveway, so far-so good. We drove a few miles. I had put a leash on the little Yorkie, Rusty, as we named him—just in case he would get loose. I would have a better chance of catching him with a leash, as he is noted to be a "runner." He was quite active in the back seat and several of the other dogs were restless. Mickie was in the front seat on Mom's lap, but not comfortable. Her white dog, Annie, was in the back seat but wanted up front. I made it about five miles and pulled off the road. Rusty had wrapped his leash around the head rest several times and had himself in a hangman's noose hold. He has been through and around the inside of the car at least fifty times in the short time we have been in it. He is agile and quick. He is curious and busy. He has craved attention and lacks any training at all. He was rescued from a family that left him run the neighborhood, and no longer wanted him.

He will "run" at any chance, and at this time, he isn't sure of his name, his owners, and he certainly doesn't know where his home is yet. I got into the back seat and untangled Rusty's leash. I had to be careful opening any car doors with five dogs inside. I certainly didn't want to be chasing any dogs, while my dependent mother was left in the car. I was also aware that she may open a car door and release some active canines. I then put Mickie in the back seat and left Annie get up in the front with Mom. Things seemed a little more settled this time, and I removed the leash from Rusty's collar. We pulled back onto the road and headed for the airport, for the second time. With the issues that have occurred in the first five miles, I should have considered what the remaining one thousand miles may hold in store, but right then, I just needed to get to the airport. The young man who would soon become what I called my "relief pitcher" would be arriving soon.

The roads were fine, with little traffic as we arrived at the Airport. I pulled into the short-term parking lot and parked right across from passenger pickup, but up one flight of stairs. It was a handicapped parking space, so we were very close to where Bri would be coming from. I sent a text to my son as to where we were parked and awaited his arrival.

My Mom kept asking, "Where is he?"

I walked restless Rusty around in the parking garage, while we waited on Bri. I had locked the car doors and stayed quite close to the parked car. When I saw him cross the street, I go to meet him. I give and get the most loving hug, then hand him the car keys and I climb into the back seat. He walks around to the passenger side, opens the door and hugs and greets his grandmother. He is not late. His timing is perfect. He climbs behind the wheel, and I relax.

I had packed the car with only enough space in the back seat for one person. I had several carriers in place and hoped the little dogs would lay up by the back window. I packed many sandwiches, snacks, drinks, and candy. Bri's sister had bought him a hoagie for the trip. We were set for a well-planned trip, or so I thought. Why wouldn't it be like a well-greased machine? Well, let me think. A small compact car packed to the fullest. Three generations in the car, along with five dogs and one of those people adjusting to a brain injury. What could possibly go wrong? Well, as it has been said so many times, famous last words. Murphy's law is alive and well, and apparently a big part of this car's infrastructure.

In hindsight, I didn't realize that the circumstances, in my mother's world, is seen differently. Upon our arrival at the airport, I turn the keys over to a young handsome man who just came off the steps onto the first landing. Then I disappear into the back seat with the five dogs. What was going through her mind, I hadn't considered? Apparently when I climbed into the back seat, I was out of her line of vision. This meant I was no longer there. Considering Mom's altered mental status, I should have given that concept just a little more thought.

Now that the trip is behind us, I could list all the supplies I needed and didn't have and addressed all the issues that presented themselves that I was not prepared for. But that would be hindsight, and it doesn't change the outcome. I have asked myself, "Judy, what were you thinking?" "Judy, were you not thinking?" "Judy, why did you not rethink this?" My optimism was impressive, but common sense, where were you?

Travel Officially Starts

We only have about a thousand miles ahead of us. Hopefully it will not be as eventful as the thirty-six miles I have already traveled this morning.

Bri drove us out of the airport garage and started the trip to Florida. He doesn't need a map or a Garmin, as he has made the trip so very many times. I had put a small change purse in the console with money and change for all the tolls during our trip. I got all five dogs into the back seat so as not to disturb the driver and we all got settled in. I am asking him about his flight and Mom is listening, but not entering the conversation. She is frequently looking over at the driver, but not asking any questions yet.

Bri talked off and on with his grandmother. I felt relief as soon as he took over the wheel and the car. I was relaxing and feeling quite tired. I have been driving with Mom and the dogs in the car for over two hours now, along with untangling, sorting, rearranging and changing the placement of the dogs. I felt myself get drowsy and enjoyed relaxing into a nap shortly after we started our trip. Two dogs were on the back window, one in the little kennel behind the seat, and the other two were close to me. I had packed the back seat on one side and only left about one-third of the seat for sitting. That also included the cooler at my feet and the food bag against the door. Naturally I have kept the people food away from any canine discovery. Did I consider riding in this small area for eighteen to twenty hours? I missed that thought. Notation made for the next trip.

Bri turned to his grandmother and thanked her for paying for his flight. She then started asking some questions—beginning with an inquiry as to when he is to get back on the plane and where it was going. He tried to explain that he wasn't getting back on the plane, so he didn't know where it was going. Confusion appeared on her face. He attempted to explain how he flew up from Florida, just so he could drive her car back down. He told her that he was so excited that she was coming to Florida, and that he "waited and waited and waited" and finally he just had to come up and get her. She responded with simple answers, all the while, trying to sort through the information given to her.

I forgot that Bri had not seen his grandmother since her surgery. He was not aware of the changes that had taken place in her mental state. What was I thinking? Rather, what wasn't I thinking about. I couldn't even stretch my legs out or reposition my way of sitting. I had packed the car to not allow that. Did I not remember that I would be in the backseat of the car for over eighteen hours?

Experience is a hard teacher because she gives the test first, the lesson afterward.

As the trip continued, Bri decided that it was best if I didn't take over driving. It was our original plan to alternate driving when he got tired. He found out that the five dogs became an absolute problem when I got out of the car and left them behind. I was advised to stay in the backseat until Bri got Mom out for one of our toiletings. I watched from the backseat as he tried to explain to his grandmother that I was staying in the car. Now she hasn't acknowledged the back seat even being attached to the front seat and part of the car. Myself, and any dogs back there with me, did not exist. He was trying to explain that the dogs would stay with me, until he got her out. He had a bit of a problem getting her to let go of the car door which she hung onto. He did manage to get the deed done so he could shut the door. After he had finally got her out, I slipped out so I could take her into the bathroom. As I quickly learned, the reason for this stop was no longer necessary. Whether it occurred in her confusion of leaving the car, or the fact that she stood up after sitting for hours, I don't know. Maybe it was because this man had taken her out of the car and was trying to keep her out by shutting the car door. How she must have been frightened. It's easy to forget that her understanding and comprehension has changed.

She told me she was "holding it okay, until" she stood up. When in the bathroom, she didn't have to go anymore. I had then assumed that she had already emptied her bladder. I was standing with her, with just a blouse and jeans on. She had on an undershirt, flannel shirt, short sleeved sweatshirt and a cardigan sweatshirt. I took off her outer sweatshirt, and then her short-sleeved sweatshirt. I put the cardigan back on her and placed the short-sleeved sweatshirt between her legs. I pulled the sleeves up over her butt and the rest covered the entire area between her legs. I then pulled up her panties and jeans and asked her how it felt. There was no longer any wet clothing against her skin. She said it "feels so good." If it hadn't, I would have found her dry clothes somewhere in the packed car. I was just thankful that it "felt so good." I should have known better. Each time we asked her if she needed to go to the bathroom, she would say that she didn't. She has done that at bedtime, and as soon as she is settled in, she needs to get up and go. I will know in the future to recall her need to toilet by a schedule, more than her answers. For every trip following this one, I will also pack extra clothing in a convenient bag with easy access. You would have thought with all the planning I had done for this trip, I would have had a spare outfit easily available. I didn't.

Life lessons keep knocking at my door, so I'm just going to leave the door wide open. Why not, they are going to knock till I let them in anyway.

In all, we had three stops for gasoline, and two that Mom and I got out to go to the bathroom. Bri and Rusty had several more stops due to Bri's sipping energy drinks and Rusty's age and restlessness. At one time, when Bri was out of the car, Mom asked me who he was and if he had a family. I could see the confusion was increasing, for now she didn't even know who this driver was.

She refused to nap, telling me she doesn't ever sleep in the car. She would ask why the road just keeps going and going. She looks ahead and says, "It just keeps going." Other times she wanted to know why we were stopped and everyone else was moving. I thought about that for a few minutes. Yes, it did look like we were sitting still as she looked out the car windows. Everything appears to be moving past us, meaning we must be sitting still. At this point in our travels, her reasoning is starting to make sense. I have learned that it is easier for me to climb into her world, than to expect her to understand mine.

I'm beginning to see things through my mother's eyes. Her eyes are wide open, so it should be easy, but Bri's and my eyes are barely able to stay awake. How does this lady do this? She should be sleeping and dreaming of a better time.

She is starting to question the seat belt. She is riding in the passenger seat in the front, so the seat belt is necessary. She wants it off. She is trying to figure out how to get it off. She tells me she "needs room for the baby, so it has to come off."

It has been dark for some time now, and the true nature of what is referred to as "sundowning" is occurring. Confusion and restlessness are escalating. I have found that eating and taking time for snacks does change her focus. Brian has decided that he will drive straight through, as our passenger is not sleeping, and her agitation is increasing.

He can see that she isn't going to relax and remember, we have five dogs within the confines of our crowded car. When riding, the dogs tend to go dormant. As my mother's agitation and confusion escalates, the dogs are picking up on her affect. This is causing a problem that may be difficult to intercept.

We have traveled a little under eighteen hours. Thank God for my son's ability to drive the distance, keeping the goal of "home" safely, but as soon as possible.

Life is not a matter of holding good cards, but sometimes playing a poor hand well. You did real good, Brian, God knew we needed you. May I also say he was confident you would handle the assignment well.

ARRIVAL TO FLORIDA HOME

We have arrived at home. Home never looked so good. Turning the dogs loose into the enclosed back yard, I watch with wonder as my mother tries to adjust to the present situation.

My son decided to drive straight through after encountering several unplanned events. Toileting at the truck stops was more of a challenge than we were prepared for. The dogs were not programmed to need to toilet at the same time. Mom had said she never sleeps in the car, and she held true to her word. Her eyes were wide open, while Bri and I were ready to sleep. Her questions during the dark hours of the night showed she was unaware of where we were or why we were there. She didn't really know Bri or myself, and I was trying to keep the dogs in the back seat to keep from distracting the driver.

I realize if I am not within my mother's visual field, that I am nonexistent. I also kept her beloved dogs out of the front seat to keep from distracting the driver. I take a moment to imagine how she may have felt with a strange man next to her, and the person and dogs she was familiar with not present. Vision is diminished in a small car after dark. My mother's vision was already compromised after the blood clot years ago. I don't know how much the cerebral issue and seizure activity have affected her vision. I also know that impending darkness causes the traditional sundowning effect on our mother. Now I put her in a car where she doesn't know where she is going or why. Well, Judy, again I ask myself—what were you thinking? Maybe asking myself if I was not really thinking things through is a better question. Regardless, the questions that I had not answered correctly are now in hindsight.

Now we are in my home and my mother was up several times to the bathroom. When she got up, she walked to the doorway and by the look on her face, I knew she didn't know where she was or which way the bathroom was located. I look back the hallway, as I see the little Yorkie Rusty's eyes fixed on the hallway. Suddenly his ears went up in attention and his eyes zeroed in on Mom. I walked back and said, "Do you need to go to the bathroom?"

She said she did and asked, "Which way is it?"

Each trip to the bathroom was a repeat of the same. When she tried to stand, she became quite dizzy and sat back down. The dizziness appeared to scare her. She sat for a few minutes then stood up again. I held her steady for she was quite wobbly and weak. She kept leaning far to the side, trying to hold onto the walls. When she was back in bed, she was very concerned as to what was wrong. I simply explained that we had limited our liquids for a day or so, so we were probably dehydrated. I told her everything would be better in the morning, that I had requested a "brand-new day." I told her we would drink more water tomorrow to fix the problem. She seemed to accept my explanation and went back to sleep.

I had left the light on in the bathroom and told Mom to just go toward the room with the light. She could be standing one doorway away, and still she didn't know where to go. Her own home was not familiar to her, so my home presented her with the same problem. I also wonder how Bri will manage our new situation. He hasn't been around his grandmother since her altered mental status. We are now in Florida without any other family.

When she was ready to get up for the day, she sat at bedside and was looking for her clothes. I walked back and sat down beside her. I thought that she had a look of concern. I ask her what was bothering her.

She looked at me for a short while, and then said, "Do we have to do that again today?"

I asked, "Do you mean go for a long ride in the car?"

She answered positively, and then said, "I can't do that again. I just can't do it."

I assured her that we were not going in the car for a long ride again. There was no need to explain that the driver may need to sleep for a whole day, and the passenger in the backseat was totally exhausted. All she needed to know was that she didn't want to "do it again"—so we won't.

She asked me, "But how do we get to your house?"

I said, "Mom, we are at my house. We are here. This is your bedroom. We are home." She seemed so relieved. She just said "oh good, good. I'm so glad."

We discussed how tired we felt, and I explained that we were just going to rest and relax today. I said we could take as many naps as we wanted. She agreed and we then walked to the kitchen for coffee and cereal. She later told me that she worried all night, thinking that we had to take that long ride again today.

I have explained over and over how we had Brian fly up to Pittsburgh so he could drive us to Florida. She wanted to know when he had to go back. She didn't seem to understand that he could fly to a city with a one-way ticket. I ask if she remembered me getting out of the car and letting him get in the driver's seat. She said she did. I told her that Brian then drove us down here, to Florida, so we didn't have to drive by ourselves. She said she understood that.

Then she again asked, "But when does he have to fly back?"

I told her that he came to Florida with us, and that he lives in Florida.

She then said, "But when does he go back? He has a job, doesn't he?"

I explained that he lives in Florida and that he works in Florida. I told her that he rested yesterday, and that he was already at work today. She seemed surprised that he was already at work.

We had breakfast, her usual cup of coffee and bowl of Frosted Flakes. I then walked her around the back yard and left her taste a tangerine picked right off a tree. I pointed out the rooftop across the highway, explaining that it was Brian's house, where we had dinner last night. She needed my arm or held my hand throughout our entire walk. We then sat in the carport in one of the lawn chairs.

Later Mom and I were sitting in the living room talking. I ask her what she thought was happening when we were in the car. She said that she felt we were not taking her where we said. I reminded her that I do not lie to her, and I told her we were going to my house.

She said, "But how would you feel if you didn't have any idea where you were, if you didn't know any of the roads, and you knew you were going somewhere. You just didn't have any idea where you were going."

I said, "That must have been scary, Mom."

She said, "Yes, it was, very scary cause I didn't have any idea where I was."

I asked her if she thought we were taking her to an institution? She said she wasn't afraid of that, but she just didn't know where she was and knew she couldn't find her way back home. I assured her that I would be with her, and I would not lie to her.

Second Full Day in Florida

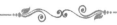

Mom woke up this morning, very dizzy with a bit of a headache. I helped her to the bathroom, gave her breakfast with two cups of coffee. She went back to bed. I don't know if we may be a little dehydrated from the trip, or as a coffee drinker, is she missing some caffeine? She only drinks coffee, so I'm going to increase liquids today. She slept for about two more hours, and then sat at her bedside and was trying to put her jeans on. She is still feeling dizzy. I helped her get her jeans on and her slippers.

She said, "I think I'm going to lie back down."

I helped her lay down and informed her that we have nothing going on today so she can rest. She lay down with her dog Mickie right beside her. She keeps trying to move about on her own, and I sure don't want her to fall and injure her head. I've caught her leaning way down to pet or talk to her Mickie. She leans way over to pick something up off the floor. As many times as I caution her, it doesn't stop her from doing it again. While she's lying in bed, I can relax a bit.

Mom woke up again and came out to the living area. She is still feeling dizzy, but no headache. Her balance is really compromised. I fixed our lunch and encouraged her to drink a glass of water. I gave her some dog treats to give to the dogs. That action caused an encounter between the two little male dogs, Ricky and Rusty. Now Mickie is intervening. As I separated the two little dogs, Mickie was already joining in on the fight. It was then that Mom got up and tried to pull Mickie away. Her collar came off and Mom fell back on her butt, the back of her head bumping into the table. I told her to sit still until I got the dogs apart. I put Ricky in the carrier and held Rusty until Mickie calmed down. Then I put Rusty outside into the fenced in yard and commenced to help Mom up off the floor. She denies any injury. She hit the back of her head above her neck on the table. I can find no sign of an injury. Thank you, Guardian Angels, again you were on duty. Just two days here and she has already fallen.

Murphy's law has rode to Florida with us. I should have prepared for that since Murphy was with us during the entire drive. In fact, Murphy was already in the car in the first five miles when Rusty wrapped his leash around everything and anything in the back seat. Toileting the dogs was not easy as Rusty seemed to need to go every two hours, and the other dogs weren't trained to toilet on command at the same time. Now we haven't even discussed the toileting of the humans or the need to refuel the car. Yes, Murphy was definitely in the car.

Sometimes you have to let go of the picture of what you thought life would be like—and learn to find happiness in the story you are actually living.

I must purchase a landline phone before tomorrow morning, as I have the cable and internet technician coming to hook up our TV and laptop. I feel I need to have a landline in case I need to call for help for my mother, and the cell phone is not charged. I know that most everyone is thinking that I need a landline phone because I'm always losing my cell phone in the house. Mom didn't want to leave the house because of her dizziness. She said she would lay down when I was ready to leave. I helped her lay down in bed, had all the dogs kenneled and accounted for, and told Mom I would lock her in the house, and she didn't need to answer the door. She agreed.

When I came back, I saw that Mom was up. She said the dogs were barking and she was trying to find them some treats, but she couldn't find them anywhere. She had broken up Oreo cookies and offered them to the dogs, but they didn't want them. I showed Mom where the dog treats were so she could find them the next time. I brought home our supper and she ate well. She had a cup of coffee with her supper. I was also feeding the dogs and another disagreement occurred between the dogs, but I intercepted before it got loud.

Since rescuing Rusty, I now have two small male dogs that seem to be disagreeing. Mom was beside me in the kitchen and she lost her balance. I caught a hold of her just in time to prevent another fall. I walked her to the dining room chair and asked her to please sit down. She obliged me, at least at the time. She is so determined to become independent again. Maybe she doesn't realize that her condition has changed dramatically.

Last night when we were sitting on the sofa, she asked me if she would ever be able to be by herself, like she was before. I explained to her that our plan was to get her there. I told her we could be more active in warmer weather here in Florida. The more active we are, the stronger she will become. It will help her balance and endurance as well. I explained that knotting quilts, washing or drying dishes, dressing herself, it all helps with the fine motor movements of her right hand. It seems things need to be explained multiple times and then repeated. If it eventually makes some sense to Mom, I will keep repeating and repeating.

We had grilled cheese sandwiches for supper yesterday, and I heated up some minestrone soup. I fed the dogs, and then walked over to the table with Mom. She was trying to cut up her cheese sandwich with her spoon. She had spooned her soup all over the sandwich and then tried to cut it up. I helped her cut it all up and she ate her soup drenched sandwich with her fork and spoon. Since this recent condition has occurred, my mom has invented different ways to eat certain foods. I must say that I had never watched any-one spoon their soup all over their sandwich until today. But then again, I watched her spoon apricot jelly on mixed vegetables, then on her mashed potatoes and then on top of her favorite sugar wafer cookies. I've seen her put cottage cheese over her pizza. I would guess that these practices may be the way new recipes are created. Soon, with the proper marketing, you may see my mother on TV with her own unique cooking show. I can assure you, without even seeing the script, that her recipes are unique.

I saw on the news this morning that it was "heart" awareness day, since heart disease is the number one killer among women. People were asked to wear red on this day. I didn't think too much more about it, but did decide to put on a red jersey, since I had that option. There will only be my son and my mother in my daily circle, but I will know I have on red for a reason.

Later in the evening, probably the 6:00 PM news, Mom and I were sitting watching the TV. Mom told me to look at the TV and see that all the women had on red dresses. She wondered if they were told to do that. I looked at Mom in amazement, as she had noticed that all the newswomen were dressed in red. This to me was another remarkable step in her progress. Usually she just looks at the TV but doesn't seem to be paying much attention to what is on the screen.

I said to Mom, "Look at all the men, you will see that they have red ties on with their suits."

She agreed that they did. I then explained to her about the "heart awareness day," knowing that my explanation was deeper that her level of understanding on this day. Each of these observations are a small unnoticed step in everyone's daily life, but in my mother's life, it is a big step.

Mom was still sleeping, or so I thought. All the dogs had been visiting with me on the sofa. Since there are three doors to the outside in the open great room in my house, I have slept on the sofa. I couldn't go back to my bedroom at the back of the house. If I woke up and found my mother and five dogs missing, because she found access to the outside doors, I wouldn't know where to begin. I didn't sleep well, but that's not unusual. There are too many thoughts and decisions going through my tired mind. I started to look through the guide on the TV network to find some shows that Mom may be interested in. I then went back to check on her. I found her in my bedroom, naked from the waist down, except for her knee socks. I smiled and asked, "Mom, are you lost?" With that she turned around with a pair of my blue panties in her hand. She said she "had messed her clothes and she was trying to figure out how to "put these on."

I told Mom she was in my room, and that the panties were mine. She looked around the room and asked, "Didn't I sleep here?" I told her she hadn't, but if she wanted to, she certainly could. We walked out of the room, past the bathroom, and into her room.

She seemed relieved, when she recognized the bed she had slept in. Several times during the day she referred to the fact that she was in the wrong bedroom and couldn't find her own. She remembered it.

Six Days in Florida

I finally have internet, cable, and a home landline. Mom cannot get used to a cell phone and she can't hear well on it. Often it is held upside down, backward, or not approximated to her ear and mouth. The landline is so she can keep in touch with family up north. All incoming calls are free, but I only get so many minutes with outgoing. I've told my sisters they must call here.

My landing in Florida has not been easy. Mom was so confused and disoriented for days after we arrived. She fought sleep the whole way down, stating she can "never sleep in a car." She told us she has always had problems with car sickness. Complicate that with five dogs, a packed car, and her grandson doing all the driving, I couldn't find a place to hide. She kept wanting to go home, especially when it started to get dark. She literally kept forgetting that there was a back seat in the car, which was where me and all the dogs were. She got upset, feeling we were taking her somewhere else, and Brian kept going "down this road, but never gets to the end." Compared to the short trips she has been used to on country roads, I have to admit the highways Bri traveled on were roads that truly never had an end. There were no stop signs or traffic lights. This would make the road appear endless.

It was not an easy trip. We, the driver and I, have agreed that this trip cannot be made in a car again. I need to be in Mom's view and able to take care of her during the ride. Toileting at a busy rest area is next to impossible. The walk into the facility is too long, making the reason for the walk unnecessary in the end. No, I need to correct that statement. Toileting at the rest stops or stations are not an option. Mom needs to be able to toilet in a very short distance. I never thought to use incontinence briefs for the trip. There we go with hindsight again. I thought I had thought everything through.

This was the first few days, she was always lost, couldn't find the bathroom, didn't believe where we were, wanted to know if we had to "do that again to get to where Judy lives." Add to that a couple falls, one bumping the back of her head on the dining room table, and about 20 near-falls where I kept her from going down. She kept getting up on her own, determined that she could do it. She already has a bad skin tear on her right hand and a very large bruise on her left arm from a fall at her house. Then the other night she became so nauseated. She lost all her color and sat with a bucket on her lap for hours. Finally, she was able to sip ginger ale and then I put her to bed. I questioned every act I had made in bringing her to Florida. I haven't established her with any physicians in Florida yet. Bri and I are the only two who know her and her entire history currently.

Don't stand shivering upon the bank, plunge in at once, and have it over with. I would say I've already jumped in—and it sorta feels like the polar plunge they do on New Year's Day. Let's hope there are warmer days ahead.

I took her to the walk-in clinic. They diagnosed her with middle ear dizziness and vertigo. He gave me a script for Antivert, but it's over the counter. I got her started on it and she's doing better. I took her to Walmart, and she pushed the cart, which gave her help for her balance. She's already fallen twice since we came to Florida and I'm still dressing the skin tear on her right hand from the fall up north. We did have a better day today.

In the darkest hour the soul is replenished and given strength to continue and endure.

I told Mom I wanted to go to the habitat for humanity and Walmart to look around.

She said, "You go ahead, I'll stay here."

I said, "oh no you won't. I'm taking you with me." She quickly agreed. I feel she declined because she knows it is an effort to take her anywhere, and she was "letting me off the hook." She doesn't understand that these outings are to help her gain better balance, more endurance, and help to build up her tolerance for activity. It is difficult to walk her in the yard, as it is very uneven and irregular. It is monotonous to walk any length of time in the house. Walking through a store gives many distractions and the walking becomes a fun outing instead of a means for exercise.

She walked through habitat with just the assistance of me holding her arm. We then went to Walmart and I put Mom behind a buggy in the parking lot, and she used it for balance throughout all our walking. She never complained of being tired or resisted walking back and forth in the store. When we finished, we went through the Wendy's drive through and purchased our supper. Mom offered to pay for this meal, which came to nine dollars and a few cents. Her offer is another remarkable step in her recovery. She is aware that food purchased in the drive through needs to be paid for.

This lady feels the only thing she can really do is wash the dishes; she is always checking the dishpan to see if there are any dishes in it. My home is laid out so that the living room, dining room, kitchen and sitting area are all open, and surrounds a large island in the middle of the great room. Sometimes she checks the sink three or four times within fifteen minutes.

This lady is a marvel of discovery and creativity. She can put her jeans on backward and wonder why her pockets are so hard to get into. She can wear her shoes on either foot. We were at Walmart and I asked her if she needed anything. She said she would like to have a toothbrush and something to put on it. I informed her that she had an electric toothbrush, a battery toothbrush, and a regular brush at home. I told her we also have lots of toothpaste, to put on it. She told me she didn't know that, because she needed to brush her teeth. Wow, if Jane were nearby, this lady would be getting a big woo-hoo.

I talked with Mom and thought it might be a good idea to send a weekly or biweekly newsletter or email up North to show her progress in recovery. She thought it was "okay." I asked her what she wanted me to tell everyone, and she simply said, "just say the truth." I don't know if she realizes just "how truthful" I can be. I also wonder if she would need to read it herself, to know what all our week had held.

SECOND WEEK OF
FEBRUARY HAS BEGUN

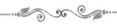

After breakfast, Mom and I were outside. I was showing her, again, where Bri's house was. I did this after she asked me where the pool was. She looked in the back yard and didn't see it. I said, "do you want to walk over to see the pool at Brian's?" She said she would. It was then that Rusty decided to get out of the fenced yard and explore the neighborhood. I must think quickly, as he is much faster than I—and I am no longer alone. I tell Mom she must stay inside the gate while I go catch Rusty. She offers to help me catch him. I can only give this gesture a quick thought, and it doesn't step forward as a good idea. Without wanting to hurt her feelings, I ask her to stay with the other dogs for now, but if I couldn't catch him right away, I would take her up on her offer. So far, she has accepted my explanation. It doesn't take me long to realize Rusty is much younger, and far faster, than I. He certainly didn't want to get caught. He would stop at every mailbox for a few seconds, give me time to almost catch up, and then off he would go again. I wondered if I went back home, if he would return? We have not been at my house very long, so I'm sure he doesn't even know where this "home" is. Also, I live in a group of streets, and close to a main multiple-laned highway. Rusty is very small and only weighs about five pounds. He would never be seen if he made it to the highway. So the chase resumes until I have him cornered in a neighborhood yard with a fence. As I carry him back through the neighborhood that we just traveled, I wondered what was waiting for me back home. I haven't met any of the other dogs running loose as I carried Rusty, so maybe they haven't been left out of the gate, at least not yet.

Home is now in view, and I see my mother waiting at the gate. The gate is closed. All looks safe and secure on the home front. Life is so good. I'm sure my mother has guardian angels. This time their wingspan had covered me and Rusty. Thank you, Mom, for loaning me your angels today. I'm sure they knew how I was trying to breath and run, neither activity coming easily. Yes, I'm way out of shape with poor tolerance for physical activity. But my priorities have changed recently. If I was truly honest, physical activity and exercise has never been prioritized on any of my lists. In fact, if I was totally honest, it is not even on a list.

In the book of life, the answers aren't in the back. Complicating our lives a little more seemed a trivial act compared to the energy and love of life we found in this little five-pound body of spit and vinegar.

I take a minute to think of mother's offer to help me chase Rusty. As I still continue to catch my breath. I can't help but smile as I think of how that may have turned out.

Mom must be seen by a family doctor here in Sanford. We were waiting in the office to see the doctor when Mom became impatient and felt we were waiting too long. She said, "come on, let's go." I told her we could do that, but we wouldn't be getting any treatment for the dizziness she was having. I then said, "what do you think the doctor is, a man or a woman?" She said she thought it would be a man. I told her I would take "a woman" as my choice and "looser buys our lunch. She agreed. She then said, "we might as well wait here as anywhere else." Now that is a profound statement coming from Mom. She hasn't had a good concept of time since her injury, but to conform to the fact that we might as well wait here as anywhere… is profound. It also demonstrates how refocusing an escalating situation that was causing increased anxiety has worked.

Finally, we were taken back by the nurse. Mom weighed 131 pounds. This just isn't right. Since bringing her home from the hospital, I have tried to help her regain her strength and build her up. We have eaten three meals a day, had midmorning and midafternoon snacks, and then a bedtime snack. During this process, Mom has gained one pound in five-plus months. I have gained twenty-plus pounds since my stay with Mom from last summer. Where is the fairness in this?

We have established a family doctor now in Florida. And Mom had to buy lunch as we were seen by a female physician's assistant.

I removed my mother's purple nail polish and trimmed and filed her nails. I then painted them a pale pink, and she was quite pleased. Bri had come over after work and changed the dressing on her right hand. Jane called tonight on the landline phone, and Mom seemed to want to talk for an extended period. She always needs help with word finding when she is talking on the phone. I'm trying to get her to answer the phone when it rings. The landline phone number has only been given to immediate family members, so that should be the only people that call.

I bought a weeklong pill holder and this morning I told Mom she would be helping me fill the containers so she would know what she is taking and why. I told her that this was another step in her independence, noting that someone could fill her container for the week, and she would then be able to take her pills properly. I told her we would learn on this dispenser, and then she would feel comfortable with it when on her own. This seems to be so encouraging to her. I don't want her to lose hope that we are striving for her independence living in her own home again.

My mother seems somewhat leery of her electric toothbrush, so I picked up a battery operated one for her today. She is managing it well. I can see why having a toothbrush that moves on its own could take some getting used to. I'm also working on getting her to put her partial plate into a denture cup to soak with the Polident tablet. I've explained that the dentist had told me that she has a "bacterial issue" with her teeth, and her oral care needs a lot of improvement. He is the one who suggested the electric or battery toothbrush to assist her with her brushing. We also purchased some chewable mints, that he suggested for her to chew two of them three times a day. We are working on that suggestion also. She says they taste good and never resists chewing them.

I have not given Mom anxiety medication at bedtime since we came to Florida. The first days were rough ones, so I didn't give her any extra medication that may have intensified her confusion. She still gets mixed up at times, as to where she is. It is easy to confuse some parts of her home with some parts of mine. Tonight, she asked me where the swimming pool was, she didn't see it in the back yard. I told her she was thinking of Brian's house, because that is where the pool is, not at my house. You can watch her process the information and try to put it in the right place in her mind. These are the times that my heart aches for her. To live past your eighty-ninth birthday, and now be trying to recollect the memories and knowledge that has come to you so easy all your life, just doesn't seem fair. But then I think of something her grandson Mark had said to me when we were discussing her altered thought processes. He simply said, "But at least we still have her." It baffles me when I think of how much this woman is loved. I'm so glad we've had the opportunity to show her. A lot of people are taken away from loved ones, before they ever truly know how much they mean to them. Some get whisked away, with no chance to say "goodbye."

We knew we were going to have to let go of our dad, when he was hospitalized the day after Christmas. We had four months to accept the inevitable, and the chance to spend as much quality time with him as possible. There were seventeen of us in the hospital room with him when he walked home with Jesus. An eighteenth family member had left work early to come to the hospital and was walking down the hallway to Dad's room. This solitary man was the most respected, admired, and loved man I had the privilege of knowing.

Mom is sleeping well here at night. She is also doing much better with telling the time of the day. I have been putting her watch on her wrist and have a clock with easy-to-read numbers. I have been marking off a calendar to help her realize the day.

We went up to the Walmart late morning. Mom chose that store to be her place to walk today. We did a lot of walking and back tracking during our shopping time. She pushes the cart to aid her balance. As I watched her in the store, I realized that she hasn't been looking around in a store for quite a while. She was enjoying herself and not in a hurry. I kept checking with her to make sure she wouldn't get overtired. She denied any problem and assured me she could walk a day on the level in the store with the buggy. There are no benches or chairs throughout Walmart. I put one of their metal folding chairs in the buggy. Every so often, as I saw my Mom slow to a stop, I put the chair out for her to sit on and rest. This happened several times during our "shoppin' walkin'" exercise. At the checkout counter, I handed the chair to the clerk and told her we were not going to purchase it. She kindly put it behind her and continued with our order. I explained to her why I didn't need to buy it, but I needed it throughout her store. She asked me to report it to the manager, because she has heard other people tell her that.

Well, in all honesty, after spending a large amount of time and energy with my favorite walking companion, I wasn't going to spend any more time within the confines of their store, at least not today. When we finally came home, I told her that she had walked for two hours with no rest periods. She was amazed. I explained how she is establishing better balance, more endurance and overall strength. She was going to lay on the sofa and nap, while I ran something across the street to Brian. I was gone about forty-five minutes. When I came back, she hadn't slept. She said she could only count four dogs and she was worried as to where the other one was.

With all dogs accounted for, I walked her back to her bedroom, helped her remove her shoes and she laid down for a nap. She must have fallen asleep right away. She walked out into the living room about 6:00 PM with a puzzled look. She said she thought she was in bed for the night, but then she heard "all the talking" and thought that she must not be. I explained that she took her nap later than usual, but she wasn't in bed for the night.

Later in the evening, she said she was going to bed. Her pj's were folded on a chair by her bed. I told Mom that she could put on the pajamas. I left her alone, then went back to check. She was frustrated. She was putting her pj top over her blouse. I helped her get her clothes straightened out by removing her blouse, and helping her put the top on over her undershirt

Sometimes I think she is gaining knowledge of her basic ADLs, and then she gets lost performing the basic routine. A few times she put her pajama bottoms over her jeans. Now I am here to inform you that is not an easy task. Another time she had tried to put her shoe on over her slipper. Somehow repetition doesn't establish the knowledge of these simple acts. Just like the way she can't find her bedroom or the bathroom, in either house, hers in Pennsylvania or mine in Florida. In fact, she seems quite comfortable here in Florida. She hasn't said anything about "going home."

I thought this day would be extraordinary and it didn't disappoint me. I don't sleep well; I only catch about three or four hours at the most. The rest is restless short napping spells. The phone rang about 8:00 AM from Millie, the neighbor. Her one finger "locked up" again while she was making her bed. She asks if she could come over and have me put it back in place. I told her I would be over in a few minutes. She had an injection into her left eye on Monday and needed to tell me about it. I listened to her rough day on Monday and gave her some support while I massaged her locked up finger and loosened it back into place. She wanted me to sit and visit, but I just felt I needed to be in the house when Mom woke up. She still has problems with her whereabouts. If only I knew what goes on in her head.

Later in the evening, Mom's dog Mickie, was stalking my dog Ricky. She does that at times, even attacking him and they end up fighting. Mickie's health is compromised with her eyesight. The vet has told me that she is almost blind. Mom pulled Mickie to her side and said, "We should go home, Mickie. I should take you home." I scooted over her comment by stating that we were at home and we have a winter home and a summer home.

She said, "Yes, but I should go home."

I didn't realize it at the time, but she was referring to going to her bedroom. She walked around the sofa in a different direction, squeezing between the chair and the sofa. She walked along the inner side of the kitchen island and stopped. She looked around and then ask me where her "home was."

I showed her how she changed her direction and it confused her. I had her back track her steps. I then showed her the hallway, with her bed at the end of the hall. She laughed and said, "How can I be so stupid?" I told her she wasn't stupid; she just changed her direction and it looked different.

Valentine's Day, Let's Make It Special

I did not have to think long, as Mom took care of the request to make it stand out from being an ordinary day. I must learn to be careful of what I wish for. I heard a thump and felt the house shake this morning. I went back and found Mom on the floor. She was seated on her left hip in the sitting position, but she didn't feel she hit her head, instead she seemed to fall in the middle of the room on the rug. I pulled a chair over and together, we got her up and onto the bed. I checked her over and didn't find any obvious injury. I helped her get dressed and helped her out to the table for breakfast.

I continue to try and explain that "dizzy" and her balance issue are two different issues. She just doesn't grasp the concept of her altered balance and her risk of falling. I continue to caution her about falling and breaking a hip, but she will not use the walker that Bri brought home from work for her use. She says that she has gotten past that and doesn't want to go backward. Again, and again I explain that her balance is altered, and a cane won't help because she needs the four legs of a walker to help her keep her balance. She thinks she needs to keep trying.

Bri came over this morning. I still need to tell her who has come to visit. He is so good with her, but he so misses the "Mawmaw" as he remembers her. Truly, I feel we all miss the "Mawmaw" that remembers us. She will describe one of the dogs and ask me "which one is that." She will describe Annie as "the white one with the spot on her back," and then ask me "which one is that?" I will tell her that it's her dog, Annie. She is constantly counting the dogs.

Until one has loved an animal, a part of one's soul remains unawakened.

After dinner tonight, I was trying to get her to help with clearing the table. She carried the zip lock bag with the onion in it, into the living room. I asked her where she was going with the onion. She looked at me and said, "the wrong way again?"

Before supper, I sat the coleslaw and cranberry sauce on the kitchen island and asked Mom to put them on the table. She worked hard at getting the silverware set out for the table. She brought back several pieces of silverware and put them back in the drawer. She then asked me how many was there? I told her, "Just the two of us." When we sat down, I couldn't find the coleslaw and sauce. They were back in the fridge. Tonight, she asked me, "Is there a bathroom on this floor, or do I need to go upstairs?" She then asked me if everything was ready upstairs because she was going to go to bed. Without going into deep explanations that our home was only one level, that there was no "upstairs"—I just answered that everything was ready for whenever she wanted to go to bed.

I showed her the hallway and told her that her bed was right at the end, and her bathroom was just beside it. I always keep a little light lit there so she can find it. She always thinks there is an upstairs. I don't know how difficult it must be to be lost all the time. I try to make it familiar; I've simplified my house and kept her bed the same place since day one. I don't think it matters, because each day is a brand-new day.

She wanted to know if there was a shoehorn. She said she thought she brought it. This little lady didn't pack one thing or offer any suggestions as to what she wanted to bring, so I know we didn't bring a shoehorn. I didn't know she used a shoehorn. I didn't know she owned a shoehorn. I was pleasantly surprised to have her ask about a shoehorn. Jane, can we give a big woo-hoo for the shoehorn? But while you're at it, look around and see if you can find one for her.

We were up at the garden center and I asked her what flowers she wanted to get to put in my planters on the porch. She wouldn't pick any, because she didn't want to take care of them, and she said we must take them back when we go. We had the buggy loaded at the Walmart, and I paid the bill. She then walked to the front of the cart and started looking in the empty bags on the carousel, ready to load more. She hadn't loaded, unloaded, or showed any interest or help during the entire shopping trip and checkout. She did push the buggy. That would be one task. When she stopped pushing the buggy at the checkout counter, she was able to consider another task. I just guided her back to the handle and told her we had everything, and we were ready to get a valentine meal and go back home. She follows all commands and just agrees. She must be so lost and fearful of not knowing who she's with or even where she is. She truly doesn't know, but her desire and attempt to show independence keeps emerging. I notice that mother. I know how much you want to help. I know how badly you try to be independent.

She asks me, "What can I do to help?" I involve her in everything. I can only give her one request at a time. If I give more than one, she stands with a very confused look that breaks my heart. Sometimes, even one request is one too many. It's then that I must show her what I mean, often leading her.

Like the quilt that she is trying to knot. I finally left open safety pins where she was to make a knot. For some reason, she couldn't remember how to follow the line across the length. She would look so puzzled, as I try to explain how she has done something all her life. It just doesn't seem fair, that she has lost so much memory so late in her life. These should be her easy years. She has been such a truly wonderful woman all her life. These past seven months or so seem so unfair.

Mom gets up about nine-ish or later and seems to go to bed at 8 or so every night.

She had put the entire plate of pork chops left over from supper right into the dishwater yesterday when she washed the dishes. I found it so disheartening when I dumped her dishpan and found tomorrows dinner soaking at the bottom. Little is surprising me these days. She has taught me to think outside the box. She has also caused me to try and do preventative damage control.

If only she knew the way I looked at her when she had her back to me. I cherish every minute—relish every experience and I smile wider than the sky.

She had fallen first thing in the morning yesterday. She apparently had been looking for money in her rain bonnet. I think she waits too long to go to the bathroom or gets distracted and then forgets to go. Today we had to help her get cleaned up and put on dry clothes. Why was she hunting for money? She says she just likes to "have some money."

Bri has an appointment with an orthopedic doctor on Wednesday so he's coming over here to fill out the paperwork Wednesday morning. He worked today and he's in so much pain. I'm afraid he's got a ruptured disc that may need surgery.

I bought some flowers and cleaned up the patio furniture today. I sure needed to work outside. I try to take Mom to a store every day and she walks all over pushing the cart for balance. It is literally the only way I can push her to walk long enough to increase her tolerance and strength. Fortunately, every store is less than two miles away.

My house is a deranged mess as I've tried to make it simple for her from the living area to her bedroom and the bathroom. Still she can't seem to find it. She feels she needs to go upstairs. She is very dependent on me, not even able to prepare a meal or do anything without constant and simple instruction. Half the time she doesn't know which white dog is hers. Sometimes she doesn't know exactly who I am, just that I am the person that takes care of her and keeps her safe. Some days are better, so I run with those days. Often, she seems to think that she's back at the farmhouse, or someday even further, at her childhood home in Kepple Hill.

I may not have gone where I intended to go, but I think I have ended up where I needed to be.

Shoppin', Walkin'

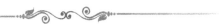

This day would be the first "close" to normal" day we have had in Florida. Now all I must do is define "normal" and then I can move forward from there. Mom woke up and went to the bathroom several times, then went back to bed. Her dogs have been in and out. This home is new territory for them also.

I have found that I need to take my mother somewhere to walk. I call it "shoppin' walkin'." The yard is too irregular, and I am not going to walk on our street. By using a store buggy, she doesn't need a walker or wheelchair currently. It helps her keep her balance, and it gives her something to lean on when she wants to stop. I had initially thought that she would look at things in the store and show some interest in the displays. Some days she does, and some days her whole concentration is pushing the buggy down the aisles. Solely pushing the buggy.

Monday Night

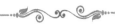

Mom sleeps until about nine-ish or so in the morning. She doesn't seem to have any trouble getting up during the night to go to the bathroom. I have a small light in her bedroom, and I always let the light lit in the bathroom. I have learned to keep the sewing room door closed, let the utility room curtains hang down instead of tying them back, and just today, bought a shower rod and one drapery panel for my bedroom entrance. I hung the rod and the one panel and keep it almost closed.

This afternoon we had gone to Walmart and she did her walking and pushing the cart. I have noticed by the end of our "exercise period," I am literally pulling the cart with her holding onto the handle. I hold onto the front corner of the cart and guide it the entire time. If she wants to stop and look at something, we stop. But I have not let her guide the cart more than a few safe feet. Somehow I picture her running into one of the displays—and then keeps on going.

She said yesterday during our trip to Big Lots, "I need to count all my grandchildren for some little things." Now, this is something, for she must feel like she is on vacation and wants to take back souvenirs. I know she doesn't mean her grandchildren; she means her great-grandchildren. Just as she often refers to "her sisters," I know she means her daughters. God bless the loving mother and woman that's lost inside this lady standing before me. I was just surprised that she remembered she had grandchildren, even though they are all adults now. Her memory surfaces at times, maybe not in the proper place, but it still surfaces. I know how many times she came home from a trip with something for her young grandchildren.

I know what she was like, her nonconfrontational nature, her selfless giving, her unconditional love, her self-sacrifice with time and ability to work at the church, meals on wheels, membership in wings," or even her existence on the bowling team. Members of wings or the church bowling team ladies would often go out afterward to a place for lunch. I see Mom's confusion with a menu now to where she might know what she would like, but always stays with a safe choice. If it wasn't a specific special like the dairy queen offers, she would usually order a BLT and coffee. I always, and I mean always, order for her. No matter how I try to get her to choose, it's always "whatever you are getting." I don't ask anymore. I take that little piece of difficulty away from her. I don't ask what she might want for lunch or supper. I teasingly always ask what she might want for her bedtime snack, often giving her three choices. I follow it with, "I bet I know your choice."

She laughs and says, "I will take my Klondike." It's a given. So I cut one in half, and we have our bedtime "picnic" in front of the TV at night.

Yesterday she stopped at the end of a counter that had some elastic bras on display. They don't have hooks or fasteners, so they can just be pulled over her head. We ended up buying two. I know she wants to wear a bra again, but I have realized that she will let it on all the time, even to sleep. This is because she can't get it back on by herself. Tonight, at bedtime, we tried them both on and she was quite pleased. She even walked to the mirror on her dresser and looked at the reflection. She was visibly pleased. She said. "I will wear the white one tomorrow." This I hung over the chair by her bed. I also hung her jeans for tomorrow, along with a shirt and short sleeved sweatshirt. She does put on her jeans, after removing her pajama bottoms, and then puts on her shoes independently.

Funny thing I discovered. She was having trouble getting her pants and pj bottoms on at the beginning. She was holding them properly, with the tag in the back. But then she would cross her legs and start putting the one leg of the pant on the crossed leg. This was the wrong leg, which then would increase her confusion, for when she uncrossed her leg to put the other leg on, something was wrong. She cannot problem solve. If she hits a stumbling block, she is stopped.

That issue came up with the quilt she is knotting. I was outside and watched her unroll the quilt on the dining room table. I saw her sewing and was so pleased that she initiated this activity on her own. I waited a bit and came in and sat down. She was putting three or four stitches into the exact same area, and then tying the knot.

This left eight strands of thread in her knot. When I tried to explain that she only needed to do it once, she said that she had to make sure it wouldn't come undone. I unrolled the first row of knots she did to show her that she only used single thread for those knots. I said to her that she was making it so much harder than she needed to. I reaffirmed that it was supposed to be fun, not hard work. She agreed, saying, "I've done so many of these."

I grasped the moment. "Mom, what's it like when you can't remember something? Does it come back after you start?" I knew I had asked one too many questions, so I waited for a response. I repeated one question and asked what it was like when she can't remember something?

She looked at me and said, "I have done so many of those," but didn't really answer the question. I have read "the notebook" and saw the movie several times. James Garner really had it nailed. I am writing "my notebook" but it's in the lost chapter area, not in the years that all those memories were made…

I stimulate her mind almost every waking moment. She never knows how many people to set the table for. For some reason, there is always more than her and me. I've even seen her look around. And it's always a question she will ask as she is going through the silverware drawer. Today for lunch, she and I had a fork and spoon. Neither of us had a knife to butter our French toast. Yesterday we had both a fork and spoon and a sharp knife. No butter knives. And yes, when she fixes her own plate from serving dishes, it is always on one side of the plate. I remember all the in-services I gave on Alzheimer's during staff development. This was such a common act. When a dementia patient was asked to draw a picture of a clock, all the numbers were placed on one side of the face of the clock. I don't know whether a brain injury responds this way also, but I know that Alzheimer's patients do.

She did ask me to trim the ends of her hair a few days ago. I was so pleased, as I was able to even the sides out finally. I also colored her hair, set it, and then showed her how pretty it looked. She was pleased. Her hair was always so important to her, even though it was so thin, and she fought with what she called her "bald spot." She always felt good when it looked nice. She commented tonight how nice her fingernails looked, because they were longer than they ever were. I must keep with the positive aspects of her appearance as she does notice.

I told her about the sad news of one of Mark's cows today. This is her grandson who bought the farm that she and my father had lived on. One of his cows had met with an untimely death. Somehow it got into the water trough and froze to death. I wanted to see if the information was retained or even carried over to another conversation. Shortly after she received the news, Jody called on the phone. Mom is getting better at "pushing the green button" to talk and pushing the red button to hang up. She was struggling to tell Jo something. She then asked me, "what was that we heard about the goat" and after a pause, "and the farm?" I told her she was trying to think of the cow on Mark's farm and she readily agreed and continued to tell Jo the news. It was accurate, after she was able to get help finding her words. It had been many years since my dad had goats at the farm. In my mother's defense, there really were two goats on the farm at one time. When Dad was no longer able to take care of cattle on the farm, he had his grandson pick up a couple of goats. They were in the barnyard and Dad would watch them from the kitchen window. I think he had a hard time accepting the lack of animals on his farm. His emphysema kept him housebound on oxygen, so taking care of farm animals was not possible.

I have attempted to keep her "word finding issues" to a minimum. Her bed is visible at the end of the hall. I keep a light on in the room, as I do the bathroom. I had found a half moon and a star, that used a night light bulb and hung on the wall. I have them hanging over Mom's bed, keeping her room alit enough to help her when she gets up. I pulled the curtains across the utility room and hung a curtain in the doorway to my bedroom. There are no doors there as yet. I also keep the sewing room door shut. Every night she asks where she goes to go to bed. I have her look back the hall. I tell her that I leave the light lit in her room, so she knows where it is. She reacts with a little sigh of relief and says, "oh thank you, thank you."

I am just confused. She could remember a bit of the story of the cow. She remembers the store where Dave buys his wife Jane's jewelry for Christmas. She remembers what kind of cake her mother made in the long loaf pan. Some is short term; some is from a long time ago. Why can't she find her bed? She couldn't find it in her own home either and she lived there for many years. I'm seeing that the place she lives is not an issue. She isn't familiar with anyplace. No place is "home" to her; at least that's what it seems like to me.

Her dog Mickie is her friend. Mickie is always by her feet or on the footstool by her chair. She talks to her more than she does to me. She always comments on how very loyal she is. Mickie has become more protective and aggressive. If she is eating her dinner by Mom's feet, she attacks any dog that bothers her. I wonder just how much Mickie understands? I'm thinking it's more than we give her credit for. She is doing well except for the fact that she appears to be almost blind. My prayer is that Mickie will maintain her health for as long as Mom needs her here on earth. Annie will come and go from Mom's bedroom. Mickie is usually there for the duration, unless she comes out to go to the bathroom on the pee pads or come and stand by the door. She isn't going to lose track of Mom again. And I have to say I did promise Mickie when Mom was hospitalized for several weeks that we would bring Mom home to her. Mickie was not doing well without Mom. She would go outside and wait by Mom's car, waiting for her to get out. She didn't want to eat. I think Mickie knows that her beloved master is home, but something is not exactly right. Something is different. Something is changed. Mickie is aware of this, but it doesn't matter to her. She will not lose track of her beloved master again.

If she wasn't my mother, it could be a skit for a short comedy sitcom. But she is my mom, so we keep humor close to our hearts.

Yesterday she walked for about two hours at Walmart. She was "dragging" by the time we got home. She napped and didn't get up until about 6:00 PM. Supper was ready when she came out of the bedroom. She always asks me, "Why didn't you wake me so I could help?" That doesn't really require an answer. I had supper prepared, ready to serve and dishes and pans washed, while she slept.

We have a weekly pill dispenser, with four color-coded tabs for the times of day. I have her remembering that "yellow" tab is for morning, when the sun comes up. The bedtime tab is purple, like when it is getting dark outside. The other two tabs are for other medication times, which are to be taken midmorning and midevening or afternoon, just on an empty stomach. She still can't remember to push down on the tab to make it open. But then the window button in her car still has her totally confused. Every day I tell her where it is. Every time we are in the car, she has her hand all over the door and handle. She slides right over the button and never retains the information of what it is.

Today she opened her quilt and I showed her how she only needs one stitch per knot. Some of her single knots have up to six individual stitches with knot on top of knot. No wonder she was frustrated.

I gave her a lap board and a deck of cards. With a little guidance, she laid the cards out properly for solitaire. She played the entire game, only once laying a nine up where the aces were to be. May I also comment that a "9" does resemble an "A"—as I have discovered while watching her play cards.

I reminded her that she needed to count out three, and only play from the card on top. She remembered and did it properly. She went back to the bed to lay down after knotting on the quilt this morning. She was tired after playing solitaire. She went back and took her nap, falling asleep quickly. She tires easily when she has to use her mind and hands at the same time.

I had supper in the oven, and she ate well. She always does. Her weight has stayed at about 131#. She no longer receives anxiety medication at bedtime.

After supper, I wiped down the card table and put out a puzzle of three hundred pieces. She helped with turning all pieces over. We worked for an hour or so, and I got the border completed. Mom would work with a few pieces, not even matching up the pattern. When we stopped for the night, she had only put in two pieces, but she laughed when she told her daughter Jane about it during their phone call.

WHERE DOES TIME GO
WHEN HAVING FUN?

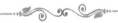

After she talked to Jane tonight she wanted to go to bed. I asked her if we could talk. I asked her what it was like when she can't remember or doesn't know something. She sat down. She said she had to work hard when we would call her "mom," after "this happened." She told me she didn't know she had daughters, but since we called her mom and we were working with her that we must be right. She said she remembers before "this happened'—that sometimes she couldn't remember names. Then it got that she couldn't remember more things. Then "this happened." She said that they fixed it without any incision. Again, I traced the incision line with my finger on the left side of her head. She didn't remember that she had forty-nine staples in her head. Her question: "Did they open up both sides of my head?"

An interesting thing she relayed to me tonight. When she can't remember something, she knows that she should remember it, but she just can't. I ask her if that is what happens when she doesn't know how to use a recipe or make the knots on the quilt. She can only say that she knows that she should know, but she just can't remember. I asked her if it becomes familiar after she starts it and she said "sometimes." I did ask her if she knew how many people were with her here in the house. She said she did and that there are just us two. I am constantly stimulating her mind. Sometimes it is repetitious, but I want to see if the answers are the same.

I explained to Mom that her use of her brain really tires her out. If she does a lot of walking, then she physically has nothing left to do any mental activities. If she doesn't walk, we had better luck with the solitaire game, knotting the quilt, or working with a jigsaw puzzle.

Bri says he is not a patient man. Bri doesn't like jigsaw puzzles. He doesn't understand why someone would cut a picture all up, then spend hours or days trying to get all the pieces back together. Yet this man would spend hours working with his Mawmaw at a table with a twenty-four-piece puzzle.

I explained to Mom that a few months ago, we would open a twenty-four-piece puzzle, and she would just gather up the pieces and put them back in the box. She didn't attempt to put them together at all. When we last tried solitaire, she didn't know how to play. Tonight, she did.

I also explained that her being tired was to be expected. I said I can't tell you how much effort and energy it takes to make your mind and brain work to do things. Her brain is trying to compensate and heal, retrain and relearn, and it is exhausting her physically. She didn't think it could happen that way.

She spends a lot of time watching me or trying to find me. She needs to be encouraged, and encouraged, and encouraged some more. Otherwise, she tells me she just doesn't want to do anything right now.

We are all broken. I'm told that's how the light gets in.

On this day Mom slept till almost eleven thirty. I kept checking on her, and she was fine. She just said that she was tired. I had tried to find a way for Mom to identify the time and date. I purchased a clock with large numbers and the date. The light was not on all the time, and you had to push the button on top to illuminate it. She was doing well pushing the bar on the top. It just wasn't helping her with identifying the time and date. At bedtime she asked me where her "crazy clock" was. I showed her where it was sitting and told her to push the button on the top and it would light up. She pushed the button at 8:11 PM.

She said, "It's eleven to eight, and then it will be March."

I started to laugh, and she joined me. I said, "You're exactly right, Mom, and then it will be March." What a truly pleasant way to tuck this lady in bed for the night. Laughter, a kiss on her forehead, and the promise that "tomorrow will be a brand-new day.

We do not remember days—we remember moments.

I had talked to Mom the last few evenings as to getting a sponge bath. She declines an evening bath and chooses to wait until morning. She doesn't initiate too much on her own. I must take her back to the bathroom and set her up for brushing her teeth. I keep hoping if we do it long enough and repeat it often enough that it will become something that she will do on her own. I am an optimist. I think positive. I try to stay consistent. We will "assume" that it may just happen, and we all know what happens when we "assume." I'm sure I will not be disappointed.

Mom did come out for breakfast in her pj's. She did not have her shoes on. It told me that she "remembered" that she was going to get bathed this morning and have all clean clothes on.

I tried to have her fix her own breakfast. While we did the dishes, I showed her where we would put the small dishes, her coffee cup, and the box of frosted flakes. She is still working at figuring out how to use her medicine dispenser. She is starting to remember that the yellow tab is for morning medication. That would be a "WOO HOO," as Jane would refer it to.

I always fill the pink thermos with coffee. It lasts her most of the day and is still hot. One thing is working out. She doesn't have to reheat a partial cup of coffee many times a day. This is a Gold Ring. We've grabbed one as our world spins round and round.

I ran to the Home Depot and left her at home today. I locked her in the house, and she was going to lie on the sofa and wait for me to return. She was not going to open the door and worry about doing anything for the dogs. When I got home, she had made herself half cheese sandwich. The bread was above the toaster oven in full view. The cheese was in the cold cut drawer in the fridge. I was so pleased. I noticed she had used Caesar Salad dressing as the condiment on her sandwich. The knife was still lying on top of the open jar. She just may be paving the way for new recipes. It could happen. I never tried

Caesar dressing on any sandwich, so how could I make a judgment. Now I have seen her stir her coffee with the mashed potato spoon. I'm not saying that this may catch on. But then again, as I keep telling my sisters, you just can't make this stuff up. Some days the box of chocolates are a sample pack. Other times I think we are dealing with a 25# box like they put out at Christmas.

As of today, I have a child gate in the doorway of the kitchen door. I have a pet gate in the front door and pet fencing all around the front porch. I bought some U nails today so tomorrow I will attach the fencing to the house and the porch poles. Hopefully Bri will feel good enough by Saturday to put a railing on the carport steps and a railing back the hallway to assist her where she walks. The gate and fence will prevent five dogs from leaving if she opens the front door. The child gate on the back door is held in securely.

I am still trying to convince her that her bedroom is her home here. The bathroom is the very next door. I hung her clothing over the quilt rack, like she does up north. She insisted that someone comes in and sleeps in the single bed in her bedroom. I sat down and talked with her. I showed her the clothes hanging in the room are all hers. The dresser is hers and her other clothes are in the drawers. I walked around the room and showed her that it is her place. I assured her no one comes in and sleeps in the bed. For one thing, we live with five dogs. Surely one would bark with a visitor. I did tell her we shared the room when we first came down until she became a little more familiar with our relocation. She always makes sure her dogs go with her when she goes into her bed. She doesn't usually know for sure about the "white one," but she always knows Mickie.

February Moves to an Apple-a-Day

I am so blessed. I didn't have to wait very long to be made aware of it. I never do.

When we were shopping, Mom had wanted to buy cooking apples. I had bought an apple shaped pie dish, and we talked about making a pie. She picked "Granny Smith," and she didn't feel one bag was enough, so we bought two. Mom has always packed apple slices between her two pie crusts. She never liked making a skinny pie. Those apple slices were always piled high.

Well, today was the day. We had bought a paring knife when we were out the other day. I got two bowls and the apples. Mom sat down and started to peel one of the apples. I watched as she slowly worked at the skin on the apple. She kept changing the position of the knife she was holding. Then she would try holding the apple at a different angle. She worked at the skin of the apple, and it was a difficult task for her to peel it. She told me my knives were dull. I left her try a few different knives. She finally told me that the apples were too hard. I told her we could let it go for now, because we had plenty of time to make the pie. She put the half-peeled apple and paring knife down in the pan and surrendered it quickly.

Another of the times that she cannot recognize that her right hand cannot use the paring knife to peel apples. We will go with a dull knife and the apples are too hard. Is it right? Maybe not, but it's a protective answer. In my memory, this woman has been a pie baker her entire life. This day her memory fails her. She has no answer for what needs to go in with the apples that are pared, sliced, rinsed, and in a large bowl. I can tell she knew she should remember. She also isn't aware that the strength and coordination in her right hand is not what it used to be. Writing, or paring apples, is an ability that apparently will not return. So this time, and for the similar issues that will occur in the future, the apples were too hard, and the paring knife was just too dull. Okay, the reasons are all valid to me.

She did make a choice as to what type of egg she wanted for lunch. She chose scrambled. With this, I put the raw eggs in a cup and beat them with a fork. I added a very small amount of water and beat them again, while I waited for the skillet to get hot. Mom watched what I did. I asked her if she wanted to scramble them in the skillet. She watched as I poured the raw eggs into the skillet, stirred a few times with the fork, then handed her the fork. I cautioned her about getting burnt on the hot skillet. She stood, holding the fork, and then said, "I don't know how to do this." I took the fork and showed her how to turn the eggs over. She looked confused. I got a spatula and showed her how to turn them over as they cooked. She asked me to do it. I prepared the eggs and then lifted them to the plates. She carried her plate of eggs to the table, along with a piece of toast, and we enjoyed our lunch.

I keep trying to find an action or task that kick starts her memory of eighty-nine years. She gets puzzled with putting three pieces of silverware at a place setting. She doesn't know how to make an egg in a skillet. I asked her to please bring me the remote for the TV, that it was laying on the dining room table. She went from the dining room table into the kitchen. I waited patiently, as she carried in the can opener and asked me, "Is this it?" I just responded by telling her that it was the same color, and I would help her find it.

I was working with some cleaning projects a few days ago. Although I have everything toxic out of reach and out of sight, I had the gallon of bleach sitting on the sidebar of the sink. I found the gallon jug sitting politely in the refrigerator, apparently chilling nicely. I realized that it appeared to look something like the gallon of milk, so I won't let that happen again. My mom's innocence currently in her life never ceases to amaze me. We have reversed our roles. She certainly does need constant protection and supervision.

She talked with "Woo hoo," alias Jane, the other evening. After she hung up, she asked me who that was. She told me she couldn't put a face with her. I told her that Jane was her second daughter, and I would get a picture of her on my phone, which I did.

She looked at her picture and said, "That looks just like Jane."

I said, "It is Jane, Mom. That's who you were talking to on the phone."

She said, "No, that one looks just like my Jane, not the other one."

Where does one go with an answer? Again, I had nothing. I found it best to abandon this conversation and move on.

Bri has a painted saying on the wall in his room. It says, "Walk a day in my mind, and you won't ask." I can't imagine what it would be like to live a day, or an hour, in my second mother's mind these days. Every night she wonders where she will be able to sleep, reminding me that she also has her kids and her dog, or the chickens that slept with her the night before. She always asks if there is a place for her to sit at the dinner table, and if there is enough food. I really hadn't worried about not having enough food for us all, since her salad consists of three small pieces of lettuce, some parmesan cheese and one crouton. It takes her all day to drink a 6 oz glass of water. She doesn't finish her pint of coffee throughout the entire day. I'm seeing that her frosted flakes for breakfast and her lunch are her best meals of the day. I'm seeing that getting her to eat much for supper is getting more and more difficult. Her answer is always that she has already eaten today. Her appetite was so good for so long, but I see things changing. I must be more cautious of what she eats now, as she eats so little. Since she no longer gets 250 cc of fluids with the daily IVs that she had been receiving, the ongoing battle to get her to drink enough fluids has been stepped up.

I had made her half sandwich for lunch a few days ago. I found half of that sandwich "hiding" behind one of the dog dishes on the counter. It could never have found that hiding place by accident or coincidence. I was going to question the dogs, one by one, later to see if they witnessed anything concerning the hidden sandwich. I'm thinking if it had been hidden on a lower position, the evidence would have been a canine meal, and never been discovered.

A ROUGH THURSDAY

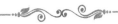

Rough night. Rough evening. Mom is confused, more confused than usual. She thinks she is at the neighbor's house. She thinks she left the dogs alone "over there." She wants to go upstairs. She doesn't know why she is here and who decided for this to happen. Her dogs are right in front of her and she thinks she left them "over there." She is looking directly at Mickie and asks, "Is that Mickie?"

She wants to know why she can't do what she's doing here—"back there?" I so much want to ease her frustration. She denies being frightened, but I don't see that in her face. She takes both of her hands and placed them on the side of her head. She lowered her head and just shook it while making exhausting noises with her mouth. I knelt on the floor in front of her. I told her that I had spent seven months with her up in her trailer. She asked why we couldn't still do that and why are we here? I explained that this was my home, and we were spending time here while it was so very cold up north. I know that concept is giving her problems, for every day she looks for the snow.

I left her alone for an hour or more today. I said we would try it and see how things go. She assured me that she would be fine and didn't want to go to the pharmacy, Lowes, etc. I told her not to open the doors and she didn't have to answer the phone. She had just finished breakfast and has no interest other than sitting in front of the TV. She assured me she would just sit and relax. When I came home, she was waiting by the carport door. She cracked open the door and asked if she could let the dogs out. I hadn't got in the gate but told her to let them out.

117

She was frustrated, I could tell. I sat her down at the carport chair and table and asked what was wrong. Just then the landline phone rang and she hollered for me to "get that, get that—it's been ringing, and I didn't answer it." Now I already know that to leave her alone, I must shut off the ringing of the landline.

She told me that she didn't have any food for the dogs-and they probably wanted water-and they wanted out-and she didn't let them out, but they wanted out. She had tied one curtain back with my sewing tape measure; one was tied back with a tea towel, so they could see out above the futon. One blind was pulled up at an angle and another was pulled halfway up. There was a half-eaten peanut butter cup on the counter. She said she had eaten some cookies and a few other things but was overly concerned because she didn't have anything for the dogs. I had put two in my bedroom and put the gate across. She said that they wanted water and they wanted out but she didn't let them out. She explained how she felt so bad and tried to help them. Now I know that if she would have been here with me, she eats her breakfast and then sits around doing nothing but following me and asking me what I was doing. She sometimes wants to help; other times she refuses any suggestions. I know if she had just spent time sitting, that the three dogs in her living area and the two in my bedroom would just go dormant. I don't know how I could have seen this behavior coming. She must have been in total turmoil the whole time I was gone.

We ate lunch and I told her I was going to replace some dead plants and plant a few more. She went back to her bedroom and I tucked her in for a nap. She always makes sure her two dogs are with her, even if Mickie is the only one she truly knows. Annie cuddles close to her and she lovingly rubs her head and kisses her nose. Mom does not know Annie, but Annie knows her.

My son stopped after his doctor's appointment, and we were talking outside. He was in a lot of pain from the ruptured disc in his back and couldn't get comfortable. He said he was sorry, but he needed to go home and lay down

My next-door neighbor asked about my mom, and I just stated that she wasn't the mom we had before the surgery. She asked if it was short term memory problems, and I confirmed that was partially it. Word finding and word searching was also a problem.

Brian walked my mom across the yard to meet another of my neighbors. Brian is so very proud of his grandma and never ceases to proudly introduce her to anyone. They talked for a few minutes and then Brian and my mom walked back to the carport. He then decided to walk home, so I continued to burn up the sticks and plant the few plants to replace the dead ones.

I saw Mom walk about on the carport and then went in the house. I finished up outside and told her that our supper was being delivered. Now this hasn't happened since we came down here to Florida. It often happened up north when my sister Jane would send up supper with one of her grandchildren or bring it herself. Often, she ate with us.

Tonight, our supper was delivered. I took the bag in and sat it on the table, then went to clean up. I told Mom to set the food out of the bag and she could set the table. I started fixing dinner for the dogs while she tried to set the table. She sat the containers on the table and opened one. I reminded her to get the plates. She got two plates from the recently dried stack and sat them on the island. I asked her to set them on the table, along with the silverware which I laid on the table. I could tell she was confused. I tried and tried to get her to sit down so her dogs would eat by her feet. She kept fussing with things but was not accomplishing anything. I finally got her to sit and started showing her what supper was. We were eating Mexican fajitas. Mom had no idea what I meant. While I fixed it, she asked me what type of food this was, and I answered that it was Mexican.

She started to cut her fajita up, but it wouldn't cut with the butter knife for her. I cut it all up and told her to add more sour cream as she wanted. Apparently, she wanted a lot of sour cream because she kept adding it to every bite. She finished it, not truly understanding it, but she told me it "wasn't bad." I laughed and asked her what would have happened if she sat that in front of my dad for a meal. She made the motions of sweeping it off the plate onto the floor. She said nothing else. Now the Dad that I remember would have never swept any food onto the floor. As I think about him, he would have patiently eaten a small amount, then would have hoped there was another choice for the rest of his meal.

She doesn't talk about Dad. But then she doesn't really talk about us girls. I am constantly reminding her who Brian is. She does enjoy talking about her own Dad and sisters. I need to let her do this more, but not tonight. Too much is going on inside her head. I don't need to add melancholy to that now.

And tonight, after long discussions and the feeling that we needed to call Jane so she could talk to her and reassure her that everyone knew where she was, I helped her dress for bed. I walked her to her bedroom, and said we soaked your feet last night, how do they feel? She said that they felt good. I tucked her into bed and kissed her forehead, as I do every night. Her dogs were with her and I assured her that all us girls love her very much. She just said, "I know you girls tell me that."

I so want to ease her mind. I told her that her brain is healing, and she is remembering things and questioning things now. She admits that she is more confused tonight and doesn't know why she can't go back to the other place now. She doesn't call it home.

I told her that this is our home for a while. She has her bedroom and bathroom and her dogs. It doesn't seem to be enough. I said, "Mom, you were confused when we were up at the trailer. We thought the nice weather and getting out more would help you get better." She kind of yelled at me and said, "who decided this?" I told her that all us girls and she had decided, and I didn't bring her here against her will. I told her we would be inside her trailer during this very cold weather if we were up there, and that she was confused when she was there also. She spoke loudly and said, "But not this confused." Again, I remain silent. I don't want her to be defensive. I don't want to increase her agitation. I find that by not continuing the present conversation, her own mind will refocus on something else.

I just want her to go to sleep. I want her to wake up to a better day. This is a night of true "sundowners" syndrome. Some days just can't be fixed, and the best to wish for is to start with a brand-new day tomorrow. I think all the extra people here, her meeting the neighbor; the extended company, has all complicated her quiet world. In meeting my neighbor, another experience has been added to her world. As we sat in the living room, she was searching for "all the dogs" because she had left them at the neighbor's house. They were all within sight. They had never left the fenced in yard, yet she still felt she left them at the neighbors. She looked directly at Mickie as he lay on the floor by her feet. I said, "Look, Mom, your buddy is right here waiting for your next move."

She looks down at her as Mickie looks at her in total love. Mickie's big dark eyes are looking directly at Mom, as she spends most of her life doing.

Mom is looking back, but then asks, "Is that Mickie?" I assure her it is, and then she speaks her name. Annie isn't recognized by Mom, but Annie knows who she is. Mickie seems to be the only constant in Mom's life, but tonight she didn't know her either. But I can assure you that with her devotion, Mickie knows her.

I spent seven months with Mom in her mobile home. She didn't know where the rooms were. She didn't know the dogs. She is doing nothing different here at my home than she did up north, but I am. I have been outside and making up for the months I didn't see my own home. I have been using good energy on my yard and flowers and vegetables. I can refresh my head and heart with physical work outside. I can clean and get things put into place, making things very convenient for Mom. I keep hoping that repetition will finally pick up some of the activity. I've hesitated to give Mom an Alzheimer's test. When she fixes her own plate, all food is kept to one side. She is doing better with telling time, but having a real problem with whether it's am or pm. After she awakes from a nap, she feels she's in a new day. She always thinks there are three people here when she sets the table. She can't explain why and I don't push her. She will always look around when a reassure her it is only us two. It seems she must visibly see an empty room, before she acknowledges it is just us two.

Life is funny, isn't it? Just when you think you've got it all figured out…Just when you finally begin to plan something—Just when you start to get excited about it and feel like you know what direction you're heading in—The paths change. The wind blows the other way. North is suddenly south. East is west…and you're…lost.

Most people take for granted the ability to follow more than one conversation at a time. In my mother's world, she hears a word or two from each conversation, but doesn't know how to set them apart. The multiple words are put together into a nonsensical grouping. Today there was a lot more chaos than usual at our home. The phone rang, and she didn't answer it while I was gone. The fact that she couldn't give the dog's some food, or that they couldn't be left outside while I was gone. She met people that she didn't know. She was put in a place that was way out of her comfort zone. She doesn't have a concept of time. It could be ten minutes or ten hours, but it seems the same to her.

I had put the TV on an acceptable channel, and Mom had apparently been watching something. She was trying to explain to me that the "mystery" was happening and that they didn't know what was coming. Some people did know, but she said it was a mystery. She said she was trying to follow it, but she doesn't know how it worked out. She was watching the news with me at this time, but I couldn't fill in enough of the spaces to put her story together. It could have been on the news or a sitcom. This is good news to me. She is listening to things on TV and following the theme of the story to a degree. She is trying to follow storyline instead of just gazing at a funny sitcom.

The other morning, she awoke at 7:00 AM. She was changing into her jeans when I told her the time. She was surprised, for she thought it was later. She said she was dreaming. She was planning a party for Jeani and her husband and she had so much to do yet. I asked her if she got the party all finished and she answered that she had a lot to do yet. I advised her to go back to sleep and finish the dream and all the work, then she could get up. She felt that was a good idea and climbed back in bed.

I've been telling Mom that we will soon be to the end of February. That means we have been in Florida for one month. I sat with my coffee and evaluated how this month has been. She doesn't seem homesick, for she doesn't call anyplace "home" right now. She doesn't seem any worse or better except we get out much more. She stops to look at things and people in stores. She can push the buggy and walk for two hours before showing tiredness to the point that she wants to go home. Her appetite may have slacked off slightly, for she never seems to be "hungry." I discussed that she must drink more, for some days her fluid intake is less than a pint. She doesn't understand the pill dispenser for self-use yet. She always thinks she has already taken her pills—and when she naps…it's always a different day. Time is a scrambled area for her. When I ask her if she wants to help with the dishes and she is watching TV, she answers that she does. But she doesn't get up, but if she is able to see me washing dishes—she offers to help. She admits that she just wants to "watch" things and doesn't want to participate.

Brian physically goes after her to involve her—and she never refuses him. She knows him most of the time, and I think she always recognizes his smile, his neon work shirt, and his gentleness to her. I had told her about his visit to the hospital to get cortisone shot into his spine for the pain he has in his leg and back. She has asked me how "the boy that had the surgery is." Names evade her very badly. We tell her who someone is when they call. We explain who visitors or neighbors are. I did that with everyone up north. She always felt someone overstayed their visit. She has a limited amount of tolerance for a visitor in the house.

When the man with the roofing company came to review my choices and selection of roofing, she stayed in front of the TV. When he finally left, I told her we were ready to eat a hot dog. She informed me that "he stayed an awful long time." I asked if she thought he overstayed, and she said, "I'd say so."

Sometimes I find solving her problems to be so simple, but to do this I must climb into her world. I must let go of the way I would think and listen to what she is saying. Her dilemma is usually simple, and without going too deep, so is the answer.

Some days I amaze myself.

Other days I look for my phone while I'm talking on it.

123

What a Truly Long, Shortest Month of the Year

She still doesn't recognize Annie. She still mixes up everyone but Mickie. Mickie was the dog that she had at the farmhouse. Annie came after her other little dog, Billy, had to be put down. This all occurred at her mobile home, next to the farmhouse. I wonder if this is the where the line on her memory sometimes stops.

She still tells me she knows she has four daughters, but only because we told her she did. She says that we called her "mom" and she figured we knew what we were talking about. She doesn't talk about our father, her husband. She talks about her own father.

I feel there is an improvement since the antiseizure medicine was decreased to once daily. She is not as sleepy. She interacts more and finds herself laughing more often. I can't wait to eliminate the medication all together, but it must be decreased slowly. She asked me tonight, "I am home now, aren't I?"

I said, "You are at my home, and we are lucky to have two homes."

She said, "But I want to go to my own home."

I said, "You can, it's right back the hall. Mickie and Annie know where it is."

She seemed relieved and said, "Okay, just so I can go home now."

I must refocus this lady while she is pleased with the most recent answer.

I said, "Let me see your fingernails."

I realized they needed to be filed and polished. I told her we were doing her nails tonight and she was happy. After I had removed the old polish and repolished one hand, I asked her for her other hand. She crossed her legs and was trying to lift her leg up to me. I said, "No, I don't want your feet at this time. I want your other hand, the one that's flying in the air over there." As I reached over and got ahold of her hand that was flying through the air, we both started laughing out loud. Mom said, "oh, I don't know."

Find the wonderful in today.

I thought she was going to sundown again tonight, but I reverted her to "going home." I walked back the hall to her "home" with her. She asked me if I was going to be alone in my place tonight and did I have all my doors locked. I assured her I had already locked all the doors. I asked her if she had all hers locked and she said, "Yes, I do. I always do." I left the conversation lay as it was. I continued to finish her nails and offered to do her feet. I told her she may want to wear her sandals. She assured me that her balance is not good enough for any other shoes. She has acknowledged her present problem with balance. Hey Jane, that would be another one of your "Woo-hoos."

We are expecting Jody to arrive tomorrow. She is flying down to spend a week with her mother and myself.

While Mom was fixing some things in the kitchen this morning I was out on the carport. She came out and told me there was an animal out there eating. I looked and found nothing. I did see the cement base on one of the corner posts in the direction she was looking. I explained that the cement was gray and looked like an animal. She accepted my explanation.

After supper, I said, "Let's walk out back and check out that thing that looked like an animal." She agreed. As she went down the steps, she remarked at how nice they were. We walked around the fence line and talked about things in the yard. She kept counting the dogs and asking if they all came with us. No matter how many times I told her there was one on the porch she couldn't see her, so it wasn't a reality at this time. She only knows Mickie. Sometimes she doesn't know her. We had a very pleasant walk and talk. I asked her if she was content and she said that she was. I told her the dogs are so very content and she agreed.

I had her make the potato buds tonight. It was time consuming. I got out a pan and the measuring cup. I got out the margarine and cut a two-tablespoon piece. I explained that she needed one and one-third cup water. She said that it wasn't very much. She had measured one-third cup water. I explained that she needed one full cup to add to her one-third cup of water. It took a little while for her to fully comprehend what I said.

She then asked, "You mean I need a full one of these?"

I said yes. I left her go and then realized she had filled it up and put the proper amount in the pan. I handed her the margarine and she put it in the pan. I handed her a small one-third cup measuring cup and asked her to dry the one cup measuring cup, which she did. I told her she had to bring the water to a boil. She turned on the burner and then watched. I told her she could get the one-third cup milk and have it ready. This she did. I then explained that she could get the full cup of potato buds and have it ready. She started to do this, and then I realized she was putting the buds into the cup with a large spoon. I asked if she wanted some help and she did. I helped her fill the cup up so she would be ready. Finally, she was able to put the milk in the pan, and then add the buds. She stirred them up with only one command at a time. This was to be "instant potatoes," usually done quickly, usually.

I asked her to help me with the cottage cheese and fruit cup. She gets a little confused with what gets taken to the table and ended up taking the dish plus another fruit container to the table. She feels useful.

Last evening, I had asked her if she could finish the baked beans and she said she could. After she put them on her plate, she took several spoons of soft butter and put them on the beans. She then stirred them up and ate them. Sometimes she does things to her food that is totally new to our memory. I'm just not sure that a cookbook of her "inventions with food" would be a best seller. I'm quite sure it would not end up on Oprah's best seller list.

She bathed herself in the bathroom today and then asked me where her toothbrush was. I walked back and showed her. She then took care of her teeth, after helping her with the denture bath and the battery toothbrush. I then put her personal care items in a basket and told her she could put them on her dresser, and she could bring them into the bathroom when she needs them. She liked that idea. I hoped it would give her a feeling of ownership—when they would be visible in her bedroom.

I was filing her nails tonight and the TV was on. The voice came from the TV stating that "it seems that we are slowly getting older."

My mom said, "Or sometimes we get old faster."

I looked at her in awe. I said, "Mom, you caught that." That is so good and we both laughed out loud. Yes, I was in awe. She was following a storyline on TV. That is another "Woo-hoo" event Jane. Give your mother the "Woo hoo" cheer.

I turned her bed around in her room. I asked Mom to come back and tell me how she wanted her bed. She said she wanted it with the head of the bed against the wall so it would "make it easier to make it'-per her words. This I did and involved her in the arrangement. Today I looked back and her bed was made really pretty.

She walked to the door of the utility room. She asked what this room was. I explained that it was the utility room with the air conditioner and furnace, the washer and dryer, and the hot water tank. She said she thought the washer and dryer was in the other room. I assured her it wasn't, that it had been in here.

I thought she was in a very alert state this morning. I told her I had ordered something for her, without her knowledge. I told her I had wanted to order a hairpiece to pin into my ponytail to dress it up a bit at times. I told her I had found a wig that was amazing, so I ordered her one in her color.

She said, "Oh, good, I'm so glad. I will gladly pay you for it." I was so surprised. She was so happy. I found the sight and was pulling up the picture. She asked if it was short and I said "yes." I found the picture of the style and showed her all angles. She was so happy. I showed her the "light brown" color swatch. She was pleased. I told her it may be here in a week. I told her the price and she commenced to tell me she used to have one and it might still be "around here somewhere." I can't remember my Mom ever wearing a wig.

I have learned to seldom use the word "impossible."

She's so lost. She doesn't talk about her mobile home. She doesn't really know where she is. I have referred to her bedroom as her home and it seems to settle her down. She accepts it. I've seen her going through her hanging clothes or looking through her drawers. Today she had her jeans rolled up a bit. I told her that she had culottes and shorts up in her room. She didn't seem to be aware of this. I told her to come back and I would show her. We walked back and I showed her the clothing that was hanging up. She gets confused when she thinks of where her things are, or what she brought with her. She doesn't get the whole idea that it is snowing with freezing rain where the girls are. I have quit referring to it as up north. I don't want her to be mixed up as to where she calls "home." I've told her we are very lucky. We have a winter home and a summer home.

I have a fountain in the dining room with a lot of round rocks in it. I watched Mom picking up several and rolling them over in her hands. I waited to see what she did. She said she thought they were potatoes until she picked them up. I just smiled. I plugged it in and showed her how it worked, with the water cascading down. She touched it and said, "As long as it doesn't freeze." My smile continues. In fact, my smile felt like I was smiling out loud.

I have never loved this lady more. All that she has done raising her daughters. All that she has sacrificed. All that she has given. It is tangled up inside her right now. I don't know if what I remember is injured to where it will not return to her. I don't know if it is just not receiving the stimuli needed to come forth and maybe the networking will find another path to follow. But I do know one thing. Just as she did for us every day of our lives, I will not give up. I will not quit. I will always be here for her.

A mother's heart is the child's schoolroom.

Mom went to bed about nine thirty tonight. She put on her pajamas. I had soaked her feet and clipped her toenails. I like to pamper her and spoil her, then she feels pretty. Jody is still staying with us. She tried to help Jody with making YoYo's tonight. She wanted to be able to explain how to do them, but it wasn't quite right. She's made so many, in earlier years, but some parts of her memory just don't surface.

She loves having her fingernails filed and painted. She gets compliments on her nails and it makes her feel pretty. Today I also colored her hair and then set it in foam rollers. Jody, Mom and I sat out on the patio today. When her hair dried, I took the curlers out and she combed her hair. When she came out to the dining room, I asked her how she liked the color. She said she had fixed her hair but didn't look at the color, then she laughed.

There is no such thing in anyone's life as an unimportant day.

She's laughing out loud more and more. I have completely stopped the antiseizure medication now. She isn't napping well in the afternoon, and she stays up later at night. Jody is here, and I'm not sure if she stays up so she doesn't miss anything or for other reasons. She seems to like turning on her dresser light and making her bed, looking things over, combing her hair, and fussing with her belongings on top of her dresser. Today she had on three short-sleeved shirts, topped with a short-sleeved sweatshirt when she came out for breakfast. She has accomplished the activity of dressing herself. It fact, you could say she has herself dressed for about three or four days—all in one morning. It reminds me of an action my daughter, Heather, did as a child preparing for kindergarten one day. She came out from the bathroom. She said she was supposed to brush her teeth three times a day, so she did them three times that morning, and now she was done for the day. If my mother follows in my daughter's footsteps, one of these nights I will find her totally dressed, laying on top of a bed already made. She will tell me she is dressed and ready for the next day, and she has her bed already made. Heather felt it would save time in the morning on school days. I think, if I remember correctly, she did that one day.

You don't stop laughing because you grow old.
You grow old because you stop laughing.

Yesterday Jody and I picked out and purchased three long sleeved cotton shirts, and 4 summer tops. We tried the shirts on her and they all fit. Then I put the peach colored top on her and it was so pretty. She said she had a lot of clothes upstairs, and that she didn't need more clothes. That was before she looked them over and tried them on. She seemed tickled to have some new very summery clothes.

Mom had been in bed since 9:30 PM tonight. I heard her door open a little later. I met her in the hall. She was dressed in a flannel shirt and her jeans. She greeted me pleasantly, until I told her that it was only 10:45 pm. She looked at her clock and thought it was morning. She had totally removed her pajamas and dressed herself. She seemed embarrassed that she had made an error, but we laughed it off. I asked her if she was that rested? I ask her if she wanted to stay up. She adamantly said, "No," and she climbed back in bed with her clothes on. I covered her up, tucked her in, kissed her forehead—for the second time…and told her "good night."

Earlier today, she was sitting at the table. Jane called and Jody brought the phone over to Mom. She did well talking to her, but there was no specific facts given. She was trying to tell Jane something we had done. She didn't ask-so I watched her and waited. She was trying to tell Jane about our lunch, and that we had leftovers from yesterday. She said "Judy" a few times, and then "not Judy." Then she asked who the "new girl here" was? I answered that it was "Jody, and she said "yes," then she continued with her story. Her third daughter has now become the new girl here.

Blessed is the influence of one true, loving human soul on another.

I was busy trying to put things in their place, after Jody and Mom had gone to bed. Jody was sleeping in my sewing room; Mom has taken possession of the front bedroom. It was about two hours since she had gone to bed. I heard Jody's door open and then close. I then saw Mom at Jody's door. I walked back the hall, and Mom said she had thought it was her room, until she stepped inside. She had been to the bathroom and got confused with the three doorways when she was returning to her room.

She came out and asked if she had her own shoes on, or someone else's? She said they felt "big." Jody informed her that I had cut her toenails last night and probably that was why, her feet were shorter. Mom accepted Jody's explanation.

130

I had picked Mom up some lighter white socks. I'm sure that they left more room in her shoes. It reminds me of Jody telling her boys, when they were very small, that we would sit on the back-porch swing and watch the dinosaurs walk up the road. She told her two small boys that you could see the tops of their heads as they went down the road. I still remember the look on their small faces. I probably had the same strange look on my face when Jody told Mom her feet were probably shorter.

Mom has made coffee, even though her thermos was almost full. She hunted till she found a small pan and put water in it. She turned on the burner, then put coffee grounds into the water and had stirred it. She was drinking the coffee with all the grounds in the mix. I try not to "undo" or correct some of her actions, but this one I couldn't watch. I told her I wanted to refresh her cup. I dumped her brew and added coffee from the thermos. She told me that it tasted better.

I came in from outside and told Mom I was going back to take a bath. In front of the bathroom I saw a very smashed pile of dog poop. It was tracked into the bathroom and then out the hall. I came out and told Mom I needed to check her shoes and explained why. All the treads in her shoes were filled with poop, but she had no idea. I removed her shoes and cleaned the treads, along with cleaning the hall. I am so glad that shoes can be washed, just as I've had to wash her slippers on some days.

Mom still can't tell the dogs apart. She knows there are five dogs, but then she also knows there are seven. Almost every day, Bri drops his dog and a friend's dog off at our house on his way to work. He then stops after work to pick them up and take them back to his house. I don't waste too much energy counting the dogs. It seems they are always very close to my mother or under my feet.

I had her helping me with planting flowers. She picked the flower for me to plant. As she did, she tried to remember what the flower's name was. After I planted one area, she held the garden hose and watered it well. She said she would do the second area later, when the sun wasn't shining on it. She said she loves to paint, but she declined painting today. She said she would watch me.

I've heard it said that you are not to worry that your children don't listen to you. You are to worry that they are watching everything you do. In a reversed world, I am the one being watched by the parent. Imagine that.

We called Jean this morning and Mom sang "Happy Birthday" to her, all the verses. I sang quietly alongside her, for direction only.

As her shoes were drying in the laundry room, she came out with her new sandals on, along with her thin white socks. She kept them on all day. You can tell she feels good when she has something done to her to make her look good.

We put her clothes away into the large wardrobe in her room today. She thought they looked very good. She wanted the doors left open, as it makes it easier for her to find what she wants. She seems so pleased with her room. She makes her bed every day and keeps her sheet and blanket even on her bed—at least most of the time. She keeps her shoes on the little white shelf next to her door. Last night I replaced her nightlight with small blue bulbs. She seems to like the subdued blue tinted lighting in her room. It's not a bright night light, yet enough that she can go to the bathroom. She did drink a little more fluid today than normally.

Yesterday Brian stopped and was so frustrated. He is having a lot of trouble with his painful back. He kept saying he felt so "useless and worthless." As he finished his statement,

Mom said quietly, "So do I, Bri."

Neighbor Millie told me that she comes out and sits on the patio when we leave her alone. My mother had told Jane that she locks the doors when we leave.

She made a decision today. I asked if she wanted a baked sweet potato, or a white potato with our meatloaf for supper. She said she wanted a sweet potato. Give her another of those special "woo-hoos" Jane.

We were expecting visitors since a few days ago. Mom's niece Sue, her daughter and her family, and her nieces" close friend Annie, were coming from Delaware. They were visiting family in Florida and wanted to see Mom. Mom got up this morning and questioned the fact that we hadn't gotten anything to set out for them, either lunch or snacks. She had come up with this idea on her own yester-day. When anybody would come to her home, she would always have "something" to put out for company to eat or drink.

She worried until we had "something" so we could serve our guests. I had told her before their visit, that we would get some food or munchies for them. This satisfied her. She was still in bed when I ran up to Walmart. I bought hot dogs and buns, potato chips, and numerous kinds of cookies. When she came out of her bedroom, I found she had already gotten dressed and made her bed. She already had her shoes on. Before she even ate her breakfast, she brought up the fact that we needed to get something before the guests came. I told her I had taken care of it and showed her the purchases. This thought and concern carried over from the day before. I usually tell her we have a brand-new day, but today we have a continuation of yesterday. And that is okay. In fact, I think it is fine.

Interesting day. I told Mom that her concern for something to serve to our company—was a step forward that she wasn't aware of. The fact that she didn't know who was coming or know anyone when they did arrive was secondary. She was a gracious hostess as far as greeting everyone and joining in on conversation. Sometimes there were multiple conversations going on at once and Mom would become quiet. She stayed in the same seat their entire visit. Annie and Sue kept up conversation with her. The guests had just ate break-fast, so preparing any food for them was not going to happen. We did serve multiple kinds of cookies and refreshments. Brian stopped during their visit, and Brian then took the guests to his house. It was perfect timing, because Mom came in the house and went directly to her room for a nap. She did sleep. I knew she had some concern because she didn't sleep well the night before.

I've been probing Mom's brain and memory. I have come to realize that name recall is on the lower part of my priority at this time. She will say, "I can see their face, but I can't come up with their name." Her memory is also intermittent, which is a little unnerving. We can take one step forward, and I delight in the progress. Then at another time I feel the slipping steps going backward. For example, tonight we sat at the kitchen table. I wanted her to know the few facts in her progress recently. I told her about her concern to "have something to serve them," referring to our 6 guests that came on Saturday. All her life she has had something "to serve" guests when they arrived. She had told me once, "I may not have anything special, but I can always make grilled cheese sandwiches." I explained to her that her worry about not having something carried over into their day of arrival. Her follow-through onto the next morning was another landmark in her memory recall of the actions that came so easily to her all her life.

These little things don't stand out to her but she just looks at me as I tell her. She said to me, "No one tells me anything unless I ask. I don't know what happened. How long did you stay with me?" Another curve ball from my mother. We jumped from the company to a totally different situation.

I did tell her that we have all explained it to her many times. Every time she asks, one of us has explained it all. I asked her if she remembered what we have told her. It seems that she has very limited recall of our entire time after surgery. She says she remembers she agreed to come down here for a few weeks, and she needs to go home. She has begun to recall my explanations of where her home is. She knows it is a place between the farmhouse where she lived for forty years, and Jane's house. When I say she "recalls," I am referring to her memory of our explanations which have occurred over and over. I am not referring to any memory of the initial happening.

I brought a tablet to the table and listed the months. I explained how many months I spent with her last year. She seemed appalled that so much time had passed. I told her that I am prying and searching her memory and brain so I can find her. I told her that she must work on using her memory and brain to get it stimulated and up and running. I told her I can't climb in there and put things in order, so she must bring everything out so we can sort it out and put it back.

She looked at me and said, "I'm in my eighties and doing this?"

I could only look at her lovingly and say, "Yes, Mom, and if we don't do this, you will still be in your eighties. You have never been a quitter, and you have good health otherwise."

She said she knew that, and that she was not a quitter. I pulled out the speech therapy sheets that were too difficult for her to do a few months ago. Jane sent them down to us. She went through two entire sheets, writing words. She wrote a little better at the start of tonight's study sheet, but it faded as she progressed down the sheet.

Life shrinks or expands in proportion to one's courage.

I drew another picture of what the surgeon did and why the incision line is sensitive. The porter's salve has taken the irritation away, so she isn't worrying about it anymore. Her understanding of the past year, since she fell on the ice by her porch, and the wreck where she totaled her car, is lost. She does remember our attendance at Sara and Ty's wedding, but I'm not real sure it isn't our telling her. Tonight, she wrestled and stretched her memory as far as she could but I'm not real sure that she truly remembers.

She doesn't talk much about Dad. I asked her if she remembered her life with him. She says "of course." but then she becomes quiet, rather than talking about him. She remembers her childhood, her parents, her siblings, but she could only name Mark & Matt, the twins, as far as Jane's children. She also recalled Sophie and Sam as being "the twins" of Jane's—but she didn't refer to them as belonging to Janes" daughter, Jenny. I'm thinking I need to draw a graph of her family so she can see a visual. As often as she sees Brian, she asked me "who" that was, when he stopped in for a few minutes. The short-term memory is such a problem. Teaching and telling and training get frustrating as each day we start over. I removed two kitchen cabinet doors so she could see what's inside them. These are the cabinets that hold the dishes and glasses used for setting the table.

She feels her walking and balance has gotten better. I told her that is why we go to a store and she pushes a buggy through it. It isn't easy to get her to walk much at home, but she will push a buggy through a store over and over. It's sort of a sneaky way to push her to walk, but it works. When I find something that "works," regardless of how simple, I run with it. This morning, for example, I told her we had to go to the UPS store, the post office, and then we could walk through a store somewhere. She told me to "go ahead and go, because I can get it done faster" if she doesn't go. I hear what she isn't saying.

I said, "Maybe I could, Mom, but we aren't on a time schedule and we want to get in some walking."

I told her to put on a little lipstick and her shoes, and then she would be ready. She has a band aid on her right hand, and one on her head. I have caught her so many times from a near fall, but she is also aware of her problem with equilibrium. She walks with caution but refuses to use the walker or even a cane. When walking in open areas, I keep her arm or hand until we reach a buggy. She talks about how she can't even drive her own car, and she wants to do that. I just don't see that happening, for several reasons. One would be the sensory problems she is experiencing with her equilibrium. The other would be knowing where she is, or how to get home.

We talked about her marriage, and how they traveled to Cumberland, Maryland. Dad's parents went with them, and she said that he had relatives there. She could name some of her nephews and nieces, especially her sisters' twins' names. She recalled that she, herself, had a baby born at home, and then another one decided to have her baby at home. Apparently after she had Jane at home, my dad's sister had her youngest baby at home.

She was dressed in her pajamas, and I had tucked her into bed, kissed her forehead, and covered her up. I was in the living room when she came back out and asked me to unhook her bra. I explained that there were no hooks and we removed her tops and then her bra. She loves the new bras we got, and even loves to sleep in them. She has done that for several nights but thought she should take it off for tonight. I've tried to get her to remove her bra at night, but she refuses. I feel this is because she can't get it on without help in the morning. She usually is dressed, has her shoes on, and frequently has her bed made before she comes out of her room in the morning. She told me she never knows what to wear in the morning, so I suggested we lay her clothes out at night. She said she has never laid her clothes out the night before, so we did it tonight. I am just wondering if she will remember that we did it in the morning. We shall see.

Today, Brian joined us for lunch. I had made hotdogs, and we had potato chips. When she heard he was coming, she said we would be having potato chips and cookies for lunch. I told her she couldn't tell Jane that, or she would think I wasn't feeding her mother properly. She just laughed. She helped with setting the table but more importantly, she helped clear the table afterward also. She questions where things go, but she seems to know what goes in the fridge. The paper plates are in the same place and there is no door on that cabinet, but she still didn't know where they were.

Getting Mom to drink adequate fluids is an ongoing task. Some days she barely gets one pint of coffee into her body, so I started giving her water to take her pills, instead of applesauce. Every night closes with half Klondike. Every morning starts with frosted flakes and coffee. The other two meals are varied, and she never complains. I am so fortunate that we pull on humor, and she never shows any meanness.

Well, it happened, exactly what I was dreading. We had such a good day. She was knotting a quilt, and had done about 7 complete rows, needing occasional help on the ends, and sometimes help to keep her from jumping around. She works best from right to left, so she always needed help with repositioning the quilt on the table. Sometimes she would take a stitch off the straight line, going about four inches down. It didn't cause any problem, so I told her we were not removing them, as she wanted me to do. I just informed her that we don't "redo" something that is okay. Years ago while baling hay on the farm, the workers put the bales on the wrong side of the barn. Dad always had a pattern of where the new hay went so he could use up the old hay first. The workers on the truck were about to remove all the bales and put them on the other side when Jody told them. "No, we don't redo hay bales. Jody took charge of the situation and had it handled, with much less work. So, Mother, "we don't redo yarn knots either."

Moms eyes tired and she went back to her bed to lay down. She came back out within the hour and restarted her work on the quilt. There has been so much improvement in her functioning with the needle and crochet thread since we last attempted to do it. Mom doesn't see the progress, because she still sees how much help she needs and how often she asks me for assistance. She is threading the needle quite well. She is putting one hand down under the quilt when making the stitch. She can lose her focus easily working with multicolored patchwork squares.

I have her lay out the twenty patches that she wants in the quilt, and I keep them in that order. She then decided what color of yarn she wants to use. I will help her with decisions, but these ones she makes herself. I tell her that these are the quilts for her grandchildren, so she must design them. We are working on Christmas gifts, and this makes her happy.

I don't remember if I recorded it, but yesterday I asked her if she knew how to use the toaster. She said she didn't, so I called her over to the toaster. I showed her the lever and how I put two slices of bread in. She watched closely. I told her it would pop up when it was done, and then we could put it on a plate, and she could put the other two slices in. She followed the instructions closely, and did put the next two slices of bread in. She stood by the toaster and watched, until it popped the toast out. She had a good feeling of being useful and helping with our lunch. I asked her to put a cupful of dog food in each of the dog bowls and showed her the bag of food. She dispensed it as I had asked, so she was involved in the dog's dinner also.

Several nights ago, I think it was Saturday night, she had asked if she could give the dogs treats. I explained that she could always do this, but just not to give them people food. They can always have their own treats. Apparently, I didn't think this through enough. Ricky was on the back of the sofa, and the other 4 were anxiously waiting her next move. She kept trying to give JoJo a treat, which she would carry a few feet, drop it, and then have another one of the dogs snatch it up. This always happens, so I continued to work on my project. Then I heard the starting of a dog fight. Mom had offered Ricky a treat, He didn't take it right away, so she laid it down for him. At this time, Little Rusty hopped up near the food. Rusty just loves life at his eighteen months of age. He is busy, he is curious, and he wants to be in every body's space. He just loves being loved.

But when Rusty got near Ricky's treat, Ricky growled first. It is then that Rusty sees this as a challenge and his testosterone kicks in. He grabs hold of Ricky's ear or skin and latches on. As the fight has started, Mickie has arrived and attacks Ricky also, going for his stomach area with open jaws. Now we have Mom involved, as she tries to get Mickie out of the area. She is reaching for her collar and calling her name, but the three dogs are like a whirlwind. I have Rusty by the back of the neck, but he won't let go of Ricky. Ricky is crying and crying, and Mickie is coming at him with open jaws. Mom gets a wound on her hand, resulting in blood on her shirt. I have several new open areas from someone's teeth during the match. Finally, Rusty's jaws let go and they are all separated. The only ones with injury is Mom and I. Apparently, Mom laid Ricky's treat down by him, which he did not eat. When Rusty came near, he growled, and the challenge began.

Again, I explained why I put Ricky up on the island in the kitchen to eat. She remembered that I did that with "one of them." I told her that I separate them from feedings or treats—because the two dogs attack Ricky when he gets some. She feels bad because she just wanted to give them a treat. She can't tell them apart, other than Mickie, so she never knows which one is aggressive and which one is the victim. She does know that Mickie is her loyal dog, and she always runs and gets involved in the fights when they start.

I'VE FALLEN AND I CAN'T GET UP

I didn't have enough Milk for Mom's breakfast in the morning. I was outside watering the vegetables and started watering the flowers. I asked Mom if she wanted to ride up to Walgreens with me. She declined, so I decided to run there by myself, since it is only about half mile away. I asked Mom if she would want to finish watering the new grass. She wanted to do that and walked over to the place where I was holding the hose. I told her I would only be a few minutes and left her with the running hose.

I came back but didn't pull the car into the carport. I pulled the car into the yard, and the headlights landed on Mom. She was seated on the cement edge of the carport. I took the milk and some new cookies into the gated area and sat them down. I walked over to Mom and said, "Did you sit down willingly, or did you end up on the ground by another reason?" She told me she had fell, and she tried to get up, but she couldn't. She was having intense pain in the right knee, thigh and hip area. Any movement increased her discomfort. I couldn't see any visual misalignment, but it was very hard to do any type of physical exam. She was embarrassed and distressed that she had "messed herself" after she fell. There wasn't anything visible, so I tried to ease her mind. There was no way that I could clean or change her at this time.

She didn't want me to "call the boy" because he shouldn't be lifting, but I told her I needed to call him, for he would want called first. We were able to get her into one of the patio chairs and off the cement. That was as far as her pain allowed us to go. It was obvious that she had broken her hip. So the next call would be 911. I went to get her ID cards, her medicine bottles, and a sweatshirt while 911 was called. The two young men that arrived with the very large ambulance were very gracious. They did have some difficulty getting her up and onto the cart. She was having so much pain, it showed all over her face. She didn't say anything, but the grimacing spoke loudly. I rode in the front of the ambulance and the young driver turned the camera so I could watch Mom's face the whole trip.

The attendants in the ER were very pleasant. The one very tall, very large man had a good sense of humor. When Mom gave them permission to cut her pants off, he told her he loves to do the cutting-and he did. He used his pink handled bandage scissors to cut them the whole way up the front. They had started an IV in the ambulance, so they gave her IV Morphine and Zofran soon in the ER—so she could be transported to X-ray. Brian and a friend were with us in the ER very soon after our arrival. They had brought Mom's car so I wouldn't be left stranded at the hospital. It's good they did, since she didn't get to a room until almost 3:00 AM.

When she came back from X-ray, she was still in a lot of pain. She was given more pain medication, but it didn't seem to affect her very much. There were no beds available yet, but we were told they would be keeping her. It was busy in the ER with the arrival of two very involved patients. I sent Brian home and told him I would keep them updated.

The doctor came in and told her she had a bad break in her right hip. Apparently the "ball" had broken off and the long femur bone was pushing up into the socket area. He felt that she would need a total hip replacement, because of the type of break. They were making a referral to the surgeon, but he already had a full operating schedule for the next day. He said he would order her something stronger for pain. A Foley catheter was put in place, and she was typed and cross matched for blood, should she need it in surgery.

It's been said, if your mind goes blank, be sure to turn off the sound.

I'll just quietly step back God…the field is yours. I put my most precious patient back in your arms. Hold her gently.

The nurse administered Dilaudid IV for pain, and then put nasal Oxygen on her because her pulse ox level had slowly dropped.

She was resting and sleeping very soundly, finally getting relief from pain. When the nurse drew blood, Mom never flinched or moved. Finally, she was comfortable. An IV was running for hydration, and she was to have nothing by mouth.

Finally, she had a room and that's when the emergency room attendant pushed her cart upstairs. He was a very personable man. I stayed with Mom until she was settled in and sleeping. I gave the nurse a report of her difficulty with word finding and explaining herself, along with the short-term memory problems. They were going to call me if they had any questions, or they needed me. The nurse was giving me directions to get out of the hospital and to my car. She told me I could have an escort to my car if I was frightened, or she told me that the attendant would walk me to my car. She said he's big enough that nobody would dare mess with him. I always walk to my car with the key positioned between my two fingers, and one finger on the alarm button. I don't think I'm ever frightened.

When I drove home, somehow, I missed our road and ended up down on Reinhart Road. I just made a U turn and came back to Vinewood drive. I parked the car next to the gate and opened the house and left the dogs out. The lights stayed on in the car and Mickie just stood at the fence and watched and watched. She had seen me, looked around, and had not seen Mom. She stayed outside longer than any of the other dogs, so I had to call her in by name. She would look at me, then look back at the car and not move. She broke my heart, as I had seen her watch for Mom not long ago. We talked and I told her I would bring Mom home—just as I had promised her the same thing several months ago. I find myself talking to my mother's dogs. I find myself assuring them I would bring her back home. They say you get what you expect.

I lay on the sofa with the TV on. Mom's two dogs act so differently in her absence. Annie was wound up and kept jumping up on me. Mickie lay down on the floor in front of the sofa and that's where she slept.

You can't stop the future. You can't rewind the past.
The only thing you can do at this time…is to press "play."

This is Thursday—March 26. This would be Mom and Dad's wedding anniversary.

The third day in the hospital, now the day of surgery

I asked her this morning if she knew what March 26 was, she did not. She was more upset with the "dark complexioned man" that bathed her this morning. She said he "threw" her arms around and then "threw" her legs around. With the IV running, nasal oxygen on, heart leads on her chest with monitoring, an indwelling catheter, and that's not counting a broken right hip joint. I'm not sure how much "throwing" could have been going on.

The nurse did tell me he had just given her pain medication when I came in about 5:45 AM. It would be my guess that she needed something to "defuse" her agitation. She is smiling and she talked quite well. She will not move or let herself be moved in bed. Any movement causes her pain. She is talking about the pain across her bladder area, rather than any hip pain. She then informed me that she must "cut back" on eating, that her belly is getting big. When I questioned her, she said that she could "feel it, cause it's getting bigger."

Her face looks good, the fluids have filled it out. She has also been receiving an additive in her IV, so her labs must have shown some possible dehydration. She is receiving an antibiotic for a urinary tract infection.

Thank you for all the things I never said,
because I thought you knew.

I may break up my visit with her today, since she is post op day of surgery. I may go home and take care of some things at the house and spend time with the dogs. I'm not sure her bed will be functional for her situation now. I will follow through with that. It is probably too low for safe positioning after her broken hip. I had her in a low bed, to decrease the chance of her falling from the bed. I guess I will be investing in a new bed soon.

Just six months after my mother has cranial surgery, we have settled into the south. There was no cold weather, and we could be outside anytime we wanted.

But now let me think this situation through. I have a brain injured eighty-nine-year-old woman who fell and is in uncontrolled pain. She is admitted to a strange hospital. She was taken away by men she didn't know in a well-lit van she hadn't seen before.

My son works full time and long hours. I have six dogs at my house.

All other family are presently about a thousand miles away. Let us open another interesting chapter in the life of this other mother.

Trust God for the unexpected and let him surprise you by doing the unexplainable. I bought my daughter the book,

"Hello, God, It's me, Margaret," *she quotes it to me often.*

Now it's my turn, "Hello, God, it's me, Judy."

Many older people who fall and break their hip, do not recover to their previous physical state. My mother is about to be anesthetized again. This may alter her mental abilities, again. She is going to be afraid. She is going to think I have placed her somewhere, other than our home. As in the movie with Forrest Gump, Life's box of chocolates presents itself again.

She left her hospital room at 6:35 AM, and she was back in it before 9:50 AM. She's a little "loopy" but can't believe her hip doesn't hurt anymore. She remembered the pain. I am there when she leaves the room, and when she returns. She wants to know how I know everything that goes on, did I get a notice?

In the name of God, stop a moment, cease your work, look around you. Don't miss moments like this—"did I get a notice?"

Surgery went well, and she now has twenty-seven staples in her hip. She has a brand-new total hip joint.

She keeps taking her pulse ox off, and the machine keeps beeping. She wants to know if that is the house phone? She tells me she can't believe all the commotion that goes on in here, referring to the hospital, with all the exchanging of recipes. I asked her to watch for some good recipes and get a copy. She said she would. She is so awake at times, and her face is animated. It relieves my heart to see her free of pain even if for a little while, after the past few days. The nurse came in and ask if she was seeing things. I told her "not that I've noticed, but she's quite entertaining." Just then, with eyes wide open, she excitedly told me that she just saw her dog jump up on the shelf across the room. I stand corrected, nurse. My mother just saw something that I didn't see, and I was right beside her. I tried to imagine a dog jumping up on the hospital shelf, but this vision belongs to only my mother. I've heard it said that kids say the darndest things. Thus, so does my mother.

No matter how many times I put her pulse ox on her finger, she keeps taking it off. This causes her machine to beep constantly. I guess I might as well get used to hearing it.

We just discussed her lunch, and I had the nurse order cream of potato soup with her lunch. I know she won't eat much, but maybe she will be more alert for the evening meal. I plan on going home after her lunch and see what my house needs for preparation for her discharge. I will spend some time with the dogs and do some cleanup. Bri may shower after work, and then come over to see her. I continue to listen to her machine beep, as I have put her pulse ox on at least ten times during the visit.

My home is only a few miles from the hospital. I can go back and forth easily, taking care of our dogs, yet not leaving Mom alone for very long in the hospital.

I know she is going to be frightened if she doesn't see me. She is going to find herself in a strange bed in a strange place with no one that looks familiar. I had given her my word I would not leave her. God willing my health will allow me to keep my word. But for this period, it must be my choice to stay with her, especially at night. She experiences increased confusion as dusk settles into each day. Who will tell her that tomorrow will be a brand-new day? Who will hold her hand when she doesn't understand what is happening? Holding her hand has become a very comforting gesture. Her anxiety eases while her hand is held. Brian discovered how easily she relaxes when he sits with her and just holds her hand while they talk, while they watch TV, and even while they nap. She seems to put her trust in the person who is holding her hand, and she then lets go of all the confusion and changes that have taken place in her world. Now, with her dog sitting on the shelf across from her bed, maybe her world won't be as frightening. This situation may need reevaluated. Each day may not only be "brand-new," but it may also be entirely altered from what we had known.

I have climbed into my mother's world many times since our worlds changed. I realize that there are now multiple people who enter her hospital room and give care, bring food, take vital signs, give medication, change dressings, clean her room, etc. Then complicate this group of people with the change of shifts which bring a whole new group of people into her room. The mother that was admitted may not be able to find her "safe space."

It seems we lost control of the afternoon. I had discussed Mom's preexisting altered neuro status with so many staff members, and there is always a new staff member in charge of my mother. It took one and a half hours to get pain medication for her. I explained again, how the scale from one to ten does not work for her. Again, I told them how her condition is a right hip repair, but also an altered mental status from her cerebral bleed of seven months ago. Now add the recent anesthesia and pain medication to this lady. I was ready to write a big note and hang it on the wall, when the aid brought the charge nurse in. I reviewed the way Mom must be addressed, and without using complex questions. It was easy to demonstrate how asking very simple questions could result in an answer. Just try to explain to medical staff how her automatic answer to "do you have pain" will receive an answer relating to that very second. She can show signs of discomfort for an hour or more, but when asked about pain, her focus will be on trying to give an answer that she thinks the questioner wants to hear. Asking her to rate the pain on a scale of one to ten may be needed for their medication chart, but it is not understood by this patient. She may give them an answer, but only so they will quit asking, and it will not be accurate.

She is very restless. She hasn't napped since she came back to her room from surgery. I have a feeling she is going to have a very interesting evening. She is constantly handling her iv tubing, her nasal tubing, her hip dressing and the name bands on her wrists. She is pulling her gown off and rolling it into a ball. She keeps her eyes shut and is reaching into the air. When I took hold of her hand and asked her if she was reaching for me, she said, "Yes, you stinker." She's been laughing and smiling a lot today. Isn't medication wonderful?

Let the adventure begin.

As I stay with my mother, she told me she walked "way down there" and got some M&M's but left them there. I asked her if she walked down there by herself, and she said she had. I asked her if her new hip was working well, and she told me it was. I inquired about the M&M's and why she didn't bring me some back. She said she would the next time.

She held her hands up high in the air. I asked her what she was doing, and she told me she was "making some plywood." When I inquired more and told her I didn't know she could make it, she assured me she could. She said she had made two jars full.

She has bright yellow socks on, since she is a fall risk. She was looking at her feet with a puzzled look. She said there was corn on the cob on her feet. It took some explaining for her to realize that they were socks. She has alternating compression pads on both lower legs.

She is fiddling with everything. She has removed her hip dressing twice and altered her nasal cannula and iv tubing. She has removed her gown and messed with her Foley catheter, pulled at her heart monitor lines and played with the monitor leads.

She's reaching for her toothpaste, says she had it, but she forgot where she put it. She's very pleasant and smiles at the staff when they address her, but usually don't know what they are saying or doing. She just watches and gives a little laugh.

It's 5 am and Bri has texted me that he stopped at the house and toileted the dogs. I've bummed a cup of coffee from the nursing station. I almost inhaled it. I'm going to have to find the coffee place this morning, because one cup was just a teaser. As I sit here on the cot that I slept on last night, Mom moans and talks and mumbles off and on during her sleep. She has told me that she always dreams.

Sometimes she tells me what she was dreaming, like the night she was planning a party for Jeani and her husband. She said she had a lot more to do yet, so I told her to go back to sleep and get it all done. She said "okay," and she went back to sleep.

The lab lady just came up and drew some blood from her left arm. She then turned out the light and told Mom she was done and maybe she could go back to sleep. Mom told her that she thinks she can.

PALM SUNDAY

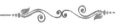

Where do I start to explain the last few days? I had come in yesterday morning, shortly after breakfast, to see how Mom's night went. She had been left to feed herself, which meant she didn't eat much at all. She had a red allergy wristlet on, but no one could explain to me what she was allergic to. It wasn't there last evening when I finally left to go home. Did they ask Mom a question and get an answer that wasn't accurate? The allergy bracelet doesn't have anything listed—just that she has an allergy. After inquiring with several staff members, they decided to just cut off the allergy bracelet. I requested some pudding and fed Mom a vanilla pudding, which she ate. She still has a maintenance IV running, since she isn't eating or drinking adequately. Brian came in today, and was going to be here for her lunch, so I left to try and obtain a bedside commode and maybe work to arrange her room at home. I need to make adequate space for her to move about with her walker, have a bedside commode in her bedroom, and add an elevated seat in the bathroom.

I was successful, I found both at the habitat store, and one is far from being clean. Amazing what a little Clorox water will do to freshen and disinfect the apparatus. I unloaded it and left it on the patio until cleaning can happen. I also found a salmon colored bedspread at good will, so I went to Joann Fabrics and found some salmon print material on the red tag counter. I will make some fresh drape/curtains for Mom's room and hang them with a lace panel. Mom should like that. The paint color in her room is called "sandy feet," pretty much a Florida happening.

I started getting texts from Bri. It seems that Bri is having some problems being "firm" with his grandmother. She wants him to take her home. She isn't eating very much for lunch, and he doesn't know how to "push" her. Therapy was in and walked her about the room, and he was concerned about her pain. He was having problems separating from her, as she wanted to go home, and she wanted him to take her.

It's not about how much you do,
but how much love you put in what you do that counts.

I told him I would be right in, but I hadn't been home yet or left the dogs out. I arrived in her room and Brian introduced me to the nurse in the doorway as "his mother." She and I had already met in the morning, as she came on duty at 7:00 AM. I walked over to Mom's bedside and she looked agitated. She wanted me to take her home. She asked me if I had a car and I informed her that I had her car. She said, "Let's go then." I explained that she had to stay a few more days, to get stronger, receive some Iv's, establish some therapy and allow me to get the house prepared for her arrival. I told her I had to get ready for the day they toss her out, so I can catch her.

Just now, the lab lady came to draw blood. After she left, Mom said she didn't know why there were so many different costumes in this place.

I told her that this lady's only job was to draw blood. Her nurse was in and discontinued the IV. He also changed the dressing on her right hip. The incision looks great, with all staples intact. She still has the heart monitor on, but it seems that every time she gets up on the potty chair, some of the leads become disconnected. She is transferring well and holding the weight on her feet and legs. She has been up about three times this shift, and now we are going to have to encourage fluids and eating more. I know that when they bring the large full trays, the sight alone can be overwhelming. Smaller, more frequent meals would be so much better, like we do at home.

I have tried to explain to Mom that I will stay through breakfast with her, but then I will go home and spend time with the dogs. I also need to clean some equipment and prepare the house for her discharge. She agrees. I was talking with the nurse when I said that the nights seem to be a lot tougher on her. The nurse agreed. Per usual, she is doing the "sundowning" come dusk as she often does at home. She becomes frightened with all the strange faces and feels that she must go home.

I'm going to try and stay home today probably knowing that I will be back here tonight. I just can't bear for her to be frightened at night and be alone. I've seen the fear in her eyes when she doesn't know where she is or why. A few words that "I am right here" and letting her grasp my hand is such an easy fix. It's an easy fix for both of us, as I wouldn't be able to be at home during the night and not have her with me.

Finally discharge day has come. We get to honor our word. When she asks us to take her home with us—we will do just that.

Mom is back home with me, what an interesting roommate I have.

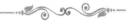

It is now April Fool's Day. I wonder who decided that only one day a year should be set aside for foolish behavior? Maybe someone that didn't find "smiling" to be easy?

Mom was helped up to the potty chair about eight forty-five, but she wasn't ready to get up for the day yet, so she went back to bed.

She became restless about 11:00 AM, so I helped her get up for breakfast. When she laid back down earlier, she had pajama bottoms on, and now she doesn't. This lady has a new total hip, staples, and just got discharged from the hospital. How did she get those pj bottoms removed while lying in her bed with a recent fractured hip? She doesn't have any idea how or when she did it. She doesn't even know "who" did it. She walked out to the breakfast table and ate her usual breakfast. She walked without any sign that she had major surgery. When she finished breakfast, it was eleven thirty, so lunch is not going to be a problem today.

Mom kept reaching down under the table. She was talking to Mickie. After she finished breakfast, she stood up and was bent way over. I went in to caution her about bending over, as we were trying to keep her right hip in good alignment to heal. Mom seems to forget about her fracture. She asked me how she broke her leg. I explained the surgery and even touched the incisional area with the staples still in place. She truly doesn't remember any of the hospital stay. She asked me where she fell. I pointed out to the little garden and told her she was watering the grass. She told me she reached for the pole but fell and hit her hip on the edge of the cement. She seems to remember some of the fall, and the ambulance ride.

I know that she had pain medication several times for her obvious pain on arrival at the emergency room. Then she had stronger medication before she was taken to the X-ray department. I know that they were not able to do the surgery the following morning. This meant that they had to treat her pain, and I'm not sure how well that went. The surgeon already had a very full schedule…and Mom has a urinary tract infection. They needed to get some antibiotics into her system to combat that infection before involving another situation.

Mom admits to some burning when she would pee before she fell. I have instructed her to tell me when she has any changes in the way she feels. She said it had only hurt for a few days—but it's been a week now, and she still has some burning on urination.

She has been telling me she has some soreness in her mouth. I don't see any signs of thrush or irritation. Tonight, she took her partial dental plate out and left it on her dresser. She wants to see a dentist and find out what she can have done. She then asked me if I thought it would be worth it. I told her, "Mom, anything is worth it if it makes you feel better about having it done." I then asked her if her teeth were hurting her. She was trying to ask me about the dentist in her hometown that she has been using for years. She thought he may have a practice down here also. I assured her that he only practices out of one town. She then asked me who my dentist was. I told her it was a clinic just down the street and then I asked her if she wanted to be seen by them? She quickly responded that she would. She said that she has a big hole in her one tooth, and they are all in terrible shape. She wants to find out what they think and what her choices are. I pulled the sight up on the computer and found out that they offer a free exam and X-rays if you have no insurance. They have an office here in town. I mentioned this to her, and she wants to find out what they say. I told her we would make her follow-up appointment with her hip surgeon first and then go from there. She seemed surprised when I told her she still has staples in her hip that need to be removed, and she may also need a follow-up X-ray to confirm the proper placement.

She just got out of bed, semi closed the door, walked right past her walker and was going to straighten up the room. No matter how often I explain, no matter how often she scares me she seems oblivious to what I say. I guess I can explain it best by stating she doesn't remember the hospital stay or the surgery, so it didn't happen. She is acting and walking like she didn't have a broken hip. I have told her over and over, that she is breaking all the rules. I should be trying my best to make her get out of bed, but instead I am trying to prevent another accident. She will not call me, she will not call out, she won't do anything to alert me, because she doesn't want to be a burden on anyone. So she gets herself out of bed on her own. She then forgets that she needs her walker. She truly is the most magnificent post-op hip surgical patient I have ever witnessed. I know it is because she isn't aware that she broke it, or had it repaired. She needs so much prompting, so she doesn't take off walking without her walker. She has no understanding of the danger of another fall, so I know it's my obligation to keep her safe, so she heals perfectly. Her future mobility surely depends on the care and preventive caution used during this recovery. I'm watching the room monitor, I'm listening to all her moves, but she sure can be quiet if she wants to be discreet. I can see its totally my responsibility to make sure she heals up once and heals up right.

I am constantly reminding mother to be careful with her hip. Her response is priceless, "Why, what's wrong with my hip?" Well, Mother, apparently, there is nothing wrong with your hip. I stand corrected.

This lady is certainly a 24-7 diversion. It is very fortunate that I am retired, so I can put in those needed hours. Bri and I have developed quite a means of communication with this other mother of mine. We can live in our world yet travel into hers without hesitation. We never know where she is going to meet us, or even if she will meet us at all. My other two children, 3 sisters and entire family reside five states away, other than my son and myself here in Florida. I have sent out emails to inform family, opening the doors to our life here with this enchanting lady. That way I can keep everyone totally informed without phone calls and phone texts and running the risk of missing someone. I have taken our family matriarch away from all family up north and brought her to my home in a much warmer climate. In the short time here, she has broken her hip and stopped using her partial dental plate. This action affects her appearance drastically. A dental issue is in our future.

By composing emails, everyone will be able to share life with her and climb into Bri and my world, which always carries a safety net with it. My life is not my own right now. Mom's only been home from the hospital for two days—so she requires a lot of reminders and prompts. We bought a baby monitor so I can hear her get up in the bedroom. I heard her and went back. She had to pee, but she had the walker backward and didn't know which way to go. The potty chair is right beside the bed. She is really a big safety risk, but I'm trying. I lost a hubcap to Mom's car during my many trips to and from the hospital. I didn't even know I lost it till Bri asked me where it was.

It's been nine years since we gave my dad back to his creator. He wore out his earthly body, but his mind and brain were as acute and alert as always. As his body shut down, he knew he was going to die. He put as many things in order as he could, before his last hospitalization. He knew he would not be leaving the hospital in his earthly form, and he was right. I often think of the differences in this married couple that is my parents. My mother's physical condition seems quite good. It's her mind and brain that are not functioning and performing as they were meant to do. Dad did the very best he could with what health compromises he knew he had to accept. My mom is doing the very best she can, without knowing what or why or how. Dad had provided and protected her his entire life. Something tells me he didn't quit when he had to leave her side.

Mom and I have a long day today. She sees the surgeon at ten thirty and then the dentist at three thirty to discuss getting nine teeth pulled and an upper denture put in. I don't know how we are going to do.

DENTAL EXAMINATION AND SUGGESTION FOR EXTRACTIONS

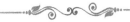

Let me bring up her trip to the dentist. Since she had her hip surgery, she has not been wearing the partial dental plate she has had for years. The mother I knew would never leave this partial plate out of her mouth. I made an appointment to have a dental evaluation. She sat in the dental chair for the exam. Her teeth were bad. The dentist informed her and I that her teeth really needed pulled. There was some that were infected, and some were broken. Adding more teeth to the upper partial plate may not correct the problem. The suggestion was to pull the upper teeth and have a full denture made. The dentist then left the room and the technician remained for questions and to finish care to my mother. My mother turned and was climbing out of the chair, stating, "Okay, thank you for your opinion." She was done and ready to leave.

I continued the discussion and explained my mother's condition, as it has been since her cranial surgery. I was informed that impressions could be taken right now, Thursday afternoon. Her teeth could be pulled in the morning and her plate would be ready and inserted into her mouth. In less than twenty-four hours, she could have new teeth, and by all the teeth being pulled, the broken and infected teeth would be gone from her mouth. I questioned how we could keep her in the dental chair for the whole extraction without her having pain or confused anxiety. I could just see her getting out of the chair part way through the whole procedure and announcing that she was ready to go home. She has been timid about her smile

155

for years, as there were some missing teeth requiring the use of the partial plate. There was one tooth that was dark, always showing darkness in pictures when she would smile. She had wanted a beautiful smile for years. Now was the opportunity to make this happen. Just a little problem before us. This would be my mother's brain injury, which has resulted in both memory problems and confusion that interferes with understanding.

We went forward. One of us in favor of the plan, the other unaware of what all is involved. Impressions were taken. The next morning, we went back to the clinic. Mom did very well. She had all her upper teeth pulled. I had given her something for anxiety prevention—now there's a new term. The teeth were very bad. The denture was inserted into her mouth and we were to return the next morning to have it removed and her mouth checked.

The evening wasn't bad. We have found mashed potatoes with chicken soup over them works well. So does milk shakes. She really didn't have a lot of discomfort, and I am so glad.

I'm not afraid of storms, for I'm learning how to sail my ship.

Easter Sunday, the last day of April

It's difficult to describe a day in the life we live. I had Mom's clothes laid out yesterday and knew she was in her bedroom getting dressed. I waited for a while then walked back. She had both pant legs stuck trying to get them both over her shoes. I don't know what kept her from falling as she had walked around the bed with them stuck on both feet. I try to make things simpler for her but she seems to find a complication to put in the way.

I am a strong woman because a strong woman raised me.

She has been preoccupied with her purse and money. She wants to have some money in her purse. She thinks it comes to her wrapped in a bundle. When I explain that I can use her debit card like a check, she acts like she understands. She has cash in her wallet, she looks and looks and looks. Then she closes her purse, starts all over, zippers and unzippers. She keeps telling me she has no money. I take her wallet, show her the money, and count it out for her. She doesn't know how much she wants. She just knows that she always likes to have money in her purse. She has money in her purse, but she doesn't remember. She brought her homemade purse to the kitchen table one day…and said…I hate this purse. I want my old one back. Since then, we have picked out a black purse from my closet, and she liked it. She seems to like it much better. Tonight, I took her wallet and removed all the cards. I put all her cards in a small card wallet and showed her I put it in the one zipper pocket inside her purse. I then put her cash in a little soft zippered makeup case. This I put in her purse and asked her where her cash was? She pointed to the case. I hope we have simplified her frustration with sorting things involved with her purse.

I watched her with a piece of paper, looking through all the things lying inside my desk. She was trying to find an address. I asked if she wanted to write a letter. She said "no." She was trying to find an address to someone that she couldn't remember their name. I gave her the complete list of people who had sent her cards. She said it wasn't any of them. She tried to explain that she "can see them"—but can't name them. She tried to describe this person as "living on the corner" and "close to the church." I couldn't help her with this one. I sent Jane a text and asked her to call. She was on her way home from work. When she called, I had Mom try to explain who she was trying to find. I figured that Jane would know the name of someone from church or bowling or helping hands or wings. Mom attempted to describe who she wanted. To my amazement, she was trying to find the person that handles her banking. We decided that Jane "does live on a corner." Jane was the one she was trying to get an address for. She wanted to have this person get her some money. She remembers Jane as doing all her banking previously. I remember Jane getting her cash …and it was in a banking envelope. Was this the bundle" that she remembers?

She keeps the clock at the head of her bed. It seems to give her some security as to what the time is. She may not comprehend exactly what it all means, but she has something she can look at when she wants to know what time it is. I truly know she doesn't comprehend the time on the clock with the time during the day—but it seems to please her. To me, that's quite a winner and I'll take it.

We had company from up north today. Three men, along with Brian. Mom sat on the lawn chair for most of the visit. I could see she was withdrawing a little and looked bored. I asked her if she wanted to go in and lay down. She answered me with "Yes. I have no interest in this." She needed help to get up and walk, as she had been sitting for some time. She bid the company a general greeting of some sort and then I took her back to her bedroom. Bri, again, graciously took the guests over to his house.

She does sleep a lot. She doesn't have much interest in doing anything, other than helping with the kitchen and dishes. I put the quilt away for a while. She did do better with solitaire after some verbal help.

She and I sit in front of the TV every evening. I try to find some short sitcoms for her to watch and she does. Sometimes she will even make comments as to what is happening. Last night I had the pre-Oscar show on. I kept commenting about the lady's gowns. At one time she said, "she almost doesn't have that one on." Now truer words were never spoken. A lot of women had very reveling gowns and she did notice that. I'm sure the entire male population noticed that also.

She tired more easily when we "walkin shopped" at several stores yesterday. She does need the carts for balance. She does look around when we go up and down the aisles. I just don't know how to stimulate her mind anymore. I push to keep her active all waking hours. She just seems to want to watch me or whatever else is going on. She did sit outside the last few days. She wants to be on her own so bad. We will keep working on just activities of daily living. She cooked two hot dogs for her and my lunch yesterday. She even sliced them both in half.

She gets the milk from the fridge and puts it on her cereal every morning. It's a start. It's a very encouraging start.

She is proud of her polished fingernails. Her hair is now evened out better on the sides. She combs her own hair. I bought some Rogaine for women and started putting it on her scalp the last few days. She knows why I do it. I just keep trying to make her feel pretty. She always took pride in her appearance. She still does.

She had trouble putting her shoes on this morning. That is rare. She had her slippers on and carried her shoes out. I watched as she tried to put her shoes on over her slippers, apparently for the second time. I knelt and moved her shoe off her toes. I then removed her slipper and helped her put her shoes on.

*There is nothing better on this earth than a soul
that you can connect with on every level.*

She always eats half Klondike at bedtime, followed by her medication. She usually sleeps at least twelve hours at night. I know this is a lot, but it has been her pattern since the brain injury. She takes no medication that would medicate her for sleep. It is the natural way of letting her brain rest. Her brain is trying to put it all together. She just asked me tonight where Brian parks his truck. It wasn't here. I told her that Brian doesn't live here. He parks it across the street at his own house. I told her that she and I are the only ones that live here. She just shook her head, kind of in a frustrating manor, as she often does. She often gets quiet, rather that attempt to converse or talk and not be able to find her words.

She will talk and talk to her daughters when they call on the phone. The one evening she received three phone calls in a row. By the third call, the words just weren't coming. Things were mixed up and she was getting frustrated. My younger sister wishes she had her mom back. She isn't adjusting to the version of mother we have following her brain injury. The brain is sort of like the motherboard of all motherboards. We can operate to correct and remove pressure on the motherboard. We can open the skull and work magic. We can remove the intruding source of pressure and put everything back. Surgical treatment has become such a perfected skill.

But what happens after the surgeon has done his magic, now that's when we uncover the mystery that's been hidden. The surgery offers us hope that all will be well. All will be as it was before the medical problem occurred. We give it time and energy. We trust that tomorrow will bring a better light. That our mother will show us she has returned to us. The mother that watched us grow and mature. The mother that always had our back. The mother that invested her life into helping us with ours. The mother that showed compassion at her own expense. The example that she set that couldn't be touched by any other influence in our lives.

But things do change, and we must change with the hand we are dealt. There is no redeal at this point. We gambled when we consented for the surgery that relieved the pressure on our mother's brain. We met and discussed what choice to make. We all agreed. Is she upset that we did this? I don't know. I don't know if she knows. Most of the time she doesn't know what happened or why. There are times she knows that something happened, and then there are the other times. Shuffle the deck. Here we go again. Hold the poker face. Keep the smile. Keep up the teaching and support. Always be there when she needs to know she is safe. She needs to see a familiar face when she gets "lost." Even if I am outside, she comes to the door to see where I was. Sometimes she calls me by name. Sometimes I am in the third person. Sometimes she is not exactly sure of who I am, but I am always aware of who she is. Who she was may be different from who she is now? I remember, even when she doesn't. One out of two is pretty good odds.

The best portion of your life will be the small, nameless moments you spend smiling with someone who matters to you.

A simple Tuesday and our mom is lost in her world today. At the breakfast table, she asked me if I was born in Kepple Hill. I answered that I wasn't but explained nothing further. I asked her if she was born there, and she said that she was. She explained that she was born, not in the house up the hill, but in the one down by the road. She said that her dad had bought another piece of property over from the house, and then they built a house there later.

She talked of how her dad had wanted to take her sister to the doctor because she was sick one morning. He saw that the road down by the river was flooded over. It was that night that the flood of 36 wrecked its havoc on the Kiski River. By the next evening the river was down within its banks. It was within that time frame that Mom and her father walked down, and she pulled the little china bulldog out of the rubble. She had it sitting in her bedroom up north. It's a little chipped and discolored, but it is one of her treasures. The memories that it brings to her when she looks at it are real priceless ones.

You can watch her face and know that at those few moments she is with her father at the river's edge. The serenity that fills her face as she holds onto the chipped and faded bulldog are without blemish. Oh that she could feel that good more often these days.

We have since gifted it to her great-granddaughter Sophie, who has an extreme love of dogs. She is planning on becoming a veterinarian. May Sophie feel the warmth of those memories that brought so much pleasure to her great-grandma—as she holds the elderly faded ceramic bulldog.

She sat out on the carport and watched me this morning. I came in and fixed us French toast and then we both relaxed in the living area. She nodded off a few times on the chair, and I may have done the same on the sofa. Working outside had made me very tired and achy. Mom may be tired from disinterest in most everything. She doesn't appear unhappy. She doesn't appear to be discontent. I am much more content being able to work around my own home, since I really hadn't got settled into it. It seems I spent more time up North last year than in Florida.

I asked Mom to cut up some leftover meat and cheese, along with some turkey sandwich slices. She cut them very finely. It took a while, but she did it. I then mixed them in the dog food bowls. Mom said they were getting some of the "good stuff" today.

After Brian and the neighbor had left tonight, Mom watched a little TV, then walked back to her bedroom. She looked it over and then said she was going to get ready for bed. She usually says something about going up and watching TV on her own TV until she gets tired. I explain that I only have one TV, and it's here in the living room. This always seems to be "news" to her. I know she "sundown's," and it's a true sun downing syndrome. Maybe if I close the blinds and keep the house lit, she may adjust easier. I will try that tonight.

She watched TV most of the time today. It was rainy and she was cold. The furnace was on, but the carport door was left open while Bri worked on a sturdy banister on both sides of the steps. It was a beautiful job, and very sturdy.

New Carport Banister

When it was finished, she tried it out. Pictures were taken and she remarked about how nice it was. When I tucked her in bed tonight, she asked if Brian had left. Then she asked if he had gone to his own home. I assured her he had and that I was sure he was stretched out in bed from all the work he did. She said "okay" and snuggled down in the covers.

Never forget yesterday, but always live for today, because you never know what tomorrow may bring—or what it can take away.

If you want to be listened to, you should put in time listening.

My niece, Julie had told me once, "While you up at 3:00 AM, and God is less busy, say a prayer for me." I liked the thought that went along with her request. It's what I call "a keeper." It's true Jul, I think 3:00 AM is a good time for a chat. I had thought that God was not as busy at that time, but I truly believe that it is me that is not so busy.

Mom seems bored. She wants to do something. So I bring out the quilt she had been working on…now for months. She looks it over, unfolding and refolding it as she explored it. I walked over where she was now. She says she wants to "finish" it today. I have taken all my stabilizing safety pins out and placed a safety pin everywhere where a stitch should be. I explain it to her and there is no acknowledgement that our previous system will work. I explain that she is to make a stitch where every safety pin is. She felt that seemed simple enough and it worked fairly well during the rest of the day as she missed some and doubled others…but she followed really well.

The following day, we run to several stores shortly after her breakfast. We went to "Books a million" and she seemed so surprised at how big it is. We have a $5 gift card that expires in thirty days, a receipt that gives us a free cookie. So I tell Mom, we are going over to Joann's and then coming back over here to sit down and have a cookie and an iced coffee. She is quite agreeable.

After our walk to Joann's, we return to BAM for our cookie. It is the first time we have ate anything outside the home since her new denture. We get a large warm chocolate chunk cookie and an iced mocha caramel coffee. We sat at the little table and chairs and Mom seemed very content. She ate the entire warm cookie without a problem. She did say that she had some problems holding the dental plate in place. I will call the dental clinic the first of the week and see what they say. As she sat comfortably working on her cookie and drinking her coffee, I walked back to the magazine section and pick up a few that was related to making cards. I have tried to find the book on verses for cards ever since I passed on it some time ago. One of those regrets. When I return with the magazines, Mom is not ready to go yet, so I check out while she sits. I realize she needs these outings and socializing...but sometimes it is hard to get her to consent. I told her we could take out cups and leave and she seemed surprised that we could take the cups with us. I said, "sure, they can be taken out." We walk to the car for our next venture and she asked several questions about the last store. She seemed a little confused that we ate there while other people were reading and doing other things there also. She thought the books I bought for Sam and Jeff looked like new. I told Mom they were new, because we were in a very large book store. I find it amazing that the combination book store/coffee shop is something incomprehensible to Mom. I don't have much of Mom's attention in this environment. When she says, "I don't like to read," she truly doesn't and has no desire to be in a book store. Her father loved to read. She has told me that when she had to do a book report, he read the book, and helped her write the report. Mother dearest, you have a past!

For several weeks we haven't worked on quilt knotting. Since Mom had her teeth pulled and the dental plate put in her mouth, we have kept things less stressful. She had enough coping lessons just getting used "to this thing in my mouth." That will be data for another chapter.

Mother's Day Letter?
It Is What It Is

I started this entry as an open letter to my sisters for Mother's Day. I knew they would have especially missed their mother on a day made tribute to all mothers.

Dearest sisters and family,

I wanted to share some of my time with our mother since you weren't able to actually be with her on this day.

I leave our mother's room and walk to the sofa. I sit down after helping her lay down for an afternoon nap. She very seldom lies down in the afternoon anymore, and when she does, often she doesn't sleep. She may lay for half hour, and then she gets back up. I try to encourage her to rest, so she can stretch out her hips and back. I kissed her forehead while reassuring her that I wouldn't let her "sleep too long." I promised her that I would wake her "before tomorrow." Her afternoon nap only means that when she does awaken, it will be tomorrow for her, a whole new day. She was tired, as she had seen the doctor this day and also did a lot of walking. Medical appointments tire her more than a usual day of "shoppin' walkin'," because it is different. It takes her out of her comfort zone.

There are more people in our house than I've met, and there are other girls that intervene in Mom's daily activities that I haven't crossed paths with yet. No matter how many times I explain that it is only her and I here, that there is just two of us, in her mind, she seems to feel there are more of "them" here. I'm not sure when they come in, or when and how they leave, but "they" are always involved with doing everything for Mom. She has told me that there are more people here because there is so much to do, and everything gets down. It's just a few words in a sentence coming from our mother, but it carries volumes to me. I take it as a compliment, and I run with it. I would like to take a day off and let one of the "other" Judy's in our house take over for a bit, but those other people don't make "themselves" known, at least not to me.

I listen to our Mom talk to you girls on the phone. She wants to talk and convey information, but for lack of memory or quickness of thought, she just "fills" in the blanks. Where some of the comments come from, I don't have a clue. I evidently was out the days that all those people brought in all those material scraps for us to use up. I would have liked to thank them, and the chopped-up chicken with torn up bread in soup served over toast—I promise you I never made that either. I do know she dreams every single night. I do know that if she talks too long, her conversation content declines, and she is harder to understand and follow. Remember, even talking with her girls on the phone is "work" for her brain.

I finally admitted defeat in the use of the telephone handsets with the green "to talk" button, and the red "to hang up" button. We now have a telephone with a curly cord and a base that is connected with a phone line. This means she only has to pick up the receiver and talk. No buttons present, so no button pushing required. Problem solved.

The Pirate game was over the other night when they "got their ninth out." Mom doesn't understand why the Pirates have started "dragging" the game out to nine innings, when they "never played that many before." They also "change the rules as they go," and "mess around a lot." Our mom watches the games every night with me. She never knows who's winning, she never knows the score, and she really doesn't care. She just watches the action and listens to the announcers. She knows what is happening, at the time, but then it gets lost somewhere behind closed doors. Sometimes verbal stimuli and clues can stimulate her memory, other times "not." I have to call her attention to "her boy" and she watches more closely when he is up to bat. She is an avid McCutheon fan—referring to him as "Cutch." Her comprehension and understanding of the game is difficult to assess. Brian asked her who won the game today. She said, "we did." Then she turns to me and asks, "didn't we?"

There is a lot she doesn't remember, and she says she really doesn't recall it. She only knows it because we told her. She still has so much trouble remembering that she has 4 daughters. I am constantly naming family members, asking questions, and reminding her of things that had happened. I honestly think there is some improvement in that area. She does ask about them when that particular sister calls.

Our mother has no pain. None! I am so grateful. I know this for sure as I watch her move and I watch her face. There is no sign of discomfort or limitation. She woke up with a slight headache several mornings. We discovered it may have been a caffeine headache. After a cup of coffee, problem solved. Her worries are based on simple activities of daily living. She is not mean. She is not angry. There is no agitation. She laughs a lot. She laughs out loud, and it's genuine. Her smile is beautiful. It was a long row to hoe after her dental extractions. Her confusion with what was in her mouth, and how it hurt when we took it out, even to the point of fainting in the process, has all cleared. She has come a long way, even though she doesn't know it, but she is so very proud of her smile now. She told me her teeth never showed when she smiled, like mine did. She looked at herself in the mirror and said, "now they do." She always commented on Brian's smile. Now I tell her to smile, like Brian smiles. I never knew she was so conscious of her smile and tended to keep her lips closed. But I still have to help her brush her teeth properly. It's a new lesson very time.

To even attempt to imagine how her mind now thinks, is out of my realm of understanding. I told her we were eating tomatoes from our garden in April, and they wouldn't be doing that up north. She agreed, but for her own reasons—not because of the winter weather in Pennsylvania. She told me that was true—because they don't have April up there...

She truly leaves a little sparkle wherever she goes.

She had another surgical follow up appointment for her fractured hip. I introduced her to the surgeon, since she has no recall of him. She also has no recall of her hospital stay or the few weeks following her fall and surgery. She had no idea I spent nights on a roll-away bed in her hospital room. I do know one thing, as I have been with her through the whole recovery, she sure has set the bar high for the next eighty-nine-year-old that breaks a hip. It certainly is not "the end" as we have heard from many sources when an elderly person falls and breaks a hip. It is a whole new beginning. From the time she came home with staples in her hip, she didn't remember that anything had happened, so she just resumed walking as she had before her fall. She didn't understand the need for a walker when she had already "weaned" herself from it. She didn't know that we were dealing with a whole new issue.

I explained that "Mom, since you were sleeping when he operated, I wanted you to meet Dr. Reed. He's the one who fixed your hip." She was very gracious as he greeted her with a salutation and a smile. The office staff was watching the doctor—and then the ball dropped. She looked at me in total innocence and asked, "What's wrong with my hip?" As Dr. Reed and the office staff smiled, I just said, "See what a good job you did, Doctor."

We don't tell time down here in Florida like you guys up north do. Everybody else turns their clocks back and we don't, per our mother's request. That is too confusing for her. I let her go with that, as it gives her a reason for not being able to totally understand time.

I wish I could record a single day with the antics of our second mom. She doesn't really like getting up early. If nothing is going on, she often lies back down if she awakens too early. She has no problem falling back asleep. She comes out of her room dressed, as she has all of her life. Her coffee is on the table in a thermos along with her coffee cup and a dish of frosted flakes. That is still her favorite breakfast. She does use a fork to smash the flakes before she puts the milk on. She is still adjusting to her upper denture.

My hands are stiff and somewhat swollen. They have scratches and cuts all over them and up both arms from working outside. My muscles are also feeling stiff and swollen. I take a step and I feel I need to push a little harder. I tend to walk on my toes on my left foot. I twist and turn and stretch in different direction, trying to break loose and move more freely. I ask mom if she has any discomfort or pain. Her answer is a simple and clear answer. "No, none." For this I am so grateful.

Mom's hair looks real neat and cute now. She has a permanent that evens out the looks of the sides. She combs her hair every morning before coming to breakfast. This is a habit she became used to living in the two-story farmhouse. She would get dressed before coming down the stairs every morning.

I told her we needed to go shoppin' walkin' this morning, as we haven't the last few days. She doesn't argue. We go to Goodwill, and this time we look for some shirts for Brian. Mom has on a pair of her capris, and she wears them well. We go to Kohl's next, as I am looking for a good nonstick set of cookware that will work for me the rest of my life. Mom was amazed at the store. We took the elevator up to the second floor, as she was pushing a cart. She kept looking around, telling me that it had everything. She told me she's never been in a store this big. We look at cookware, but I don't make a purchase. The saleslady tells me the truck is due in tomorrow, but they never know what they are going to get. We leave the store as Mom continues to be amazed. I don't know where her memory starts or stops. Has she never been in a store so large? Has she never been in a store that carries everything?

Mom smiles a lot, giggles more than I ever remember, and laughs out loud. I always remember her with the quiet hidden laugh, the stifled sneeze, the contained and controlled emotions.

We have gone through Wendy's drive through for our lunch. Mom gets her zipper case opened to pay for lunch. It comes to eight something, and I hand Mom back the change from her ten. She always seems surprised that it costs so little. I just explain that I'm a cheap date.

Life is beautiful. Every day is like opening a sealed envelope. Every morning has the ability to be simple. She likes to sleep in. I fill her thermos, sit her cup on the placemat, and put frosted flakes in her bowl. She gets the milk from the fridge without any problem.

She is dressed when she comes to the table for breakfast. We review the plans for the day. She always insists I eat with her and she shows absolute relief when she finds out that no one is coming this day. I like to go out and work in the yard in the early morning. We haven't had any rain, so watering is such a refreshing thing to do. I've also been transplanting some red tipped plants with very jaggy leaves so my arms and hands are a collection of scratches.

I did Mom's fingernails last night, a pale lilac color that matches her new glasses and sunglasses. They looked so nice. She is so proud of them when they are polished.

We watched the noon news and the soap operas and then loaded the five dogs, Mom's walker, and Mom into the car. I have asked my vet to see all the dogs, as they need flea medicine and my three need rabies shots.

We were early. I left the car running and left Mom with the five dogs in the car. I went into the office to make sure I had all the paperwork done. Laurie, the receptionist told me the Doc wouldn't be back from lunch for another half hour. As we worked on updating the records, he walked into the office. He asked me if I had five dogs for him. I told him I had five dogs and one mother. He said he didn't count my mom. He then told me to bring them in.

As I got a few of the dogs out of the car, Joie slipped her collar. I reached to grab her in the parking lot and had her in my arms just as Rusty made his escape. I chased after him, Joie in arms, when he decided to stop and leave his mark on the street sign. I then stepped on his leash and retrieved him. I walked in with three leashes with a dog on the ends, one dog in my arms, and guiding Mom, who had Annie with her with her walker. Just as we got to the door, the doctor met us and tried to pick up Annie. That didn't work, as Annie panicked. I then took Annie, bringing my count to five. The Doc then assisted Mom and her walker to get into the office. He invited her to have a seat in the waiting room, and the rest of us went into a little office.

The visit went very well, after we were in the confines of his office. We now have enough flea medicine for a year for each of the five dogs, three have got their rabies update, the newest one got a q tip up his butt to check for heart worms. I paid the bill and we were ready to make our escape.

We laughed once we were all inside the car—and all were accounted for. It wasn't negotiable, it was going to be a straight shot home.

I was relieved and I was tired. I had Mom's two dogs with me, so I was able to get flea medicine for them in pill form. Her doctor up north refused to give me pills for fleas. I asked Mom if she was game for strawberry shortcake for supper. She was. I asked her to stem the strawberries while I fixed the dogs food. I watched as she stemmed, then washed and sliced the strawberries. She then added sugar and left them set.

As we set down for supper, she informed me that "the grapes were hard, but after I sliced them and added sugar, they softened up." I'm beginning to wonder if my ease in climbing into my mother's explanations will affect my social abilities in the future? I do it so easily I'm concerned I will forget how to talk to an average person. I already know I can talk to an exceptional, special, astounding, awesome person without missing a beat. Bri has joined me in this talent. It works so well in establishing a comfort level to this lady in our world.

I think Bri and I have chipped stepping stones out of stumbling blocks.

We will do what we need to help this lady feel she is "home."

We are moving into May.

I was outside early, working up a sweat. Mom's coffee and frosted flakes are at her place setting, for when she arises.

I listened to Mom talk with Jane last evening. She talked and asked if everyone was okay? She asks how her grandson was, the one with the broken leg. She had remembered that one of the boys had broke his leg from a previous time? She even answered questions that were asked of her, like what we had to eat for supper and did we go out and about today.

After Mom hung up the phone, she turned to me and asked," Was that my Jane I was talking to?"

Life is fun, and always full of surprises.

I can't assume she won't leave the yard, for she goes down the three steps and out to the carport by herself. I can't assume she won't open the gate and dispense 5 or more dogs into the universe. She went to get the mail for me one day, walked right past our mailbox, crossed the street, and opened the neighbor's mailbox. Of course, I was watching and monitoring her. I must remember her eyesight is also based with one eye and half sight in the other. Peripheral vision is altered.

We were watching a pirate game. I asked her "do they have someone with them when they travel that does their laundry?" I found it a good question after watching one of the Pirates slide onto a base. I heard her say "They probably do because they have someone that does my laundry." I looked over at her, and my gaze just wandered over her beautiful face. Then she added, "I guess it goes in with the care that I get." Sometimes I just don't have a comeback for fear I confuse her more, or maybe confuse me more?

It is comforting to know her laundry is included in her care. Again my mother, I have nothing…your explanation has left me speechless.

Bri invites her to the kitchen table every evening when he stops after work. He tells her if they go to the table, that "food will appear." She believes that the food comes from somewhere—just when they sit down. We live in such a wonderful place. It is a magical world on Sunset Drive.

Now mother has decided she don't want to go to bed. I need to problem solve this issue. I may not require a whole lot of sleep, but I need her to require an earlier bedtime—for my sanity. Last night she was determined to sit on the sofa with me all night, so I wouldn't be by myself. She adamantly refused to go to bed. I had to get Mickie to intervene for me and show her that she wanted to go to bed and needed Mom to lead the way.

Dear Lord, I am now talking with the animals, and making sense of it. This isn't the first serious talk I have had with Mickie. I think she realizes we are both trying to find the same lady.

I don't understand Mom's fixation on moving her money about in her room. This wouldn't be a problem, except when we are ready to go somewhere, I will be waiting beyond the normal length of time because she can't find some money to take. Even when I ask her why she keeps moving it, she says she doesn't know. She has money in a bank envelope that I find in different places. We've simplified her purse with a zipper case for her money. I found the zipper case on her dresser with coins in it. When I asked where her money was, she said she didn't want to take a lot with her. Again, I asked where the bank envelope was. She didn't have an answer. I looked in her purse and found it folded up in her purse. Even though she didn't want to take much with her, she had all her cash with her—but without her knowledge. I can't seem to make things easy for her, or us. I don't want to seem controlling, for she is my mother. She is an adult. She does like knowing she has money in case she wants to buy something, but the ongoing search to constantly find things seems to be just one small battle in an ongoing war.

We went to Goodwill for our "shoppin' walkin'" today. Mom is looking at things more than she had. She picked up a ceramic cat from a top shelf and looked it over, then placed it back on the shelf. We continued down several more isles, and all at once she left my side and said, "I have something to do." She came back with the cat carefully placed in her buggy. She showed interest in something, and then backtracked to pick it up. It was another landmark move in her recovery. It may not seem remarkable to most, but for Mom, it truly is. When we went through the checkout, she paid for her purchase herself, and then handled it very carefully.

Again, we went through the drive through and brought our supper home. We eat cheaply, tonight it cost a little over $7 for us both. After I ate, I went outside to water the bushes on the far side of the lot. During the time I was there, Mom came outside several times, once even walking to the other side of the shed where she could see me."

MEMORIAL DAY

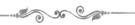

Another day with our mother and me. Mom asked if there was three to set the table for. She was talking to my sister, and I heard her explain that "both" of them had one shot in their foot. She said it still hurts them, but so far "they" both only had one shot. I don't know where this other person hangs out at. I am often correcting Mom, stating there are just two of us here, she and I. I am "them," or "they" or "someone," possibly other names also. "They" just don't come to mind right now. Now after I figure out who "both" of them are, I need to research who got a "shot in their foot"? I am having problems with plantar fasciitis in my left foot. While at the doctor office, I refused an injection into my heel and chose to work with it in other ways. Mom remembered my options. Sometimes conversations get scrambled together, making for interesting info to pass onto family.

I needed to put some flower bulbs into the ground tonight. I asked Mom if she wanted to help me, I would take a chair out where I was working, and she can help with the water hose. She did walk out, but Annie jumped up in her chair and she didn't want her moved, I worked at loosening the ground, so I could set the bulbs. Meanwhile, the neighbor brought her two dogs out into her back yard and the five dogs living in our yard went nuts. Mom kept trying to quiet "Mickie" down. I watched her walk into the house and open the back door. I waved to her and she waved back. I kept digging and placing the bulbs. Soon I watched her walk out toward me. She asked me how many dogs we had. I said I had one out here with me, and I could see two at the back door and one on the carport. She said,

"Five," and walked back toward the house. I will wait a short time, and then follow through with whatever is going on inside the house. Hopefully number 5 is inside the house.

I wish I could figure out the problem with counting inside Mom's head. She cannot tell time, no matter which clock she looks at. She told me tonight she was staying with me tonight. I told her she was, but she was sleeping in her bed. She seemed surprised and stated, "Are you sure?"

I said, "Yes, Mom, you are right back the hall. I will be fine." She feels she has been staying with me to keep me safe?

Earlier today I was asking her what she was expecting when we go up north. She was hoping she was going to be staying by herself. She said she hoped she could. She said she had stayed there by herself before, and she wanted to do that now. I didn't have anything left to discuss on the subject. She doesn't have any concept of what the time of day is, no ideas of what to prepare for any meal or breakfast, no knowledge of just how many people are here in the house, who I am, which dogs are hers, and she even tried to write down how to feed the dogs yesterday. She started the directions by writing "five dogs." At night, she doesn't know just where she will be sleeping, or if she needs to go home. She doesn't know how to call out on the phone, but at least I have her answering the one phone now. She has not been able to master the remote, even to turning the volume up. When I looked to see what the problem was, as we were now on channel 9999, she had the wrong end of the remote aimed at the TV. She cannot push three numbered buttons fast enough to bring in that three-digit channel.

Just yesterday, she found out where Brian lives. She was in awe when she found it out, as she had felt he lived down this road. Even though we have walked over there, and I have pointed it out more than once every day, it was total news yesterday. Today she stood by the back door, without the porch, and commented on the breeze that comes in that door when she has it open.

The dogs started fighting in the middle of the night, and Mickie and Annie came out of Mom's room barking and running. Mom was not far behind, but by then I had it under control. All day yesterday she told me she needed to take her dogs and go home, because they were being bad. We talked a little, as I reassured her that it happens because dogs are pack animals. I also wanted her to know if she was going to go home, I would be going with her with my three dogs anyway. I told her that I would feel so bad because she left, yet I would be taking her there and taking my three dogs, so the situation would be the same. She is feeling bad, I'm feeling bad, so we are both feeling bad and we are in the same fix. She decided that we might as well just forget it then. I agreed, and the subject was changed.

Quite a long day yesterday as men were working on leveling the floors

Workers were at the house for eleven hours. I fixed Mom's supper at 8:00 PM last night, took a package of sausage out of the freezer and broke it up in the skillet to brown. Mom wanted just one little pancake. So I made her two. She loves putting strawberry syrup on them. We held off supper until the worker guys left to go home. When she realized that we had sausage with our pancakes she wanted to know how I came up with a meat that quickly. She didn't think I could put a supper together that quickly. I can only smile, for I know exactly where I learned to pull that trick off.

Today, I planned to have egg salad sandwiches for lunch. I ask Mom if she wanted to make the toast for our sandwiches. She quickly came into the kitchen and wanted to know how to do it. I took four slices of bread from the bag and showed her where to put the two slices in the top of the toaster. I then showed her the lever on the side, that she needed to push down. She stood in front of the toaster, until the toast popped up. She took the slices and placed them on a paper place and brought them to me. She said "Look at these, they are beautiful." I agreed with her, and then told her that she needed to make two more, so they better be beautiful too.

She said, "Or I might get fired."

I assured her that could very well happen.

She put the bread in the toaster and then she was beside me, watching me make the sandwiches. I looked to the toaster, and asked Mom to tell me what was wrong with the toaster. She walked over, and said, "I forgot to push it down."

I said, "You are certainly right."

She pushed the lever down and then watched it until it was finished. We will see if she remembers how to make toast sometime in the future.

Courage doesn't always roar. Sometimes courage is just a quiet voice at the end of the day that says, "I will try again tomorrow."

A quiet day sure became busy. I took Mom to have her upper denture realigned this afternoon. I told her we needed to take a load of stuff up to Goodwill, and while we were there, we could look around for a good used left foot for me. She thought for a minute, and then she laughed. Sometimes she comprehends my subtle humor easily, and the next time—something more obvious misses the connection.

Her denture needed realigned, but it is sometimes hard to get a good read on Mom when it comes to such things. Until just a few days ago, she hasn't been able to remove her own denture and put it to soak. She tells me it keeps falling down, but when I remove her denture, she fuses because she is expecting pain. She hasn't completely understood why they left her in so much pain for so long, when they could have just fixed it this easily. Explaining to her that she had nine very bad teeth pulled and had the denture put in her mouth immediately following the extractions, is all news to her. She doesn't understand why they would do it that way when it hurt so bad. She realizes it doesn't hurt to remove her denture now and thinks they could have done it that way before. I have nothing. I can only agree with her at this time.

Tonight, as we sat on the sofa and resumed the regular conversation of where she would be sleeping, and how she didn't plan on staying here this long, and how she doesn't like leaving me alone "out here by myself," or did the other people go home? Brian stopped by after his meeting. When he started to walk home, I called Mom to the carport so she could watch where he went. She keeps telling me that "all this time, she thought he lived on down this road. She has asked me how big his house is, or how close those cars are that she sees. When I tell her that she stayed there with me when I lived with him, the most confused look comes over her face. I know she has no memory that she can pull to the surface. I describe the bedrooms and the screened in porch and the hot tub, but nothing clicks any recall. I told her we walked back and forth before she broke her hip…that is all news to her also. If I could just climb inside her noggin and rethread some of those neurons so they can find the right passage when called upon—if only. But then I might change something that is working at its best right now. I guess it's better to leave well enough alone.

Sitting on the sofa, I asked Mom what it's like when she can't get her thoughts to work well. I asked her what has been the hardest part since her head surgery—that she has had to deal with. She again explains to me that she didn't know all that was happening. She only knows it, because we have told her. She tells me that sometimes she knows she should know something, but she just can't remember. She told me that she was talking to "her Jane" tonight on the phone, and then all at once, another Jane came on the line. I asked her if that is what happens when there is more than one of me? She looked so puzzled. She feels that I have been here part of the time, and then the other one comes and takes over. She can never name the other one, but I lose my identity midaction, just like Jane lost hers tonight midway during her conversation. She did tell me that when the girls call, they always give me their name.

Mom wants to try to live by herself when she goes up north. She said she has done it before, with her three dogs, and it worked well. Already I see the "dog counting episodes" to be traumatic. She wants to try it so bad. I told her that she definitely needs a dog fence, and she told me she already had one. She does not. She continues to be so confused as to the difference in time from here to the north. No matter how many times Jane will confirm that she has the same time as we do—she can't grasp the concept. She never knows where to look for the time, without total prompting…even though there are clocks everywhere.

She has ventured to try and find good shows on TV by using the remote. That usually doesn't work out really well, but she is trying. I keep telling her that the worst that can happen, is we need to reprogram—but the best could happen, and she could find a good show. Now if she gets the right end directed to the TV—we will have gained a lot of ground.

She still thinks that there is more than one of "us" alternating with staying here. She can't explain why going home sometimes means walking back the hall to her bed, and other times she feels she should have left earlier because she didn't plan on staying. She doesn't want to leave me alone in the living room, because I will fall asleep out here by myself—but other nights she will actually walk back to her room by herself. She will always have her shoes blocking the door open, so "the dogs can go in and out"—I think it's because she doesn't want the door closed between her and I. Funny thing is, since the guys have been leveling the floors on the house, her door won't shut anyway. I guess some things are just meant to be.

We discussed her being alone in her home, and what would happen when she gets a little mixed up with where her bed is, or how she is to get home? I told her that one time of that happening is one time too many, because it would probably scare her like it does here. I told her I just walk her back the hall and we find her bed. We talk for a bit, and I tuck her in, and she knows she is safe in her own bed. I told her that our goal is to get her back to her home, but safely. She said she can get her own coffee in the mornings, and I say, but that's because it is made and in the pot or in your thermos. I tell her that the fact she is thinking along these terms and questioning how she can do it—is a step in the right direction. I also tell her that it takes time for things to heal, and it's still early. Again, she tells me that she didn't even know that "all that was happening"—I reassure her that it did, that we were all there, even her three sons-in-laws—and she has come a long way. She just shakes her head.

Today I walked her into Goodwill, look at her face, and her pretty purple sunglasses are on her face upside down. I can't stop laughing. I tell her why. She tells me that they are working fine. I tell her, after I regain some composure—that she finds a new way to do so many things. Who's to say the way we are used to doing them is the only way. I remember a quote from Thomas Edison—He didn't fail to discover electricity a thousand times, he just found a thousand ways not to discover it. We need to write a book.

I try to climb inside her head when I see a certain look come across her face. I worry that those neurons are connecting to the wrong live wires and she gets lost in the wrong place. We have tried 30 ways to knot a quilt, as she has done all her life. We still have thirty ways that don't work. I now have a quilt across the length of the island. I have removed the safety pins. I have it rolled from both sides, so that she only has a narrow work space. She has a neon pink square to use as a guide. She won't work on it unless I am close beside her. She says she "gets in trouble" and can't get it figured out…and she is right. I have to reguide her every few stitches, to keep her in line. She was so upset the one day that someone had come in and just put stitches everywhere…and she hated that. I have nothing to say. Bri might have a good alarm system in my home…but it sure don't keep everyone out. Even the dogs don't bark when other people show up.

I showed her how to make toast again yesterday. I had to show her how to push down the lever again today.

Pass that box of chocolates, please.

I baked a spaghetti squash. I showed her how to remove the spaghetti with forks. She did a great job…and was surprised when we added spaghetti sauce, meatballs, cheese, and fresh baked rolls to our dinner meal. Everything always tastes so very good to her. She never complains. Tonight I went into a pizza place by the shoe carnival, where we had bought her some new tennis shoes, totally against her will. They sold pizza by the piece. We brought it home and she thought it was so good.

I got her to put the cookies from a new package into the cookie jar after dinner. She asked me twice if I wanted all the cookies in the jar.

I did a lot of research on left sided brain injury tonight. I'm going to write up some information sheets to give to the family. I got info from several sources, and it is so informative. It gives some insight into things that may be perceived differently. It gives a little more understanding as to how this lady's beautiful mind is working. It also tells us we are doing well by hanging onto our sense of humor.

Mom tells the girls that "we" both are outside working all the time, and neither one of us stays off our feet. She has explained that both me and her has got a shot into our heels, but that we are still hobbling around. Maybe if that other one had left me get her shot, making two for me, there would at least be one good walking person living here with Mom. I don't even worry that I get comfortable in my mother's world so easily.

Mom loved her Pirates games. She watches the action now. She sees them hit the ball and watches them run. She doesn't pay much attention to the score, and often wants to know how long they played. I tell her the score and what inning it is…and she is content. It doesn't stay. After the game is over, she "thinks" they won…but doesn't have any idea of the score. It doesn't matter to her if they lost—just so they hit and run and slide and play. She does watch the action.

I mentioned to Mom that I had to get the dogs clipped and their nails cut. She said her granddaughter Julie used to do them. Score one for Julie. Okay, where are you Julie? I'm just a little busy here. You used to do this for Mom's dogs? Well, they are still Mom's dogs—so where are you?

My days revolve around Mom. Her days revolve around her dogs. Today she wanted to mail a thank you letter to the congregation of the church and thank them for their cards and letters. I stopped what I was doing, and we created a card on the computer. She says her writing is not legible, but she will sign her name the best she can. We got the address from Jane today…so we will put it in the mail tomorrow.

I wonder—if we have egg salad sandwiches tomorrow—if our toast will be beautiful? Mom is so pleased because her teeth show when she smiles. She said they never showed very much, like they do now. Her new eyeglasses are a very pale lilac…and they sure look cute with dark purple sunglasses over them in the upside-down position.

She's not wearing knee socks every day. She loves me to lay out her clothes. She hates to pick her clothes—she says she always has. I didn't know this. She said she could never match them up right, and just wore what she had worn before. Now I know why she would have on a dressy outfit for church, and then put on a green checkered flannel shirt over top. Now I know why she always wore polyester pants with different tops, she loved those polyester pants…in all colors. And she doesn't hesitate to tell you that she's had them for a long time. Yep, we kind of knew that, Mom.

One day left in May.

Wow, how fast the months go by. We made a thank you card for the congregation at Highfield Lutheran church. Mom wanted to thank everyone for their cards and letters and let them know how they were appreciated. She also wanted to let them know that she is doing the best that she can. We put a quote from Cary Grant in the card that seems to fit Mom's life at this time. He said: At this time in my life…I get up in the morning and I go to bed at night. In between that time, I do the best that I can."

Three workers were here to work on leveling the floors again today. Mom is more difficult to keep content when there are people in her space. It is difficult to manage the dogs, as Mom seems oblivious to Mickie's constant barking. She tells her to "be quiet" at least fifty times in ten minutes, with no follow-through. She doesn't want to hurt her feelings, she gets upset when I manage the dogs and make them listen. She doesn't like it when I bring Mickie beside me, and make sure she quits barking. Mickie usually settles right down and sleeps by my feet—yet Mom calls her and asks her if she needs to go outside. I point out that Mickie is sleeping by my feet, and she doesn't need anything—but Mom can't let that alone. The minute I moved away to get the guys some cold water, she took her leash and brought her beside herself then took her leash off.

Mom will not eat in front of the dogs. She says she can't look at their little faces and not feed them. I have tried constantly to enforce the "please don't feed the dogs people food, Mom." It's like I've never said it. Mom brings her plate or dish to the kitchen island and stands to eat, rather than sit down and eat "in front of the dogs." She claims they are hungry—that they need to go outside…that they feel bad… Mom truly worries about how they are feeling.

She feels that she knows what the dogs are thinking and communicates with them more than she does with people. I've been trying to help Mom learn some simple tasks, so she feels she is helping more. She tried to write down ways she could help me. At the top of her list was "five dogs."

Today we started with the same tasks again. I sat the five bowls on the counter, and watched Mom reach for the large bag of dry dog food. I again, showed her where the dog food is in plastic containers so she can handle it easier. I sat the white bowl on the counter, along with the plastic container of mixed hamburger with rice—and the quarter cup measurer. Mom did well with putting the dry dog food in the bowls…except she also put dry food in the white bowl also. I showed Mom that we only needed five bowls and dumped the dry food back in the plastic container. I then told her to put five measured cups of the mix in the white bowl and place it in the microwave. I told her to push the number "one"—as she did yesterday. I had to point out the number "one "on the screen, which Mom did. I explained that it heats it for one minute, so the flavor goes through the dry dog food. I then had Mom divide up the moist food and mix it through the five bowls. This she did, and the bowls were left on the island, since our dinner wasn't done yet.

Then I got out two little bowls and put some canned pears in each. I then had Mom put some cottage cheese in each bowl for our supper. I turned to do something, and when I looked back, Mom had put a large spoonful of cottage cheese on the tops of the five bowls of dog food. I stopped Mom and asked her why she was giving the dogs cottage cheese. She answered that she thought she was supposed to.

I see that Mom doesn't know when something doesn't seem right. She doesn't seem to question any of her actions or have the ability to think things through and see the end results. It makes her very vulnerable for injury or unsafe actions. It is the reason I went out and bought some storm doors for the house today. It is the reason there are child gates on several of the outside doors. It is the reason all caustic or poisonous chemicals are stored high on a shelf in the laundry room, or outside in the shed. Our mother is not safe alone or left to her own ideas. She is such a mystery.

I took Brian's truck and went to Lowes to get three storm doors this morning. Bri said "I got this, I will stay here with Mawmaw." Of course, a Saturday morning at Lowes, one man working the computer in the door department, a line to wait for his time—Two white doors were in stock, but the dark brown door had to be ordered.

The man working in this department could not have been nicer. He ordered the dark brown door, and then loaded the two white doors on a cart. He said he would push the cart to the front of the store for me, even though he already had several people waiting in line for his attention again. As I paid for the doors, he waited with the cart, and then pushed it outside to load in the truck. I thanked him for making my trip so easy, and he said he needed to get away from the computer for a bit, and get out into the sunshine. He loaded the doors for me, and told me he would call me when the third door comes in. Such a nice man, Jonathan was. I need to make sure I let Lowes management know what a helpful employee they have on staff. Too often positive comments are not made. Too often only the bad acts are brought to one's attention, or the negative actions get all the media attention. It makes a woman feel a little extra special, when a stranger goes the extra mile. Thank you.

When I got home, and walked in the gate, Mom was sitting on the lawn chair. She greeted me with, "What took you so long, did you have to get them made?" I told her that they weren't easy to make and I only got two finished. I then responded with a comment that asked Mom if she missed me that much when I'm gone. I do know that she doesn't like it when she doesn't know where I am or can't see me within her visual field.

So again, I have been reprimanded by my mother.

Mom loves to have the doors open. She is always opening them. She especially likes to open the one without any porch or landing. She doesn't get the concept of how the welcome sign goes out to mosquitoes here in Florida. I am a little surprised at this action, because she always wanted things locked up and closed down when it became dark up north. She will open the doors and go outside after dark with the dogs here in Florida. Of course, she has to go through the ritual of "dog counting" again—when she comes inside. She has told me that she would like to try living alone in her home with her three dogs—to see if she can. Already I see a problem, but she doesn't. She now has three dogs—so I guess I have lost custody of one. I wonder which one?

She did ask me this evening, if her room was "put back together." I assured her it was, that I was already back there checking it out. The working guys had to level out the floor in the one corner of her room today. But she did call it "her room"—and she loves the handrail I put on her bed, and the two layers of mattresses on her bed. I told her she was the princess and the pea—so we may have to add more in the future. She laughed. She followed my train of thought this time. She is a mystery. Her beautiful mind is full of surprises. If I see it as a mystery, I can only try to walk a mile in her shoes to know who she is these days. We do laugh…and she smiles a lot.

She does have incontinent accidents at times. Sometimes I think she waits too long or doesn't realize she has to go—and when she stands, gravity bears it's ugly face. She has been able to change her underwear and outer clothing when she has an accident. There is a step forward in self-care. There is a four-watt bulb burning at the other end of this tunnel. Where there is any sign of hope, we will be heading in that direction. How can I not? I might miss something that makes my day. And as I've said many times before…you just can't make this stuff up.

At 12:55 AM, I'm watching the pirate game, recording it for our mother. I've recorded several. They are on the West Coast, so they don't start playing until 10:00 PM. I hear the dreaded "thump." I know why I sleep on the sofa. Maybe I do need the bed in her room again. She is laying on her back on the floor. She tells me she was trying to fix the door with her shoe so the light doesn't shine in so much. She said she hit the back of her head. I wonder quickly, just for a brief moment, what the rest of my night is going to be like. Selfishly, I catch myself wondering what "my night" is going to con-tain. It brings me back to the situation at hand. I've kept Mom sitting for a short period. She is trying to tell me what happened, but words aren't readily available. She doesn't appear to be injured as I help her to her feet. Rusty has galloped back to Mom's room with me. Mom's two dogs, whether they be the white Annie and the Black Annie, or the black Mickie and the white Mickie—lay on her bed wondering what their night will hold. Mom tells me her feet were slippy. I take off her socks and put on a pair of the hospital socks with treads on them. We have corrected this problem…in hindsight. We will add this to our nightly routine. Earlier I met her in the hall carrying her upper denture plate in her hand. She stated that she had taken in out, and now she didn't know what to do with it. She asks, "Should I leave it out, or what?" Sometimes I don't think she quite understands what is in her mouth, or why.

Oh, what shall tomorrow bring? Oh, but this is tomorrow—just a very early edition of it. We have, hopefully, dodged another bullet, and we both get to skip the 911 call, and spend the night at home. "At Home"—just wherever that may be for the orbit our mother's beautiful mind travels on. I know that the words "at home"—for this daughter—have taken on the mindset of wherever my mother is. It brings to mind the advertisement that used to come over the airlines at night. "It's 11:00 PM, do you know where your children are?" I might not be able to climb inside her world and stay there—but I can keep her as safe and protected in my world as humanly possible.

At least the Pirates won, and it was a good game. They made the ninth inning interesting. I have it taped. Mom will watch it tomorrow. She watched last night's game twice today, while the guys worked here. She still doesn't know who won, either time. She always thinks the pirates won. I'm not going to alter those thoughts. She has some tough hurdles to work through every day. So as long as the Pirates are winning these games—at least on the channels she's connected to—she's on a positive path.

I was a bit sleepy. I was researching brain injury on the laptop when she fell. Adrenaline sure does kick up alertness—and all it took was a "thump." It's now officially "Sunday," a day of rest. The worker guys don't come back until Monday morning. Mom has been waking up and getting up every morning, feeling that it is the day "they are coming to work." Tomorrow will be another "practice run," and by Monday she will have it perfected. Maybe I should write a book, someday—when I have time. Right now I'm considering one of those tall orange triangle flags they use on bike riders. It makes it easier to spot bikers on the highways—so just maybe, it will make it easier to spot Mom's whereabouts. Maybe a pair of those tennis shoes that flashlights with every step. The baby monitor works well when she's in bed. She was out of view after the "thump" tonight. It's difficult to stay one step ahead of her these days. I just put a side rail handgrip on her bed yesterday. It gives her a safety bar to grab when she needs to get up to the potty chair. She had been grabbing onto the arm rest of the potty chair to aid sitting up in her bed, which wasn't real sturdy. I hadn't thought about her placing shoes on both sides of her bedroom door—in the middle of the night—after she used the potty chair. What was I thinking? Why had I not thought that she might need to do this?

Am I wrong, or is thinking abstractly getting strengthened by use?

The month of June has arrived.

The worker guys were here again this morning. Mom was still in bed, so she was caught unprepared. She was rushing to get dressed, her hair was sticking out in all directions, and she was out of her comfort zone. I helped her get dressed, explaining that they weren't going to be in her bedroom today, they were going to put the two storm doors on.

Well, that didn't happen. After they removed the door from the packing, and discovered that it wasn't going to fit in the present door frame, after they removed several pieces of trim, several screws, and frequent use of the level, they informed me that they didn't have the right supplies to do the job. They thought it would be a quick job, just in and hang the doors. Apparently, the rules of the crooked house continue to the outside of the door frames. With the door open and the dogs barking for several hours, after involved explanations of how the previous contractor had altered everything and nothing was level, after talk of how much more work is involved and they needed to get some more boards, they packed up their tools and left, saying they would be back tomorrow after the attorney comes to the one workers house for a meeting on workman's comp. Another open-ended time frame—and Mom watching from the dining room table the entire time.

Mom wanted to finish knotting the quilt on the island today. She needed help getting started, but it was going very well. She was actually moving her plastic guide in the proper direction and taking stitches in the proper place. She was rested and it showed. I kept threading the three needles and tying the knots and keeping her in the right direction. She kept asking how much more was left. She wanted to finish…but we had just started it yesterday. The only thing is, she requires me to be close by and with a watchful eye, plus threading her needles, cutting her stitches, rolling the quilt, and catching her before she would take more than one stitch at a time. I have to admit, I was tired. The guys had left without hanging any doors. I had listened to the one constantly yelling at the second one. They were disrupting an already disrupted life. I could handle it, if they would just come in… do the jobs…and then move on. As it is, they come one day, miss a few, plan to come another day, but not accomplish what they had intended to do. They spend more time explaining things to me…that I don't really care to know. I just want them to do their jobs and let me out of it. My plate is full enough right now.

Mom is determined. I needed to sit down for a bit. I needed to decide when we would be returning to the north. I needed to check airplane fares. I needed to find out the date of my oldest grandson's graduation party. I turned around and saw Mom sitting on the barstool. She looked downhearted. I ask her what was wrong.

She said, "Will you please help me finish this?"

She gets "stuck" and doesn't know which way to move her guide and pattern. This is something that she could have done in her sleep at an earlier time in her life. How frustrating it must be to not be able to move a pattern down a piece of material. How weary a person must feel when she knows she "should" know how to do something—but not be able to.

I can tell, she is tired. It is not going easily. I explain to her that she needs to rest, and we will finish the quilt after she naps. I explain that I can see how much harder it is for her to follow the guide to place the stitches. It went easier this morning, but she's pushing now…and it's become quite a hard task. She did say she would lay down, and she did. She must have fallen asleep right away. No task comes easily to her at this time in her life. She is pulling and struggling to follow the guide and make stitches. She is using her brain and all powers connected to completing a thought. Those neurons just don't have the right chemistry to make a proper connection in that beautiful mind of hers. When she is tired...I can just picture the neurons misfiring in all directions ...not connecting to complete the current, but instead shooting off like mini fireworks...and then fading away as the spent charge loses any chance of grabbing a hold of another neuron.

Sometimes I need to remind myself that this mother figure cannot return to the person she was before the injury. She can't find her way back to somewhere that she doesn't really know when she left.

Dear Time—please slow down—even just a little bit.

Every day informs me of some aspect of our mother that wasn't so obvious before. Tonight, our mother was standing by the door, and switching light switches, trying to turn off the carport light. I walked over and said, "Mom, let me show you how to do this, and then the next time you will know. I showed her the light switch that covers the light outside, and that there was also a motion light out there, that she cannot shut off. There in laid the reason for her switching the switches so many times in a row. After we reviewed turning the lights off, and then on again, I explained that the motion light was on a time delay. She waited for a while, and then attempted to close the blind on the door window. She stopped moving the lever, but she was doing it right. I encouraged her to continue, and to watch how the window will be closed. She was so truly delighted when she completed the task at hand, and it worked out as she had planned.

I explain to our mother that her brain is amazing, and that it is making leaps and bounds. She laughs at this comment, stating how far she has come to where she can turn lights off and on. I agree with her, but I am not using sarcasm. Humor still dominates our days and nights...and it works for us. She has a new appreciation for food, and different tastes, and marvels at how good everything tastes. She doesn't hesitate to try something new, like the spinach and mushroom quiche today for lunch. She always says, "Whenever you want to eat," "Whatever you are going to eat," and mostly, "I don't want to eat by myself."

Today we did her "walkin' shoppin'" and then I mentioned eating along Lake Monroe. She was agreeable to that idea, although I knew she didn't know exactly what I was referring to. We went to "the coffee shoppe" and walked inside. I told her we were going to have quiche. She said, "Okay," and then asked me what that was. I ordered the quiche, two coffees, and then two pieces of apple pie, probably "to go." Mom was surprised at the appearance of the quiche, and before the meal was done, she had eaten all the salsa on her plate, along with the quiche. She said it was probably the first time she had ever ate it…and it was so good. We haven't eaten out in quite a while, since Mom had broken her hip and then because she was getting used to her new denture plate. Today we dined outside the coffee shoppe and gazed upon Lake Monroe. Mom was not in a hurry and was truly enjoying the change in environment. I told her how Lake Monroe was a manmade lake from the St. John's river. I told her how much Brian loved this lake, and that he used to live in the apartments overlooking the Lake. She commented on a man walking two dogs on the River Walk. I told her I used to walk Ricky and Brian's dog, Lucy, in the mornings, when I stayed with Bri at his apartment.

Some parts of my explanations sounded familiar to our mother, so some of her memory was trying to kick-start. She is enjoying so much of life, as if she has been given this new gift of time. She appreciates everything. She smiles a lot.

She removed her denture, put it in the soaking cup, and brushed her lower teeth today. She then put her denture back in her mouth unassisted. This is such a big step for her. She doesn't see the whole picture, probably because of the short term memory issue. She sees that she is relearning a lot, she feels she should already know how to do these things, but she keeps moving along. I did get to explain to her how well she did working with the quilt the last few days, when she was rested. I reminded her how hard it was for her to follow the steps when she became tired. She hears me. She recalls how hard it was to do one of the quilts that "jumped" all over the place in stitches. She doesn't look forward to doing another one like that.

Mom would work hard to put stitches in half of a row and be exhausted. That would be her accomplishment for the entire day. Now she can work along with cues, with occasional help getting "unstuck." For sure, I can't walk away from her when she is doing the knotting.

She wanted to help me do something, so I had her press the hem in curtain panels that I had just hemmed. It just so happened, that she ironed the top of the panels, but ended up melting the fabric. I gave her a pressing cloth, and reminded her that she only had to press the new hem line down. She feels the dogs are hungry. I suggest she do the dogs dinner, with me close by—but nothing set up for her. It went fairly well, but when Mom forgets the next step... she just gazes—not knowing what should come from her repetition. I asked if it would help if the steps were written down—and she felt it "sure would." I will have this done. I will get a loose-leaf notebook, so pages can be added if we find this effective.

She was going to go to bed at 7 tonight. Her comment was, "I might as well." I was tired today, kind of like jet lag. I was cleaning windows and blinds and shortening curtain panels. I wasn't guiding her with every step of any projects, or explaining the story lines on TV shows, or the actions that were occurring with her Pirate games. I realized that I needed to step back in her world for a while, so I started stripping the homemade tree of broken lights. She watched every move and commented about its appearance. I then got the next quilt out on the island and started pinning the borders. She was up and right by my side, so I got the box of crochet threads out so she could pick the color that she wanted to knot it with. She was excited. She felt we had done two quilts in a single day "yesterday." Most things that happen have happened "yesterday"—in her world. She felt that "someone else needs to start making some decisions here that she doesn't need to be making them all." She also wants to know if this is one of those hard quilts with the stitches all over the place. I mentioned the fact that these were the Christmas gifts for her grandchildren, and what did she want to do for the great-grandchildren. She thinks for a bit, then states, "You said I gave them money last year, so we were going to do that again this year." I feel myself smiling inside...she recalled what we had discussed days ago. She doesn't see my smiling—she doesn't know that her brain was working with her for these few seconds. It is short lived, as she is so confused with the dogs this evening. She cannot put the proper name with any of them. She has taken them outside, and then counted and recounted—to make sure they all came in with her. She questions where they sleep. She knows that her two dogs don't spend the entire night in her bed. She is dressing herself for bed, and also putting on her nonskid slipper socks. This is a new addition to our nighttime routine, and she is following through with it.

I understand that the most improvement following a brain injury will be in the first six months. I also understand that there is very little improvement after the first two years. I watch her gather up the Sunday newspaper, and move it to another area. She is still moving her money around, never leaving it in the same place. Today it was stuffed down inside her sunglasses case. The zippered bag that we were using for her money was empty and in one of her dresser drawers. I don't know why this is such an obsession with her, unless it gives her a sense of security.

She asked me if I was staying here tonight. I just told her we were both staying here.

She said, "No, sometimes I go back to my own bed."

I take a deep breath, pause a minute, and then add, "Yes, you do."

I wonder what it will be like up north. Will anything seem familiar? Will she notice if anything has been changed? Will she be able to sleep in her own bed and find the bathroom? I have her using the potty chair during the night, right at her bedside. Still she fell in her room two nights ago. "a stitch in time" just don't work in these circumstances. "an ounce of prevention" just goes by the wayside also. It is what it is.

We are both partially broken, but the last time I checked,
broken crayons still colored the same.

I was trying to do some research as to why my mother sees me as multiple people. The studies were so deep or so statistically laced with information, that is didn't make sense in my world of questions at this time. I just wanted to know why Mom always wants to set the table for three…or wants to know if "they" went home or are "they" still here. She counted the person laying on the couch yesterday, so planned on three here for supper. I asked her to show me that person. She walked to the sofa, then looked at me and asked, "Was that you on the couch?" I told her it was, but that I had been in the kitchen for some time now. She just answered that she "didn't know that." The time of day, the date on the calendar, the score of the ballgame or the inning that they are playing…the number of people living here in this house…the number of dogs in our care…the number of dog dishes for feeding the dogs…the fact that everything seems to have happened "yesterday," verses this morning or even at the present. I can put a recorded version of the ballgame on to entertain our mother. I can change the channel at any time, and she doesn't question why the game wasn't completed, or as to "who won?"

It doesn't matter; she is seeing the actions as they occur, and then they are gone. It's a big spin of the wheel, and you just never know where it is going to stop. Is it going to stop on 100 and she becomes an automatic winner? Is it going to stop on 15, and she still feels the game is over and we have won? Did the Pirates win is not important, because the score is a number and it doesn't tell her if it is a winning number or otherwise. She will question the fact that she doesn't have any idea what time it is, or whether the dogs have been fed yet, or be looking for something to feed "these dogs, because they are hungry, and they haven't ate." The concept of time doesn't matter to her, even though she tried hard to program it in her day. She did count out all the months till Christmas when we were working on knotting a quilt the other day. She was able to name all the months following May, but when she got to December, it seemed like the reason that she had been counting and naming the months …got lost in the quest to get from May to December.

It's like the words a psychiatrist has used in describing my son's learning problems as a youth. This was Bri. He said he works so hard at reading the words set before him, that he hasn't gained any understanding of the concept of what he was reading. He was as lost as to its content at the end of the paragraph, as he was before he read the words. It seems to fit Mom's daily routine also. She gets through each day, without regard as to what we did or accomplished at the end of that day. Bri has a very easy understanding of his grandmother. Maybe he had traveled some of the same roads that she walks in now.

I do have to watch my behaviors. I was tired this week, more so than usual. I'm withdrawing from some of my ordered medication, changing my diet, and feeling more pain and discomfort with fibromyalgia and heel pain than while under the influence of medication. I was trying to get myself "recharged." Mom seemed to see my changed attention as to "keeping me from doing what I want to do" and the fact that I needed to discipline her dog, Mickie, and follow through with some training for the barking and Mickie's obsession with stalking Ricky. She was going to take her "misbehaving dogs" and go home. The downside of this was—she didn't know where "home" was, or how she was going to get there. I listened to her talk to Mickie, and tell her that she is a good girl, and that we just need to go home. I listened and watched, I wanted to see if Mom was able to problem solve beyond this. Finally I said, "Mom, you do know that when you take your dogs and go home, that I will be taking my dogs and going to the same place with you and your dogs, don't you? That means, the dogs that aren't getting along are still going to be together, and I will still be with you. That means we won't be changing anything, all the dogs and you and I will still be together in the same place…and yet you have worried about it. We haven't changed anything, and yet you are getting upset, so why don't we just quit worrying and let things settle down for now."

She thought that sounded good and said she would quit worrying then and thanked me.

She is always thanking me, especially when I tuck her in at night. I left her in the waiting room at the doctor office when I went to get my heel checked again. The doctor spent some time deciding on my treatment for today and doing some research. When I came out into the office…she greeted me by saying "I thought you went back there and fell asleep." She doesn't wait well, for anything. We were early for my appointment, and that doesn't factor any of her waiting time into the equation. Like I've said before, she hasn't regained the ability to tell the time. If we are doing something else, and she knows that we have to be somewhere at a certain time…she will keep asking me if I am checking on the time. She doesn't ask anything more…just am I "keeping a check on the time." She must feel like she is suspended in a timeless space. I quoted an actor in one of her cards...and it just keeps coming to mind. "I get up in the morning, and I go to bed at night...and I do what needs to be done in between those two times..."

Where are the goals? She does know that she has to have so many quilts done by Christmas. She doesn't remember how many, or who they are to go to—just that she has to have "so many" done before the holiday. She is so dependent. She tells me she got some bread and put butter on it, and it was so good. She said she was hungry and didn't know what I had planned. I pull her into conversations and try to make her think. Just tonight I asked her what her favorite meat dish was. I had to give her examples like pork roast, barbecued ribs or pork chops, or beef roast. She told me she liked barbequed meat, but not real browned. We still didn't name a meat.

She did pick out a shirt that was hanging on the end of a rack today. It caught her attention, and it was pretty...so we bought it. She has picked up several little Knick knacks during our trips to good will. I'm not sure what it is about them, but she gently lays them in our shoppin' cart. They are lined up on her dresser. It is an interest. I will take it. We have spent enough time in apathy land—look around Mom and see what you like.

Good morning, Brain—we are coming after you—and we are persistent. You are the controlling device of the body...you decide what everything does, how they do it, when they do it...and even "if" they do it. Well, welcome back brain—cause we know where you stay. Once in a while, we find a way to get you to answer the door. Once in a while, you hear us knocking. Once in a while—but we will take it.

It's movement in the right direction. As long as we are moving—moving forward...we are not stuck and stagnant. You are using your brain Mom, even if you aren't aware of it. When a person is not brain injured—these actions are so taken for granted. Until I climbed alongside you in your world Mom, I may have taken these small actions for granted also. I will never do that again. I realize how hard it is for you to establish any actions now. Things that you did without thought in your other life, now require concentrated effort. Some days you push the buggy through the stores on our shoppin'-walkin' trips…and just go through the motions. Then there are the days that you put three knickknacks in the buggy that you have discovered and taken off the shelf yourself. There is the blouse that you took off the end of the rack and looked it over. I needed to check the size and put it in your buggy, for it would fit you. You keep telling me if you ever get back to all your good clothes…and I keep telling you that it doesn't hurt to get something new occasionally. You really don't know how to match up clothes. You really don't enjoy picking out your clothes. I never realized that, but you put on whatever I have laid on the chair by your bed. Even this is a very notable action.

In the mornings, your pj's are folded and placed on your pillow, along with your "not slippy socks." You have put the clothes on your body that have been placed on the chair. Yesterday evening I had you remove your elastic bra and lotioned your back and arms and legs very well. Your feet got soaked and you now have a fresh new manicure. I asked you not to sleep in the elastic bra, and you could put it on in the morning. This morning you had put it on but couldn't get it right. You had it on backward—and you wondered why your breasts just wouldn't fit in. It's just like today—you put your sunglasses on when we left the doctor office. Again, they were upside down—but they worked just the same. They were protecting your eyes from the bright sun. Some actions are just too precious to correct. This time I didn't laugh. I didn't lose composure and laugh uncontrollably. This time I just appreciated the lady behind the upside-down sunglasses… and smiled warmly inside.

Your world is tough enough—seeing it from a different angle on your side of the sunglasses—may be just the right medicine at this time, for both you and me.

It's the old adage, "Take time to smell the roses" or "Bloom where you are planted." Mom, you are blooming well…some days you are a whole blooming garden. Dear Lord, may I never lose sight of this. Dear Lord, please never let me think that the small stuff don't count—cause it does. Sometimes we build our whole day on the small stuff—cause some days that's all we have. Some days that's all we need Mom. You keep making the "small stuff" so important that we don't need the bigger picture at this time. Maybe the bigger picture is too much for now. Sometimes people rush through life and miss this "small stuff." They miss a lot, don't they Mom? If we didn't take notice of the small stuff during our days—we wouldn't have appreciated the happenings of one of our days. Some days you just can't get that seat belt hooked, no matter how long you tried. Some days you just can't get it unhooked. That would be the reason you kept the scissors in the bin on the driver's door. You had a plan B— back when you were driving. You questioned the day you may not get the seatbelt unhooked, and you had solved the problem. Some days, most days, you must manually pick up your right leg and lift it into the car. Do you remember "why" you must do this? Maybe— but it's not important now. We are looking forward, not backward.

Mom I love you more than a million colors.

It Looks Like My Jane

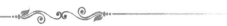

I had to run to the pharmacy late morning to pick up my script. The doctor is starting me on a cortisone dose pack for the heel spur. When I came back, Mom was in the kitchen with a slice of bread. I asked her if she was hungry. She said yes, so she got this piece of bread and put lots of this good butter on it. She did have it loaded with butter. I asked her where the strawberry jelly was? She said she couldn't find "the red stuff." I got it out of the fridge and Mom coated the buttered bread with the strawberry jelly. It wasn't toasted and she enjoyed every bite. I wonder why I cook so much when she is so easily pleased with simple buttered bread? Things to ponder.

Later in the afternoon she wanted to know what she could do to help me in the kitchen. I told her I had cooked the pork chops, so baking the potatoes wouldn't take long when we were ready to eat. I came in from outside and she had set the table with silverware. I told her she could put the plates on the table, while I got the dogs' food ready. I turned around just as she started to open the doors under the kitchen sink. When I asked her what she was looking for…she told me "you wanted me to get the plates. I said, "yes I did, but they aren't under the sink. They are right there on the open shelf above the countertop. She acknowledged that it was and reached up and brought down two plates. She wants to help, but when she does it requires prompting, clues, direction, and sometimes actually assisting. It's like when she wants to knot a quilt…I have to be right there while she makes every stitch. No matter how many times I explain that there doesn't need to be any stitches in the border—there is always at least one. She "gets stuck" and don't know what to do. She

197

waits for me to "fix" it. I keep waiting for some parts of her memory to "kick in." There is no problem-solving ability surfacing at all. She can question whether she did it wrong—but she doesn't know how to make it right. That's what makes it so scary to think of her being alone. Just when I start to think that we may be finding our way through—she looks for the dinner plates under the sink...or asks me if it's okay if she and her dogs can "stay here" tonight—or puts her bra on totally backward. I showed her the picture of my grand-son Gage's graduation with my daughter Heather and her husband Markie at his side tonight. She said she needed to send him a gradua-tion card and also to Heather. I asked why. I couldn't let well enough alone. She said "because she graduated too, didn't she? I explained that Gage was heather's son—and only he graduated this year. She corrected herself and said she didn't need to send her one "then."

Jane called her tonight, while I was getting a bath. When I came out, Mom was telling her about my doctor's appointment yesterday and how long I was there. I guess she had gone up to the desk and asked the girls if her "granddaughter" was okay? I think she was afraid that I had left her there...and it's a real worry for her that she doesn't know where she is or how to get home—or even where home is. I had asked her if she wanted to come back with me and she declined. She said she would wait out here in the waiting room. I put her on the sofa facing the TV...and asked her to please not take her money out and count it while she waited. She said she wouldn't—I guess I'll never know that part.

Back to Jane's phone call...after Mom hung up and said that was the one that calls all the time. I asked her who that was. She didn't know. She told me she couldn't put a face with her. I told her that Jane was her second daughter, and I would get a picture of her on my phone, which I did. She looked at her picture and said, "that looks just like Jane." I said, "It is Jane, Mom. That's who you were talking to on the phone."

She said, "No, that one looks just like my Jane, I was talking to the other one."

It's impossible for me to even climb into her mind for one min-ute. I don't have a good memory, but it's hard to imagine lacking one

198

altogether. I see her look at the clock often—she actually studies it. When I ask her what time it is…she doesn't know. There is a large light up digital clock under the TV, and another one in her bedroom. She still doesn't know. If she wakes up too early, and I see her sitting at her bedside. I go in and join her. I tell her if it's early, and whether we have anything going on in the morning hours. She will say, "It's early?" I will tell her what time it is…and she will often say "then I'm going to lay back down for a while." I ask her if I need to move her clock so she can see it more easily. She declines…telling me she can see it fine. I hear what she doesn't say—and I let it go. I will tell her if it's "close to noon" or "we will feed the dogs at five like we do every night" or "it's time to get into our pj's, cause no one will come to visit at this time." I drive best by landmarks, so why can't we go through days with "time marks." I remember giving in-services on Alzheimer's…and how moving a patient from their environment can affect many things. The school bus stopping at the bus stop kept their afternoon time accurate. The Mailman always came at "close to lunchtime" or the fact that the school buses didn't come meant it was the weekend…or the mailman not coming, meant it must be Sunday. "Time marks" in the day—I can do that. After all, time and dates are just numbers—we want to be more social than numerical—that's the side of the brain that we use in this chapter of our life anyway…keeping things simple and easy. Why not?

What could tomorrow bring? Some neurons fire and hit…and memory connects. Other little guys just miss fire off into the sunset.

It's Saturday; it's D-Day.

History speaks loudly; the invasion of Normandy has been referred to as the beginning of the end. Despite the heavy losses of life, it has been referenced as the turning point of World War II.

The beginning of the end—not so is life in our corner. Physical health seems good. At times, I could be encouraged to think that mental health is also. We had 3 guests for supper tonight. Mom had set the table and tried to help as much as she could. After the meal, she helped clear the table of dirty dishes and leftovers. As I walked into the kitchen, she stated that I would be putting them in the dishwasher. She was obviously having a problem remembering where it was. I motioned to the cabinets…and then held up both of my hands. I said, "These are my dishwasher." Mom seemed surprised and continued to look over the cabinets.

She then asked, "You don't have a dishwasher?"

I confirmed that, again referencing to both of my hands. We have been washing our dishes by hand for about five months now. This is the first time she has mentioned a dishwasher. She has been clearing the table after meals—another small step for some—and a giant step for this lady. Any attempt at former activities of daily living makes us a winner. There can be no downside with it. A napkin can be pushed into the top of a drinking glass—that now houses some vegetables. The little dinner rolls are wrapped in a paper napkin. The dirty dishes are stacked on a pile, and all the leftover food is scrapped onto a paper plate. Some of the things she knows what to do with… others she has no idea. She really tries—and wants to help. She feels useless but is so aware that she really doesn't know "how" to help. When I give her a task to do—there is always a pause, where you can see her trying to comprehend how to start.

Here's an example. As I type, she is leaving the dogs outside. She is trying to figure out how to turn the porch light on. The light switch is right in front of her. She has opened and shut the door about eight times, in a row. She has pushed it shut, and then locked it. She is trying to shut off the light, but the motion light has her so confused. While watching it, she has turned the light switch off and on several times. She has shut the door and counted the dogs. One dog is still outside, so we go through the whole door and light switch steps all over again. Finally, Annie comes in, and Mom steps into the doorway to look outside. Just then one dog runs outside and barks, followed by three more. I just watch—for now we have one mother and four dogs outside. Now of course, the motion light is again activated. So of course, Mom resumes shutting the light switch off and on again. You just can't make this stuff up. After what seems an eternity of repeat moves and actions, the door is shut and there are five dogs and one mother on this side of the locked door. Now she has decided to close the blinds. That goes relatively well. She has now remembered how to close the blinds inside the door. I complement her on this…and she just says, "Well, I watch people doing this, so I should be able to do it." Oh my mother, Let us remember those profound words of wisdom—let us make them our gold standard. "Watch people do things…and remember."

She has finally walked away from the door and windows and seated herself in front of the Pirate baseball game. She has started yawning, and I asked her when the Braves got three points? She asked me, "Who got the points?" I repeat that the Braves have three runs. She tells me she doesn't know, because she was busy with the dogs. I tell her that the other team is winning, and the score is 2 to 3. I'm waiting for it, because I know it is coming. It only takes a few seconds…and the question comes out. She asks, "So are we ahead?" She did see her favorite player hit a home run a short time ago. It's interesting…how she can watch the action, realize what is happening, watch them hit the ball and watch them run—and yet not follow the progression of the game. She gets very restless with the nine inning games. She feels that they "drag" them out more than they ever used to. As I sit and watch Mom, Ricky walks across the keyboard and types a few letters. I just sit in amazement as Mom laughs. I told her he typed a few letters, and just continued on his way.

She looks at Ricky, laughs, and says, "He had something to say." Now that statement alone is compound. Neurons are firing—and some are finding their target.

I got some groceries at Walmart this morning and did $100 cash back for Mom. She was so thankful when I handed it to her and told her to put it with her other money. She kept asking me where it came from. I explain as best I can. She did spend a fair amount of time in her room, before she came back out. I asked her if there was a problem…and she said, "No." I'm guessing her money is in a new place now. I'm also guessing that it is in more than one place. I'm only guessing. Her little collection of "knickknack" people are sitting on her dresser. I'm not able to figure out these actions yet.

Last evening, I had her trying on different capris and shirts. I told her we were getting her clothes sorted and making sure they fit well. She was so grateful. She fused over the clothing and how pretty the colors were. She never once got impatient with the fashion show.

201

She again tells me she hates picking out her clothes, because she's not good at matching them.

We watched the ballgame, almost side by side. She made it through the whole game, but when I said, "Well, we lost, and in the bottom of the ninth.

She said, "We did?"

I felt her looking at me and finally she asked me if I ever talk to my sisters? I told her I talk to them all the time and they also call and talk to her. She said she doesn't have a car and she doesn't drive, and nobody knows where she is. She said that they would be worried. She told me she hadn't meant to stay here this long, and she should have gone home before this. She was confused, feeling that she spends time staying by herself with someone staying at night. I assured her that everyone, even the entire church congregation, knows exactly where she is at. They all know she is here with me in Florida. She just kept thanking me, repeatedly. I sat for a bit at her bedside and told her that I always know exactly where she is, and I am always with her. She told me she had stayed overnight a few times, because she doesn't like to see anyone be by themselves at night. I explained that she is in her bed and I am in my bed, but we are together all night long. I used the dogs to bridge the gap, telling her they run back and forth between our beds all night long. I then told her that her dogs even know exactly where she is. The comfort of the dogs knowing where she is seemed to be the "cup of tea" for tonight. They were visible. They were already lying on her bed. None of this conversation had surfaced while she was getting in her pj's and nonslippy socks a few hours earlier. We had the Pirate game on, she ate her ice cream sandwich, and then—out of the blue—she's lost again at bedtime. What a helpless, scary state of mind that must be.

She knows that her mind is an issue. Today she referenced the fact that "you know how my mind doesn't remember"—or "you know how my mind is" several times. The neighbor, Millie, was over and ate supper with us and Brian. She commented on Mom's mobility after breaking a hip. I told her that Mom didn't remember anything about breaking her hip or being in the hospital, so she just continued as she had before. She just kept walking and moving like she had done previously. Millie commented on the fact that she doesn't use a walker or even a cane. I just told Millie that Mom remembered how she walked pre surgery for her hip, so that's exactly how she got up and moved afterward. Millie commented on Mom clearing the table and her desire to put the dishes in the dishwasher. I told her that Mom and I make a good team—we have good teamwork. Mom agreed but then I had to help Mom understand that I don't have a dishwasher. She always seems so surprised when she learns something new like that. Every day is like Christmas morning as a child—you may not know what the day holds in store for you, but you know that it is going to be interesting and different from all the other days. I just try to be consistent and make sure she feels secure and safe. I'm still feeling bad because of her wait in the waiting room at my doctor's appointment. I shouldn't have left her in the outer office, because I know what usually happens. She is not patient as far as waiting goes.

It's Sunday, and Bri doesn't have to go to work.

Brian came over early for coffee. The dogs barking had Mom awake. She did lie back down and didn't get up till close to 9:00 AM.

I tried to get some thoughts from Mom this afternoon. I was discussing our plans of living between our homes. I'm trying to find out what her anticipations are when we go north. As far as staying by herself—she just says, "We'll see how it goes." I was explaining to her that we got an electric stove for her home, and that we needed to put up the dog fence yet. We talked about how everything will be like we left it. I try to get her to tell me what she remembers. I already know that she doesn't really know. She doesn't truly know that her home is still there.

I try hard to make sure she doesn't feel like she is putting me out. I tell her we need to "help each other"—while she gets stronger. I brought home two small samples of wood flooring and she loved it. She said she liked the floor tones we have now, and she didn't want to lose it. I should be able to get estimates this week on a few projects. I need to talk to family…as my personal life is totally suspended. Mom will not comment on going back and forth to Florida, like snowbirds. I'm determined for her to know that I am not keeping her anywhere against her will. I asked her if she would rather have someone else staying with her for a break from me. I asked her if she needed a break from my constant company. She denies all of these, but I haven't been addressed by a name as yet. Some days she looks at me with a type of "distance" in her eyes. It's then that I can only imagine how scary it must be …looking from the other side of her eyes and not having a feeling of some recognition.

She wants so much to be able to stay by herself with her dogs. I put 6 small bags of jerky treats in the dog treat jar about five days ago. I looked today, as she got a "handful" out…and it's darn near empty. She gets treats out by the handful. But she does it so very often. Even when reminded that she had just treated the dogs, she will tell me they are hungry. They may have just finished eating their dinners, or she may have already treated them numerous times this day. She doesn't remember. She also forgets which one gets picked on when she treats the dogs. Annie knows her well and makes her feel guilty when she eats. Mom would have very fat contented dogs if she were to be by herself. I'm quite sure that she would not be able to take care of herself that well. She starts treating the dogs during her breakfast and wants to do it into bedtime. I've tried to ask her to stop, as they get up and poop during the night. My requests are insignificant. They are gone from her thoughts as soon as they are gone from my mouth. She tells me she meant to save them some of her meat at lunch but forgot and ate it all. Should I tell her again not to give the dogs her food? Have a brought it up often enough to know that repetition is not working when it comes to her dogs?

I discuss the few things we need to finish at this house, if our plans are to go back and forth. We have purchased a van that I can stand in. I will be able to take care of mother as we travel, and the potty chair will be functional in it as well. I have named it the snowbird, since it will make trips between Pennsylvania and Florida much easier. I explain that the snowbird is to make the travel more fun and stressless. I told her that we would leave her car up north in her garage, and we could drive my car or the snowbird down here in Florida. I reminded her that I have a bedroom in her home up north and she has one in our home in the south. I've told her that we hadn't planned on staying away this long, but her hip is healing well and she has all the needed dental work completed. She no longer has a rancid breath odor, as she did when her mouth was full of bad teeth. I've assured her that we will reach the goal for her Christmas gifts for grandchildren. I had picked up a few more colored bras yesterday and two short sleeve shirts for Mom. I laid out the melon printed one and she had it on this morning. I complimented her on the color and how it gives her face color. I told her I just picked it up for her yesterday at Walmart, along with a few more bras and some groceries. I had also got the $100 cash back for her to keep in her wallet. She looked at her shirt and smiled, feeling the fabric. She said, "Look, I got something new and I didn't even know it." Her naivety is so honest, but it does get tangled up with the disorientation. She has no pain…none. This amazes me. Her right knee is stiff and takes some limbering up when she first gets up. I had bought glucosamine tablets the last vitamin replacement shopping day. I will pick up her osteo bio flex the next time up town. Now I am curious to see if it makes a difference. Her appreciation of meals is so cute. We heated up yesterdays" leftovers for lunch, and then made some spaghetti squash pasta for supper. She eats so well, and always raves on how things taste. We are so lucky. The ability to taste and enjoy flavor is lost for some elderly folks. Whether it be to the medicines they take, or the downsides of aging. I don't know. I do know that we don't have an issue with it in our world. Her personality is different, but it is gentle, quiet, and happy.

A smile is the lightening system of the face and the heating system of the heart.

She's thinking that someone could stay the nights when she is up north. I have informed her that any ideas will be heard, for our goal was to get her back in her own home from the start. Several concerns:

- She is at a loss as to what to do when alone. She wants to watch what others do.
- There is always the fear of the fall. And it's so true…when they fall, they cannot get back up.

- She is moving about more. Could she actually get into the car and start to drive?
- Would she venture away from the house, without realizing that she may not find her way back?
- She spills things, and the safety factor is so obvious when she is trying to clean up the spills.
- The gas stove will be gone—that measure has been addressed.
- The dogs getting in trouble outside…the fence will be off of one door—that is the plan. They also have many accidents inside. Sometimes it hits the pee pads, other times not even in the same room. I've cleaned poop from Mom's shoes, that she wasn't even aware of.
- The dogs require clipping and nail trimming and bathing…
- She has personal accidents. I know her pride is damaged when this happens. It is the reason we have bought a second pair of shoes that she likes wearing.
- Someone coming to the home—or someone calling on the phone. She read the caller ID on my cell phone yesterday. She knew it rang, and she could read the name that was calling. This may be the first time she has even picked up my phone when it rang.
- The dogs do not move. She does not ask them to move. I have tripped over them. She goes out of her way to step over them or walk around them.
- Her balance is quite an issue. She tries to carry things, giving her no access to using her hands quickly to save a wobble. She has started picking up the little dogs and carrying them around. She carried one the whole way back to her bedroom one evening.
- Very thin skin—with many skin tears from dog scratches.
- Very minimal fluid intake. It takes constant reminding and presentation and availability to get her to drink over a pint of liquid in a day. Even her voice is faint on some days. Iced coffee has been a success as far as increasing the liquids.

- She tends to go up and down steps with the wrong leading foot. When she does this, she shows a definite weakness with the weight bearing during the step. When she does it the proper way, she does not show any leg weakness.
- She shares me with no one during most days. She requires prompting and usually assistance with personal care—and oral care. Most days she cannot remove her denture plate-even though she tells me it "drops down" by itself.
- She moves things and "puts things" away—including cash. So far I've found everything except the receipt from the floor leveling guys. I brought it into the house, before running to the bank. I haven't seen it since.

I ran to Home Depot with Brian this morning. She was finishing her breakfast. When we got back, she was washing the dishes from the night before. She had cleaned most of them and dried some. I used my large electric grill for the meat last night. It was covered with cooking grease and meat particles from browning and grilling the steaks. She had stacked all the clean dishes, plates, and even utensils directly on the greasy gridle. No connection that there was something wrong with this.

She toileted herself tonight and came out to the living room and asked if it was okay to flush the commode. She tries to use the remote and often has the wrong buttons pushed. We have had almost perfect results with the landline and single corded phone on the stand with the lamp by the window.

I brought out the third digital clock into the living room today. She can read the large numbers and get an idea of the time of day. She is always wanting to get the dogs fed, "because they are hungry."

This story is not to be about me…but it is too closely entwined… to not. I must deal with some issues that I'm trying to alter with diet and set a goal of some weight loss. It's a bit complicated when Mom wants me to eat what she eats and when she eats. No matter how closely I keep her meals and mealtimes—plus, snacks, she tells me she is not really hungry and can wait to eat when I'm ready. I also have to take into consideration, that if I am out of her direct presence for any length of time, she has looked in the refrigerator to see what I am "planning" on having to eat, or what there is to eat, and has most often heavily buttered a piece of plain bread to eat because "I was hungry, and couldn't find anything else to eat." I can't seem to get this one right. The cookie jar is full, there is cheese and crackers in obvious sight, with any simple search. But it isn't obvious to her any longer. The peanut butter jar is present. I have left so many of these things openly sitting on the counter. She can miss the most obvious. I don't know how to fix this, for her previous behavior just doesn't seem to surface. She will eat foods prepared before her and rave at their taste. She hasn't lost a bit of "taste" or "smell," as does happen in a lot of elderly or recovering patients. Just today I had a beef roast in the slow cooker. It was not done or tender enough by supper time, so I left it cooking and chose pizza for supper.

Early this evening I went outside and told Mom I had to water the shrubbery, since no sign of rain was present. I see her come to the doorway often. She sat on the carport patio for a short period of time but went back in the house. She likes being by the door, she likes the door open, but she likes to be inside. Does she get confused when she is outside, does she fear she won't find her way back inside? She did once, when she walked to the other side of the shed and couldn't see the carport door from where she was standing. Does this still come to mind when she is not in her comfort zone? Just as she can be facing the TV and not know where she is to sleep that night. I've even considered placing the TV at a different direction so she can have her room in peripheral vision—but it's not going to be in her line of vision at her other home either. Is this why she was always getting up and going into my bedroom, when up north, because that doorway could be seen from the place she sits on the sofa? Would changing the placement of anything…really change anything? Just one day inside her beautiful mind would enlighten me so. Or would it just be somewhere that I couldn't find my way back from either? Ask me how I have so much patience or the ability to work with her so constantly? I just have to take a few seconds to see where she is "stuck." I just observe, for a few minutes, to see how she is struggling to just get from this minute to the next. My life is so very easy.

I have a lot of experience in struggling minds. I sometimes see the best thing to do is just listen. Don't question. Don't give advice. Keep my opinion to myself and listen to the situation as described by the involved party. No matter what I think, I do not know how another person is feeling. Regardless of how I would resolve an issue, it may not be possible for another to handle it the same way. Just listen, just be there, don't pass judgement, don't react, and after listening—just be there.

I sat and talked with her today again. I must watch the timing for any real conversation. She wants to go back to her place by the farm with all her family. She wants to stay longer than the few days that I tell her Brian will be there. I tell her we will. I tell her we will probably be there for months, till after all the holidays. It's too much information to process properly, for "waiting" in any waiting room, or "waiting" till I come back from a short errand, has no ending in sight for her. I mowed this day, and really tired myself out. I tell Mom I need to lay down and get off my sore foot for a while. I know I will fall asleep…needing a power nap right now. I sleep lightly. I hear her move from one place to another. I suggest she lay down and take a nap with me, and then we will both be rested for the Pirate game tonight. She says she will try that, and she goes back to her bedroom. It's midafternoon, and she finds the bedroom and bathroom without hesitation. I feel her watching me, and I sit up on the sofa. She is sitting by the window facing the sofa where I am resting. She doesn't know what to do, or where to go, except to be where she can see me. She doesn't try to wake me, or disturb me, and tries to keep the dogs quiet. She often encourages me to lay down and rest because I do so much. She understands that is what I am doing.

I have told her that the worker guys won't be doing the floors on the inside of the house while we are here. Even the contractor that spent time here, realized her restlessness in his presence. She becomes quiet and tries to withdraw. She tries to keep the dogs out of his presence, because "they won't quit barking" and "they are trying to talk."

How did Mom remember to tell Jane about the waiting time at my doctor's appointment this week, and how long I was "back there"—and yet not know where to take the next stitch in a quilt? I lifetime of repeat actions does not come back in memory, but a short term one from the previous day does. Shuffle that box of chocolates and remove the cheat sheet of where all the creams are located and let me guess which one I will take a bite out of this day. You can bet it's the hard toffee one, the one that locks up my teeth for a while and requires me to hold it in my mouth for a long period of time to melt some of the hardness. It would be easier to spit this one out and start over with another choice. But what if the next one I pick, or gets picked for me, is even harder to chew? At least I know what I've got this time. That's more than my mother knows. I've kinda learned that dealing with what you have is sometimes easier than dealing with the alternative choice.

I assure her we are going up north and staying awhile. I asked her how long she wants to stay. She tells me she wants to go up there and see "how it goes." She says she hopes to stay there for the rest of her life. She says that she doesn't think it will be that long. I let her talk, without interference at this time. I don't lie to her. I don't know what these results will be. I just watch her face. She is watching the Pirates play. She has Annie on her lap, and she's softly petting her, often talking to her. She tells me all her family, and her sisters, and the farm is up there. I ask her what she wants to do up there—when we get there. She doesn't know. She is watching the TV but talking to me. I ask her what inning it is—she doesn't know.

Later this evening, she wanted "to finish this one." She was "stuck" at the end of the quilt. I got her back on track with her knotting. She doesn't want to try a game of solitaire. She doesn't want to try out our new crayons. She doesn't want to watch anything on TV, except "whatever" I want to watch. I so very much wish I could find one thing that she could do when she doesn't have anything else to do. She used to do "find-a-word" or pick up the deck of cards and play solitaire—now she just tells me "I don't want to do anything." She watches me. I try not to do anything that can't directly involve her, but it's difficult. She loves to paint, but she refuses to do any. She loves to mow, so I told her I was going to go buy a little riding mower, because I could sure use her help with mowing. She said she already had one, but her legs won't hold up to doing it now. It's an uphill climb with her…and yet we can be outside with doors open. What will it be like doing this climb in a small mobile home living room? Will the family visitors and company be a form of entertainment and activity for her, or will it frustrate her? We shall see.

I must remove her denture when I suggest she brushes her teeth. She is not good about bathing or personal care, but she does like to "wash her face" after breakfast in the mornings. If she has an accident, she will change her underwear. Otherwise, I must "suggest" a change. I take her socks off and put them in laundry each night, laying out a clean pair with her shoes. I check her clothes, and if she hasn't spilled something on them, I lay them out two days in a row. She puts on what is laying on the chair, when she gets up in the morning. She doesn't want her bra off, because she cannot put it on herself in the mornings. I take it off, lotion her back and her arms, and help her put on a fresh bra every other day. I tell her the elastic in the bras get weak, and we need to change them. She is agreeable. I soak her feet and rub to get the dry skin off, check her nails for problems and lotion the dry skin on her feet and legs. I mix up a glass of Kool-Aid and have it follow her around during the day to increase her liquids. We buy iced coffee when out, knowing she will drink it before the day is over. If I didn't push her, she would sip at a pint of coffee throughout the day, and nothing more. She doesn't even pour a cup of coffee anymore; she only puts about one-third cup in her mug at a time. I give her water to take her pills. Sometimes I just wait…to see if she initiates one of these activities herself…to see if she could be by herself. It doesn't seem to happen. If I asked her if she brushed her teeth, it always happened "yesterday." Her "Yesterdays" have been very busy—her "todays" just don't seem to have much going on. How much value does the time between getting out of bed in the morning, and climbing back into it at night—just how much value does that time have to her? It's been quite a few months here in Florida. In the times since we brought her down, she hasn't seen any winter or snow. She has broken her hip and recovered dramatically well. Mostly because, she didn't really remember that the fracture had occurred. She sat in a dental chair with a healing right hip replacement, having her upper teeth removed and a new denture placed in her mouth. The foul strong rancid breath odor has gone. The bacterial issue she had in her mouth with her decayed teeth has resolved. She has recovered from her oral surgery and is very proud of her smile. How much does she really know? Does she recall all that she has been through? Sometimes she does, other times some things are better left in the dark. She doesn't see her progress, even when pointed out directly. She just gets through every day…from morning till night—and then we do it again.

Tonight, Brian walked over for a short visit. We got Mom to walk out and sit on the patio. She told me that the car lights came on and went off several times. I was watering the plants. She thought someone was coming or leaving. She said, she waited but no one got in or out of the car. She asked me why the lights did that? I don't know how deep to go with this right now. I said, "I guess the car was just saying, "Hello, Mom." I don't have anything else to offer. I got nothing.

It's 3:24 AM. I've had the TV on, the Roosevelt story. I fell asleep earlier. I type Mom's story, during the night. I don't want to let go of this time…for something like "sleep." She got a card from a friend today. The writing was too small, so I read it to her. She struggles with reading most times. She just tells me she never liked to read. It's a little late in her life to wonder "why" now—but I still do. Why hasn't she ever liked to read? Why does she hate picking out her clothes to wear each day? Why is she so happy when I lay out a matched outfit of clean clothes for her each morning? I bought a very light weight gray ¾ length sleeve cardigan for her at Walmart yesterday. I helped her put it on, and she loved it. I told her it matched her tennis shoes and goes with her clothes better than the flannel shirt or pj top that she uses as a sweater. It's just enough to cover the tops of her arms and another layer on her back, like she likes. She left it on again all day. When Brian commented on how her clothes matched tonight, she just looked them all over, and smiled.

She talked to Jody today, and Ken got on the phone and talked to her for a while. She called him Dave, several times, and apologized. She is talking into a phone. She does not see a man in front of her, so it's easy to lose a name. But searching for names is tough for her...and when she can't come up with a name...it frustrates her. I try to help her with this, and she appreciates it. She often doesn't remember Brian's name. I don't ever get called by name. She will get my attention, which she always has. What is ahead for the next month in our lives has yet to be displayed.

Patience is not the ability to wait but the ability to keep a good attitude while waiting.

A MONDAY EVE IN MID-JUNE

Less than a month, and we should be heading North. I haven't made airplane reservations for the driver to return south. I have been talking and listening to our mother on her expectations. I'm trying to hear her thoughts, but not letting her build impossible goals when she does get "home." She has told me she would like to live in her own home for the rest of her life, but she also knows that isn't possible yet. She tells me there are a lot of kids around there, not little kids, but big kids, that would be there. She tells me her other girls are there. I have reminded her that two of her "other girls" work, and the third one is raising her two granddaughters plus dealing with Leukemia. She acknowledges this information. She feels that she was able to live by herself before and she thinks she can now. She tells me that "I guess we will see when we get there."

It is then that she tells me how she "has a dilemma tonight." She tells me that she has run out of time here and she needs to find a place to go. She is confusing me when she talks about how the other person used to come and stay at night, and how the "girls alternate." It's so real to her that I'm beginning to believe her. It's like a comment made about my cousin many years ago—"You know damn well that he's lying, but you believe him, anyway." I know damn well that there is no alternating of girls here…but she is so convinced that I am starting to believe her.

Earlier in the day she came to the doorway, held up the remote to the TV and said, "Whoever you are, can you fix this for me." She had been watching the Pirate game, but lost interest. She said all they were doing was throwing the ball at each other. It seems the games are too long for her attention span. She feels the games are over much before they are, and she can't be convinced otherwise. Sometimes her explanations of the games are breathtaking. For a lady who has watched professional baseball games for so many years—the game and it's rules are not familiar. I don't see why I will need to pay for the extra innings sports channel in the future. She seems to enjoy the half hour sitcoms and laughs out loud. I could buy a pirate baseball cd and just play it at will. After all, the day she watched the recorded game, right after the actual game—she was so happy that they won "both" games.

Tonight she wouldn't lie down on the bed until she got at least one more dog in there with her. Her two dogs had been on her bed, but for some reason she has wanted more. She can't seem to recall that she only has had two dogs that have slept with her. Last night she came out to the living room, had closed her bedroom door, and she was hunting the "other two babies" to take them to bed. She knew her two dogs were back in her bed already, so she shut them in until she found the "other two." She was "worried" that they wouldn't have a place to sleep and didn't know where they lay down at. I don't know if the little white dog is considered Annie's baby and the little black dog is Mickie's? But now there are babies in our small circle of life. Considering both my mother's age and my own, who would have ever guessed?

She wanted to feed the dogs yesterday and was working at doing so when I ran a few errands for Brian. He stayed here with her and was trying to get her to "wait" until I got home. When I returned, I stayed outside to help Brian work on my well water pump for a short period of time. I came in to check on her, and it appeared that there were dogs everywhere. She had picked Rusty up and was trying to handle his squirming, confused body and get him to stay up on the kitchen island. Even the other dogs were watching in amazement. She was talking to him, telling him to stay up there and eat. Of course, he wasn't cooperating.

I said, "Mom, you have the wrong dog."

She looked at his little face, and then looked at me.

I said, "You have Rusty…and it's Ricky that we have to put up there when we feed them." She appeared exhausted. She put Rusty on the floor, and I "suggested" we switch dogs, and put Ricky up there.

Some things I can let slide. Avoiding another canine encounter is one I will try to avoid. Bless her heart. She was in the right church, just in the wrong pew.

A Thursday in June

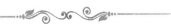

Another very hot day in Florida. I've had to water plants and shrubs frequently. The thermometer hits about ninety-five for the third day in a row. My dear little plants are wilted in despair. I do some of the watering in the morning before Mom gets out of bed. I've been moving a lot of stuff to the shed before we make out trip up north. If we get someone to put down the flooring, they will have less headache to moving all my "stuff." I finally got all the rat poop and pee cleaned from the shed. I kept telling Mom that I was going out to the "shitty shed" and clean. She would walk out several times if she couldn't see me from the doorway of the house.

I browned some pork chops and then had them simmering on the stove. I turned the heat down to a simmer and went out to do some watering. I didn't realize some of my plants were so wilted, but the heat has been intense. I saw Mom come to the back-door window several times and I waved. After I did the watering, I came into the strong smell of browning meat. It seems that our mother "turned down the heat" under the skillet when she saw it was cooking. I hurried to the stove and noted the heat had been turned up quite a bit, and the meat was browning well in very little shortening. I asked Mom if she had added any water. She told me "no," but I did turn the heat down." This is an untruth. I explained to Mom that she had turned the heat up—not down. She showed me how she had turned it toward the "off" word. That she did, but she had turned the dial in the wrong direction to shut it off. I add water and attempt to do damage control. Mom feels bad, she thought she was helping but then discovered that she really hadn't. I just refocus—and get her to start fixing the dog food. Again, I teach her the amounts to put in each dish. Again, I have her add the warmed rice and hamburger. She wants to help, and asks me how many are here? I haven't had any enlightenment as to where she always sees this third person. Maybe this is something I will never figure out. I simply answer that there are just her and I. It's then that she acknowledges that they "must have went home." That's good news to me, since I'm beginning to doubt my most recent eye exam.

She wants to finish the quilt on the island. It does not go easy. She is not moving her neon pink pattern forward. She has decreased some stitches to single thread. Why does the simple movement of the pattern and the placement of the next stitch not click into place? As it happens some days, I have to flip the pattern over every time, and still point to the placement of her next stitch. I have to thread her needles and cut and tie all the knots. She gets to the end of a row and stops and waits for me to give her direction. I try to push her a little, asking her where she is to go now. She has no idea. I direct her to the other end of the quilt and remind her that she works from right to left. She does not know where to place her pattern. I need to move her neon pink plastic pattern every time. I have to point her to her next stitch. She has doubled several stitches in the same area, if I don't keep moving her forward.

She answered the phone this afternoon and I heard her saying, "Oh hello, Julie." Then I heard her say that she was very happy with what she had. I walked to the phone and saw the name "consumer relief" and reached to take the phone. She said, "It's Julie."

When I took the phone from Mom, the caller was making arrangements to consolidate Mom's credit card balances. On another day, I may have just left them work with Mom on this subject since Mom has no credit cards—but today, not.

Again, I inform the caller to remove this number from their call list.

I'm not sure but I think I've confused Mom by talking about getting ready to go up north. She told me she has been worried about getting a place for her dogs to stay. She was fretting about this last night at bedtime also. What tipped me off was when she asked me, "When are you all planning on going up north?"

I explained that her dogs and her were also going up north. I told her we were going up to her house. I told her that my dogs and I would be following her wherever she was going. It took me awhile to get her to understand that we were taking her and her dogs up north to her house, and that we weren't leaving her here. She asked me if we were taking her car with us, and I said yes. The plan is to tow it, and all ride in the snowbird. She seemed so relieved. I've tried to get her to worry less, because everything is working out fine. I do realize that the connections—and misconnections, going on in her healing mind do not always find the best route to take. I do have to say though, that they usually find interesting alternate trails to ride down. Thank you, God, that you have found many ways to keep a smile on our faces, and an even bigger smile in our hearts.

Don't let your worries get the best of you, dear Mother. Remember, even Moses started out as a "basket case."

Like yesterday, while she was washing dishes, I looked over and asked her if she had put any soap in the water. She said that she had used the Dawn when she drew the water earlier. It was then that I realized she was washing the dishes in leftover dishwater, and it was cold. Why didn't she realize that the dishwater was cold and had no suds?

Brian stills laughs when he watched how she had the table set yesterday. She had set a small container of cold lima beans on the table, and the jar of spaghetti sauce. No rhyme, no reason. No right, no wrong. Is it a normal way to set the table? Maybe not, but who's to say what "normal" is to one person may be a planned action to another. I just record things as I see them. I couldn't make some of these things up myself—my imagination just isn't capable.

She offered to go get the mail yesterday. I haven't let her go alone since she broke her hip. She had walked right past our mailbox, crossed the road, and opened the neighbor's mailbox on that particular day. Today I left her go on her own. I watched from the window. I also watched that neighbor Millie was at her front door. She kept looking over at my house, I'm sure to see if I knew Mom was out of the yard. I watched as Mom made it to the mailbox and removed the mail. Millie, who is 92, found a reason to walk out onto her carport.

I know she was ready to step up to the plate, had Mom turned and walked the wrong way. Our mother then started looking through all the envelopes and papers. She then turned away and looked across the street and then looked both up and down the street. She was taking longer than I was comfortable. It's so tough to let a loved one take those independent steps, not knowing whether they will get hurt in the process or succeed. I started to wonder if she "lost" the direction to our house. I walked out through the gate to her car, and shut the trunk. She asked me what I was doing out here and I told her I was locking up her car.

She tells family that it has rained here today. She attempts to carry on conversations about her Pirate baseball team, not really knowing how they are doing. She hasn't watched a complete game in so long. When she does watch, she doesn't know the score, the innings, or even what the players are doing. She doesn't understand why they just start "throwing the ball at each other," or why they "talk so much when the game is not over." She feels they make up the rules as they go and change them whenever they want.

Let me see if I can document the events of just one day for my sisters to enjoy. I'm going to keep it to twenty-four hours. I shall title it : Just 24. Not 24-7, just 24.

JUST 24

After finally getting Mom to stay in bed with three dogs, she slept till about seven thirty this morning. Everybody was out walking their dogs this morning, so the dogs that live here had to welcome them all to the neighborhood by barking from the time they were in sight, until they disappeared down the block. About 8:00 AM I see on the child monitor that Mom is making her bed. She is dressed and is fussing with things on her dresser. Her clothes were on the chair, so I'm sure she has not removed her undershirt before putting on today's" jersey. I just know this is a given. Mom came out to the table and appeared fully dressed, including her undershirt that she sleeps in at night. I saw this one coming. For some reason, she never removes it. She always has on one of her stretchy bras, so it's not that she doesn't have a form of underwear on. As she sat at the table, she asked me if her pants were right. She said something doesn't feel right. She stood up and she had her capri pants on backward. The drawstring ties were dangling down over her butt. We decide we will change them—after breakfast—and put them on the right way.

She said there was a sore place in her mouth. I asked her how long this has been an issue. She told me it's been hurting for several days now…but I don't know what "several days" is to our newest version of our mother. I told her she has to tell me these things so I can fix or correct them.

After breakfast, she went to her bedroom and turned her pants around. I then told her I'd meet her in the bathroom, and she can brush her teeth. Per usual, she worked at it for a while, but couldn't get her denture out of her mouth. Again, I showed her how to tip it down from the back and it will remove easily. I put it in the denture cup to soak. She was, again, instructed how to brush her teeth and clean the areas close to her gums. As she brushed her teeth, I went into her bedroom and got the potty chair to empty. I returned the bucket to the chair and went back into the bathroom. She was holding her denture in her hand. I asked her why she didn't let it soak for a few minutes, but she said she thought it had soaked long enough. I put a little Fixodent powder on her denture and put it back into her mouth. I then got the little hand mirror and showed her how she hadn't got the food removed close to her gums. She told me she would brush them again...

After her denture was in place, she said it didn't hurt. I will keep an eye on this area, although she has an appointment in a few weeks at the dental clinic. I question Mom on her bowels, and the fact that they haven't moved for several days. She is receiving fiber twice daily to aid her movements, a bowel softener every evening, and I try to push liquids. I need to pay constant attention to her bowel activity, as she doesn't say anything until she is constipated and uncomfortable.

She wants to work on her quilt, so I put everything else aside and help her to knot. I thread her needles and instruct her with every movement of her pattern block. Some areas she takes two stitches, sometimes she is down to a single tying thread, and other times she advances the pattern down the row. When she gets to the edge of the quilt, she never seems to know where to go or what to do next. I tie all her stitches, and then clip the knots. I direct her to the edge of the quilt and place her pattern, then show her where her next stitch is to be made. We do this repetitious activity until Mom says she needs to take a break. I try to tell her to take her time knotting, because I don't have the next quilt ready to go yet. In all innocence, she asks me "why not—there is enough people working on it!" Once again mother dearest—I got nothing.

I get her a small pudding to eat as a snack. It is tapioca, which she loves. I also put half of a dove chocolate bar on the table for her to eat. She presses a few strips of material for me, and then asks if she should unplug the iron. I tell her to unplug it, and then we will get ready to leave. I watch as she works to pull a plug from the extension cord. She sits down at the kitchen table and I walk over to the ironing board and unplug the iron.

She said, "Did I unplug the wrong thing?"

I just answered "sorta," but it's unplugged now. I didn't want to say anything, as she thinks she messes up a lot anyway, but I also didn't want to forget to unplug the iron before we leave.

I suggest we go up town for shoppin' walkin', as we haven't been out all week. I suggest we eat lunch out, pick up a few groceries, go to Joann Fabrics, and be home in time to watch her pirates play ball. I want to pick her up a few pairs of nonskid socks that she can wear at night. The hospital freebies that we are using don't fit too well. Out of the blue, Mom states, "You don't have a big stick here anywhere. Why don't you have one? I always had one in case someone tried to break in. I had a baseball bat beside my bedroom door."

I look at her slowly and then ask her if she wants to buy a baseball bat during our shopping trip today. She says she does. I assure her we could certainly do that.

Before we get involved in something at home, I asked her if she is ready to go. She is back in her bedroom, going through her purse. When I walk back, she is going through her medical cards. She has laid the bank envelope on her dresser and is confused as to where her money is. I pick up the envelope and show her that she has all her money right where she put it. She is relieved.

We are getting ready to walk out the door when she turns and says, "You mean there isn't going to be anybody here when we leave?"

Again, I explain that there is just the two of us living here, and the five dogs will be fine together.

She needs help at times, lifting her right leg into the car. I also pull the seat belt out so she can lock it in place.

She does well pushing the cart through the stores. She does not do well at all, knowing what money to give to buy or pay for something. She picked two more little knickknacks at Goodwill. I'm not quite sure where or why her thoughts are on these. She sets them on her dresser when I unwrap them at home and hand them to her. We also purchased two baseball bats, one wooden and one aluminum. She seemed so relieved that we had found these "big sticks" to buy and take home.

We ate out today, not having done that for a while. I order for her. She cannot seem to make decisions, even the color of thread to use on a quilt. She has no suggestions with any purchases of food, just as she doesn't question anything I put in the shopping cart. I end up pulling the weight of the cart in the stores, so she doesn't have to push. She uses the carts for balance but doesn't really have the amount of strength it takes to push a full cart. I never get a comment of anything in the grocery store. I picked out 4 pair of socks with treads on them for her nighttime wear. She has been wearing the hospital ones and they don't fit well. She didn't question the purchase of the socks. When we went to JoAnn's and bought some quilt batting, she did pick up a few bags and look at them, when we were trying to decide which ones to get. I did give her three different get-well cards to read in the store, and she picked the one she wanted to send to her nephew, Marlin. She was so pleased with her choice of the card and laughed when she read it. She said it was "so cute."

She was standing by the wheel with all the bags at the Walmart checkout. The cashier bagged the products as she scanned them. Mom looked at her for a while and then asked if she "had checked them yet." I informed her that if they were in the bags, they were checked, and she could put the bags in our buggy. She reached right past the filled bag, took off a whole section of empty bags and put them in our buggy. She did not even realize that she had done something wrong. I took the stack of bags and returned them to the cashier's wheel. Our mother then tried to remove some of the filled bags but couldn't master getting the filled bag off the handles holding it on the wheel. She does well on the push side of the grocery cart, not so well on the bagging end.

When we got home, she placed the baseball bats behind the carport door. Now it opened to the inside, as it should. The door was left open, which meant both bats were safely placed behind the door. As I tried to think this situation through, my results left me with many questions. I wasn't sure that intruders would excuse themselves from our home and step outside until my mother could get behind the door and retrieve a bat. I was also not sure how long an intruder would wait for her to get a good grasp on the bat and draw it backward so she could get a good swing at the intruder. I also saw her losing her balance and falling from the thrust of the swing. Meanwhile, was I to be wrestling with the intruder while she got all her defense moves in place? Regardless of how it seemed ill-fated from the start, she was so pleased to have these "big sticks" now in our home. I saw this as a good resolution to a concern she had. I could only hope we never have to test the theory.

Tonight, we were watching the baseball game. She didn't nap and we were busy all day. She walked over to me and said she hadn't planned on being here tonight. She was all mixed up again with where she was to be, with the thought that no one knew where she was, that she didn't have a car, and that she couldn't drive, that her babies and kids need a place to stay also. She feels that someone used to come and take turns staying here, and that some days she stayed with them. I asked her to sit down beside me and let me do the worrying. I informed her that this is her home also. I slowly told her that we have two homes, and she has her own bedroom in both homes. I told her that the dogs are very content, and just want to be with us. Otherwise, they don't care where they are, just that we want them, and they have a full belly. I asked her if the dogs were unhappy. She adamantly said "no." I then asked if she was unhappy, and she quickly told me "no."

I explained how she is using her brain to question her surroundings, which her brain is trying to sort things out and find a place for stuff she is remembering, that her brain got squished when she had to have surgery and it's trying hard to heal. I reminded her of the writing she practices, the knotting of the quilts where she has to figure out what step is next, the walking and shopping, the dishes she washes, the search a word, the solitaire card game, and the shows and games we watch and talk about on TV. She said she knows she gets mixed up and doesn't know what to do. I reassured her that she is never away from me—that I and her dogs are always together, that I will do the worrying—so she doesn't need to. I asked her if she trusted me and she said she does. I just told her that it's all planned out, and her and her dogs will be fine. I helped her get into her pajamas and put lotion on her legs and arms. She wasn't ready to leave the

TV room yet. When she had sat for a while, I offered to take her and her dogs back to bed and tuck her in. She wants the door left open so the dogs can find their way into her bedroom. Rusty already has five toys in her bed, along with himself.

Sometimes, when she gets "lost," and after reassuring her, I just sit with her. I can tell by looking at her face, that she's not even sure who I am or how long I will be staying. I mentioned to her that we would reach the deadline of quilts by Christmas.

She simply said, "We should make the deadline, with all the people that are working on them."

Sometimes there are no words to be said. Sometimes I'm not sure if she sees all these people, or just sees me in different places, and takes it to the bank.

She has been tucked into bed, along with three dogs and five dog toys—at last count. She had Honey Crisp for breakfast, as Frosted Flakes was one of our purchases at Walmart today. She had a snack of tapioca before our trip uptown. We had string potato fries and a cheeseburger steak melt for early afternoon meal, along with a chocolate covered strawberry milkshake. She pushed a buggy through Goodwill, Walmart, and Joann Fabrics. We walked into Steak 'n' Shake and ate. She waited in the locked, running, air-conditioned car while I ran into one store to check on a price. During that time, she finished her milkshake.

We returned home and watched the 4:00 PM ball game. She didn't want anything else to eat today but did eat half Klondike as bedtime snack. I put lotion over her extremities when we put on her pajamas and not-slippy socks. With her denture held in place with Fixodent, the sore area in her mouth has apparently resolved. She is not aware of any sore place. She's had breakfast, lunch/supper combined and two snacks during this day. She's had one small glass of Kool-Aid water with fiber, medications have been given twice, Not once does she get anything to eat or drink on her own—but she asked me if I wanted her to fix the dogs' food. I helped her get the dogs food mixed and sat down for them.

I began laying out another quilt top and sewing the pieces together. Mom came over by the fake tree with lights, holding a handful of "something." She attempts to put it in the base of the tree, when I ask what she is doing. She is trying to find a place "to put this." I asked what "this" is. She doesn't know but tells me it was on her chair by the table. I show her the trash can, sitting in the same place as always, and tell her to put it in there—which she does. I look at the stuff left on her hand and realize that it is chocolate, mixed with dog food. I look at the chair and find more over the upholstered seat cushion. I remind Mom to wash her hands, and I cleaned up the cushion. I asked her if she fed the dog her chocolate. She says she did not, but neither did she eat all that was on the table. I explain to Mom that it is my guess that Annie consumed it, as she is always hunting something to eat. I also explain that it is good that the dog threw it up, as chocolate is harmful for dogs. She seems surprised to hear this. Annie's begging eyes are the reason Mom won't eat in front of her while watching TV.

Today was a little different than our typical day, as I didn't have to prepare two meals. Our most recent mother became confused tonight again-that seems to be the norm when she doesn't nap. I couldn't begin to count the number of times she opens and closes the carport door, letting dogs out or in. Often it is so she can count them. She anticipates the dogs needing to go outside to pee. She does talk to the dogs more than to any of the other people living here in this home. When I think about it, she doesn't initiate most of the short conversations that we have. I need to follow up on her bowel movements, so she doesn't get constipated again. She receives osteo bio flex for her knees, a good multiple vitamin, cranberry capsules for her urine, a bowel softener, along with a glass of Kool aid with Metamucil added. She has not lost any of her sense of smell or taste. She is always complimentary on the food.

On an abstract note, I had to tell Bri that the bathtub has leaked since the floors were leveled. I don't know what that involves, but since the water just runs across the floor and then through the floor boards to the ground—I choose to continue to enjoy my bath. I seem to be in a preparation mode at all times these days—preparing for a trip away from home for months—preparing for a possible trip to the emergency room on a "thumps" notice...prepared for my entire house to be refloored, thus in total disarray—semi-prepared for the surprises that lurk behind door number 2—and always ready for the embellishments from my choice from the box of chocolates. Bri's wording anymore is, "It's okay, Mom, we'll fix it." He, also, has learned recently that some things can be fixed, while others—not so easily. I can't begin to tell you how many times I have approached Bri about a nonworking "something" to hear the beautiful words, "Mom, aren't my days hard enough?" Apparently, I hadn't thought they were.

Mom doesn't want to color or do search a word. I pull out a crossword puzzle and tell her we will do it together. I find a question about skating, which she enjoyed as a younger woman. I ask: what is the shape of a skating rink? 4 letters. She thinks for a short time and then says: "Long?" then she says "wide?" I can see where this is going. The answers are 4 letters. They describe a rink, sort of. I will not tell her they are wrong, so I will put the puzzle away.

Tonight, while trying to comfort her worried mind, I tell her that one month from today, on this a Saturday evening; she will be climbing into her own bed in her own home. I wait for her reaction, but there isn't one. Maybe I have given her too much information at a time of the day that she doesn't process information well. She is worried that she needs to find a place for her and her dogs to stay—past that—not much more is going to get sorted properly. Instead, I change her focus. I get her pj's and her body lotion and give her some personal attention. She thanked me for taking the worry from her. I asked her if she wanted to talk to one of the girls, so she believes that they know where she is. She asks me not to report her confusion to them. She understands the questions are in her own mind, and the confusion prevents her from being able to understand the circum-stances. She has accepted the fact that she and her dogs will always have a home with me and my dogs. At least she has for this moment. This information she relays to Mickie and calls her "the loyal one."

This day is over, and we have moved into early Sunday morn-ing. I have two dogs on the sofa with me, TV is on, as is my com-puter. I should get some rest, as we have a brand-new day of events ready to dawn in a few hours. I have not taken my medication and supplements as I should, but Mom has received hers. I have not eaten healthy this day, as we ate out and had a large milkshake. My hair is up in its normal ponytail and my fingernails need filed. I didn't have to water anything outside today as we have had rain the last two days. I am moving stuff into the shed so the floors can be done when we head north—but I didn't do any of that today. Mom and I had agreed earlier that I will do her manicure tomorrow, usually during the ball game. She said that her nails are getting "a little light." Her hair was washed and set a few days ago and holds the set well since she received her permanent. I've laid out another clean outfit for tomorrow on the chair in her room. She had gotten some of her chocolate from her milkshake on her clothes today. I haven't said anything; I will just take care of it quietly.

Tomorrow is a brand-new day. Hopefully there will not be any occurrences that we cannot handle without medical or surgical intervention. Hopefully it will be pretty much the same as all the other days that preceded it. I will give simple instructions for the same daily tasks. I will attempt to protect her from any danger and try to get the dogs to move out of her path. She sat on the footstool tonight because one of the dogs was comfortable on her chair. I will hope that she doesn't let the dogs out of the gate. Simple matters have become so important in daily tasks. Tomorrow I will probably discover something else that doesn't come naturally for her, just as I didn't expect her to remove all the empty Walmart bags from the cashiers bagging wheel. Simple things that we take for granite, are things that our mother finds confusing and a challenge, and another new lesson to be learned. Will it be retained on our next Walmart visit? Only meeting all the tomorrows with a positive attitude and a pleasant smile will let us know.

Bring on all the tomorrows Dear Lord—the most recent version of our mother and I are ready for it. I've got lots of smiles from times past and memories of our first mother to last another lifetime.

Those memories involve a woman who gave of herself to everyone she knew, those kids in the cafeteria, those folks at church, on her bowling team or her weight watchers group. She was limitless in her attention to family. She didn't have monetary means to spoil, but she never thought twice about giving of her time and herself. She always took time to color, work a puzzle, or listen to family happenings. The simple fact that she is on the receiving end at this stage in her life, and that our second Mom can actually benefit from all the sacrifices that our first Mom made—it can't be any more than a well-deserved payback. Go ahead, Life, bring me a brand-new day.

Resolve to be tender with the young, compassionate with the aged, sympathetic with the striving, and tolerant with the weak and the wrong. Sometime in your life you will have been all of these.

What happened if there is an injury to the left side of the brain, as with my mother? The left side of the brain deals with language and helps to analyze information that it receives. With a left sided brain injury, you're aware that things aren't working right but you are unable to solve complex problems to do a complex activity. These people tend to be more depressed, have more organizational problems, and have language problems. A Reader's Digest version of the functions of the left side of the brain:

- Listening, speaking, reading, writing and language problems
- Memory for written and spoken messages
- Ability to analyze information
- Controlling the right side of the body, which would explain the problems mother had with her right sided fine motor movements.

With the list written out, I can see where our mother's problems lie.

July Arrives

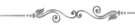

I haven't written anything for a while. For some reason I've been a little tired and energy-less. I sort of spent the last few days mostly on the sofa. Mom doesn't get into any activity unless I've directed her in that direction. If I fall asleep on the sofa, I awake to her sitting in a chair just looking around. Sometimes she is just watching me. She hasn't mastered changing channels on the TV yet. She has tried. Brian put his number on speed dial tonight, but I know Mom has already forgotten how to call him. She still needs some prompting on fixing the dogs food, and we've been working on that simple chore for months. Mom does keep up to washing the dishes. If I wash some of the pans or empty her dishwater, she will tell me that I'm doing her job. She lets them dry in the drainer or on a towel, and then I rid them away. Sometimes they are not clean, but I just put them back in her dishwater and say nothing. I've learned her eyesight is limited.

This morning she had one shoe on and was holding her other one. I ask her if she was having a problem. She asked me if these were her shoes, because the one didn't feel right. She had the left shoe on her right foot, all laced up. Sometimes I think she is advancing, and then a little glitch in her actions catches me and puts me onto the reality train. This afternoon I handed her a deck of cards and asked her to play a game of solitaire. She laid out the seven piles correctly, so I was busy at the island. I walked over to observe her a little while and noted that she had laid two Kings up where the Aces are to lay. I pointed it out to her, and she repeated a few times how she knew that—and how many grandchildren she had taught the game to—and how she should be able to remember how to play.

She watches the baseball games. Her eyes are on the TV. I explain most of the actions and point out when McCutcheon is up to bat or catching the ball. She never knows the score, or for that matter, who wins and who loses. She doesn't understand what inning they are in, or even what inning is next. It's almost sad to watch her watch a game or a show. She can get the obvious humor, but most often things must be explained to her, and then she understands.

Something isn't right. She still has some wounds on the incisional line on her scalp. I am concerned. I have increased her water consumption and been giving her Lasix the last few days. When she wakes up in the morning, her hair is matted over the wound. I try to get her to leave it alone as it is drying. She still works on getting her hair unstuck from her head and plays with the area throughout the day. She doesn't want her hair to grow into her head. I don't want to see that happen either my mother.

She had a phone call from her niece tonight. She talked and laughed and seemed to enjoy talking. She had answered the phone herself. I heard her say, "she's right here." I walked toward Mom and she told me, "I don't think you know this person." I took the phone and spoke into the phone and to Mom. I told her niece, my cousin, to "hold on a bit" and heard her laugh. I asked Mom if she knew who she was talking to? She told me she did but couldn't come up with a name. I explained that it was her niece, Sue, and then further explained that she was her sister's daughter. When I said that she was Aunt Fran's daughter, she seemed so surprised. I could see she was trying to sort out the information, so I named all of Aunt Fran's children. She was so interested in who I was talking to as I informed her of Mom's fall and hip fracture. I told her niece how remarkable her recovery from her surgery was, because she couldn't remember that she had a fall and had a fracture, so she would get up every morning and walk as she had before. She didn't want to use the walker, because she told me she had weaned herself from it before, and she didn't want to go backward. She didn't slow down from the walking and ambulation she had done before her hospital admission. She had some noted discomfort, that was eased with Tylenol. Sometimes I had to remind her that she truly had a broken hip, and that we had to take some extra precautions. I told her niece that she had "raised the bar" for an eighty-nine-year-old patient's recovery from a fractured hip. I continued to tell her niece how awesome she was and then put her on Speakerphone, so my mother could hear the conversation. My mom said she wanted to ask her about her friend, but she couldn't remember her name. I told her it was "Annie." My mother then asked, "How is Annie?" Sue explained how well she was doing and then soon ended the call.

I went back to my mending on the island. Mom came over and stood next to me, and asked, "When did I break my hip, that I don't remember?"

I'm perplexed. I don't know whether to enter this arena-again-currently. I think I will just let this question get absorbed in further conversation.

We're planning a trip up north. We have purchased a Van that is tall enough inside that I can walk around. The windows are very large so you can see out everywhere around. I have put a tray table into it, a cooler, a potty chair with camping bags to use in it. It has a TV screen for the back seat and we have put movies and comedy CDs in it to entertain Mom. The third seat reclines into a bed, so I can put Mom to bed at her normal sleeping time, and with her dogs. I have food, snacks, liquids, and spare clothing in case we need to use them. There are pillows and blankets to make travel comfortable. We have heat and air, and room for all the dogs. We are towing Mom's car back to Pennsy. Such a well-planned idea we had, and Bri had covered everything—or so we thought.

We are all packed. So far so good.

This trip was different. I didn't take Mom out of the van for anything. We had food to eat, a potty chair for personal use, and Bri walked the dogs on leashes when he would stop. We put the third seat down and turned it into a bed for Mom and most of the dogs.

WE'RE HOME

When we first arrived home and started to bring luggage into the house, I had sat Mom on her usual chair in her own kitchen. She watched as we carried in things, and then said, "I don't know why you guys are bringing things in, cause we're not staying here."

Brian asked if she didn't think this was a nice place to stay. She just continued to watch us bringing in her stuff, and she said, "It's a nice place, but it's not for me."

Bri looks at her in disbelief. He has just driven eighteen hours, and his grandmother informs him that she isn't staying here. Another day, another chapter in our lives with my mom.

July Moves On

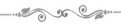

I've come to admit that my mother is a marvelous faker. She can fool the most in-tune person. But you can't fool all of the people, all of the time.

Jane brought up some groceries tonight. It was evening—almost dusk. The time was probably between 7:00 and 8:00 PM, not good times for our mother. We all three sat at the kitchen table, and this time there were actually three of us there.

We explored the idea that Mom refers to me as "the girls," or "them" or "they." It's always in the plural, never in the singular—just me, only one, not multiple people taking care of her. She asked me to "help" her out.

I said, "Mom, you're on your own with this one. I don't know, I can't help you with this one. I would like to know the answer to this one myself."

She heard Jane explain that there has only been one person taking care of her and staying with her. She looked somewhat confused. She said, "Help me with this, don't put me on the spot." She listened to our explanations, but you could tell she didn't really comprehend that there were not multiple people taking turns and alternating in her care and company.

Jane visited for a while, and then left. I told Mom to come in and sit down and watch her Pirate game, and I would get her half Klondike to eat while she did. I gave her the bedtime medications and a glass of water. She never questions the how or why of her medications, she just takes them without question. She ate her Klondike but wanted to know where the bag of dog treats were. She will not eat in front of her dogs without giving them some treats. I showed her where the opened bag was and she happily gave three of the dogs several treats. I only put one bag in her presence at a time, as when I filled the dog treat jar in Florida, it was almost emptied in one day. The more she sees available, the more the dogs get.

She finished eating and feeding the dogs, came in the room and counted the dogs. She counted to five, and then asked me, "Is that all there is?" I hear this question often, and I answered, "I hope so. Five is all there is."

She sat down on the sofa. I was really tired today. I seem to have a cough that I can't clear, and the settling in and observation has been a bit exhausting. Sometimes I do so much explaining during her days, that I'm almost hoarse by evening. Today I had brought a forty-five-piece puzzle to the kitchen table and invited Mom to put it together. I had helped her lay out all the pieces, and showed her how to lay them in groups according to their color. I had to keep helping her with the fact that the straight edges were for the sides, and show her how to build the frame. She would put pieces in place where the color didn't even match. We built the puzzle from the top down, working with the words on the puzzle, then the sky, the grass, the dogs, and then the bottom. She needed help and prompting and explanations from the start till completion. She didn't know to put the corners in place or keep the straight edges for the border. After we had completed the puzzle, she picked up all the pieces and put them in the box. She left it on the table, stating she was going to do it again tomorrow. I am so anxious to see if she initiates doing it herself. That seems to be a big problem. When I make suggestions, or bring up an idea of something to do—she waits, or maybe forgets, or maybe doesn't know where to begin—but she can't initiate it herself. This is a lady that has taught all her grandchildren, and great-grandchildren to put puzzles together.

This is a lady that I try to explain that sorting clothes, or choosing which clothes she wants to keep and which we can remove from her closet and drawers, what we need set on the table, or where and how the dishes get washed, what we need to prepare the meal, or how to put a puzzle together—is very hard work for her brain. Just as she had to give her permission to the mail order prescription company to allow me to change the address where her drugs are to be sent. The man on the other end of the phone was saying too much…he didn't keep it simple. And her face showed it. I had to take the phone and explain to Mom what he wanted from her, then explain to the man on the other end what I was doing, and then give her the phone back. Too much too quick for too long—and she falls behind. Just as when there was too much company in the kitchen yesterday. Too many conversations going on at once. She just sat there for a bit, and then said, "I am lost. I don't know what's going on." Jean and Mike had come, while Mom's nephew Allen was here talking about the farm. Mom kept up to the farm conversation with him quite well, after I had explained who he was. When Mike came, he talked of the Pirate baseball game…and she did well. When Jody and the girls came, along with me here…she fell behind. More than one person was talking at a time. I try to watch that so it doesn't happen, but I missed it this time.

At her first great-grandchild's graduation party on Sunday, I tried to make sure she wasn't left sitting alone. You also must watch and make sure she really does know who she is talking to, for she can cover her confusion pretty well—but only for so long…and then she's done.

Back to this evening. Jane had left. She said to me, "The person that was here doesn't have any children, does she?" I looked up from the TV into a face that was sincere. I said, "Yes, Mom, that was Jane. She has four children" I watched her face, as she heard information that was totally new to her. I explained that she lived right next to us, and she is the one that takes care of her money. I've had this conversation many times, so it doesn't take me by surprise. Knowing her four daughters is a big problem for our mother, and she has admitted and apologized for it many times. I tried to explain who her children were, and broke it down by families several different ways, but I wasn't connecting with her comprehension tonight. She would shake her head and look so disappointed that she couldn't grasp the knowledge that I had just laid before her.

Again I explained to our mother that she is awesome, and that she is making so much progress—but her brain gets tired. I explained that is why I insist she take a nap in early afternoon, and that it is evening and she's done a whole lot today. She bases her situation on the fact that she hasn't done anything to be tired, using physical work as her form of comparison. I remind her again that all these memories and word finding and sorting of the things she can remember and the questions she can ask of the things that she can't, really tires her brain. Jane and I had both told her that she thinks and reasons much better when she isn't tired. On her own, she got up to go to the bathroom, but headed for my bedroom. I just stated, "Not that way."

She said, "Oh shit," and turned around and headed in the right direction. When she came back out, she had on her pajama bottoms and had her shoes off. She checked on the front door and went back to bed. She put herself to bed tonight, and I left her. I checked on her a little later, but I left her do this on her own. Her two dogs were with her. I turned on the monitor and turned down the lights in the house. This was a day that I needed more rest than usual, so this was fine with me. She went to bed when she couldn't get Jane's family figured out—I think her daughter and her family is different from the lady that handles her money and gets her groceries. I think Jane has joined me in the plural sense—I'm no longer alone in my multiple personalities life.

I fell asleep in the chair again this evening. I hate to sleep when she is sleeping, it seems like such prime time to waste sleeping, but I have to be so quiet with five dogs listening to my every move, that I'm limited to my activities anyways.

I can joke with my mother, and I can use sarcasm, and she can react to it.

I casually asked Jane, "Can you come up tomorrow and help me move Mom's bedroom from where it is to the other end, and move my bedroom back where hers is?"

Mom says, "No, you're not moving my bedroom."

I kind of ignored her negative response and said to Jane, "So when she gets up in the evening and heads to bed, she will be going in the right direction."

Mom laughed, as did we. She then explained to Jane how she thinks she should go in that direction—and it happens every night, and it's never right. How does my mother get my sarcasm and humor, but often not know who I am? Ours is not to question why. Ours is just to love her as she has been gifted to us. Is there a lesson to be learned? Is there a reason why such a gentle giving woman is learning who she is and who her family is in the late stages of eighty-nine years? Are we to be seeing that she doesn't give up? Are we to learn that life is too precious to even consider any alternative? Are we to simply give back to this woman that was our mother, what she gave without reservation all of her life? As her grandson simply stated after she had come through brain surgery and was not quite the same woman that had entered the operation room. "At least we have her." You are right, Mark. What else needs to be said.

Jump, and you will find out how to unfold your wings as you fall.

Two Judys and Two Janes

Mom fell in her room, she said she got "tangled up" somehow trying to get to the potty chair.

She told Julie, "You know there are two Janes down there. that's right, she doesn't work there anymore."

I had told Mom, "Jane didn't work at the bank, she just does your banking. She worked at the doctor's office." I guess I didn't clear things up very well.

I couldn't find the hamburg and rice mixture that we had made for the dogs. It was not in the fridge anywhere. It was not in the freezer. It was not in the cupboards with the plastic containers, like the mixture was in. I asked Mom, and she didn't know where it was. I finally found it under the sink where the dry dog food is kept.

I couldn't find the seam rippers, and there were two. I had watched Mom picking up things where I was sewing and attempting to rearrange them and make them neat. I looked everywhere but couldn't find them. Mom was helping me look, for she knew she had seen them. Finally, Mom lifted her stack of quilting squares on her sewing machine, and they both lay there, neatly together.

We kill fly's, and I shut the door to keep them out of the house. I look around and the door is propped open. The dogs start to bark and bark at the neighbor's dog. Mom stands at the door and doesn't manage the dogs at all.

I told Mom she needed to drink more water. She told me she just couldn't drink any more. She tells me she's drank so much that "it's coming out of my head." The ulcerated areas on her head have started draining some serous drainage again today. It had been dry for several days. Yes, I am concerned.

Trust yourself. You know more than you think you do.

It's been awhile since I entered my thoughts on these pages. Today I asked my mom is she was ready to get her teeth brushed. She responded by telling me that she was, but that some of her teeth were broke. She couldn't explain which teeth were broke, or even how they broke—so we just headed back the hall to the bathroom. She asked me to take her upper denture plate out…a task she hasn't quite mastered with any level of comfort. I removed her denture and it appeared intact. I fixed her toothbrush and instructed her to brush her teeth, front and back. She rinsed her mouth with instruction, and I took care of her denture. As I put her denture back in her mouth, I asked if there were any that appeared to be broke? She seemed to think that they felt "okay," so goal reached at this time. We could repeat this same action again in a few hours, and again in the morning—and we would be starting, again, from square one. My mom asked me if I found the broken teeth. I told her that they did not seem broken so maybe we fixed them and then asked her if they felt good in her mouth? She said they did, and we moved forward to our next adventure.

You have to be available to the invisible voices
that are swirling around you.

AUGUST ARRIVES

We have another trip behind us as we arrive back in Pennsylvania. Her head wound has reopened. We are back in the proximity of her neurosurgeon.

There has been so much company since we came back to Pa. Mom handles visitors for a short period, then she has run out of conversation. She's recovered from her Fractured hip quite well but does have some weakness in the right knee when she gets up to walk. She refuses any walker or cane, feeling it means she has regressed to needing assistance. Meanwhile, I must have a good grip on her arm when ambulating outside the home because of her ataxia or balance problem. When in Florida, I would take her up to one of the stores and let her push the buggy throughout—while we also had stuff to look at. Here in Pennsy., there are not stores in close proximity, and driving a distance is not something she likes.

There are some memory issues that we've been trying to deal with, but not much luck in some fields. She's having a problem with remembering her four daughters. I don't know how that gets to be the very area of her brain that suffered damage, but it seems to be. She is not able to do daily activities as she had her entire life.

Everything seems to be a learning and retraining process. On Sunday, I had her sew two blocks of material together on her sewing machine and she was so proud. She thinks it's been years since we've been in her house and even longer since she's sewed on her sewing machine. It's unbelievable what can happen in one year. I must introduce her to everyone that comes and explain how they are related. She doesn't know her way around the kitchen like she did just a year ago.

One visitor came, my sister Jean's relationship. She had just left, and Mom was so relieved. I started putting Mom down for her afternoon nap again, even when she resists. She will sleep about one and half hours and then her mind will be more refreshed and better for the rest of the day. She sleeps well at night but gets up often to pee so I have a potty chair right by her bed. She fell again the other night while trying to get up to the pot. So now the pot is much more approximated to her turning from the bed to sit down. No matter how I try to protect her from accidents, she finds a new way to be a tumble bug.

I don't see how she is going to be left alone, as she has altered mental status at different times. Sometimes you think she's starting to get a grasp on things, and then you get thrown a total curve. The other night Jane came up and then walked home. Mom couldn't get the concept of where she walked to, so I walked her down. She thought that the house was Dave's and she didn't know where Jane lived. We finally settled her down with the idea that Jane lived in part of Dave's house. Tonight, Jane came up after being with her mother-in-law. Her mother-in-law was admitted to the hospital on Friday, because she couldn't get out of bed. She has Parkinson's disease, but she has been independent. Today they transferred her to a rehab nursing facility in Kittanning. Mom sees the deterioration happening to all the ladies she hung with.

She started telling Jane how she had no place to go, that she lived in somebody else's house and it was illegal. She said she was always afraid that she would get arrested. She told Jane how she would be staying at one house, and then she had to go to another one—and how other people were there that stayed all night. She said they must have been getting paid, or they wouldn't have stayed. She just doesn't know who has been with her, or even why she was with someone. She told Jane how bad it was when she didn't have anywhere to go. It's so sad to hear her tell us how "homeless" she felt, when she has never been left alone. I have been with her for over a year now. My life has changed drastically—but not nearly as much as this little lady who is so lost.

She is a sweet lady that seems to have taken over our mother's body. She is a different mother than we have had our entire life, and she doesn't remember much about raising us, although she remembers so much of other parts of her life. I showed her how to close the mini blinds the other night. She is working with learning how to put them up and down also. I've been teaching her how to sew on her own sewing machine. She now sets the table with butter and jelly and silverware. I make her coffee in the morning and put it in a thermos bottle, which she uses throughout the day for her coffee. We replaced her gas stove with an electric range, to eliminate the open flames in her house. I've been teaching her how to use the burners, and how to clean the stove with the nonscratch cleanser. It's a glass top stove.

She said, "I need to write this stuff down." I started some pages with simple directions for daily things. Somedays it's like starting all over again. Life with this sweet lady is a learning process every day, and I've been with her 24-7 except for short trips to the store. Last Sunday I spent most of the morning and afternoon up at my sister, Jody's. I was painting one of her granddaughter's bedroom. I had fixed Mom's breakfast, as I do every morning. She had made a sandwich out of some ham salad spread in the fridge for her lunch, and for supper, she found some potatoes, so she boiled two and ate it with butter on. She also had bread and butter. I suggested meals on wheels, but she became adamant, she didn't want it. It is going to happen, someday if I can get her somewhat independent, so I can come home.

Labor day last year was her cranial surgery, so it's going to be one year. The changes in that year have been amazing. I've tried to keep a record of my time with this lady over the last year, because some of the stuff she has dealt with you just can't make up.

Things are not as convenient up here in Pennsylvania. I've had a lot of trouble with my left foot, with the heel spur and plantar fasciitis. I can't get treatment up here easily, because of the type of insurance I have. I need to research how to get preapproved. I was supposed to get physical therapy and be fitted "with a boot of some kind" but our trip was the following day, so I couldn't get there.

I have had the medicine for my fibromyalgia increased, and the doctor warned me it would make me gain weight. My appetite is so increased, and my activity has decreased so much. I figure I'll never have this time to spend with my mom, and also protect her—that I will deal with the weight as best I can. She has told my sister that she doesn't know how to do things, and she really needs me. If I have a tired day and don't do much, she just moves about and watches me. She doesn't initiate any activity without my providing her with instruction, and helping her throughout. I had her make hamburger helper for our supper last night. She browned the hamburger and did well. She couldn't measure the water and milk that is called for, so I had to do that. She stirred it and watched it until it thickened, then I showed her how to shut the stove off.

Tell me a fact, and I will learn. Tell me a truth and I will believe. Tell me a story and it will live in my heart forever.

We have made an appointment with the neurosurgeon to see Mom. She has an open draining head wound and she was scheduled for a CT scan of the head.

From this report, she is scheduled for removal of hardware. She is also scheduled for removal of skin cancer by her nose. It is believed she may be reacting to the hardware used to hold the cranial bone in place from the initial surgery.

She was admitted to the hospital August 25. She was prepared for surgery again. The hardware was removed and the surgeon found the bone had to be debrided. A skin and muscle graft repair was used to close her open head wound. This makes the third time admitted to the hospital within one year. Her initial cranial surgery, her fractured hip, and now this surgery. She also had removal of all her upper teeth and replaced with a denture. Quite a record for anyone, but especially for a woman who is pushing age ninety.

HOME FROM THE HOSPITAL—
AGAIN, AUGUST 29

We just brought Mom home from the hospital on Thursday. They had to open her head up again and remove the plates and screws they used to hold the bone in place with the first surgery. They became infected. She has had a tough year. Hopefully when she turns ninety in December—we will have a new page. From the craniotomy with the large blood clot, the fractured hip, the decayed and infected teeth, the urinary tract infections, and now the infection in her head—she is amazing.

Just to clarify, having a mild head injury does not mean the person has mild problems. A mild head injury can prevent someone from return-ing to work and can make family relationships a nightmare.

The brain can be hurt without hitting onto an object. With an injury, the soft tissue of the brain is propelled against the very hard bone of the skull. The brain tissue is squished against the skull and blood vessels may tear. When blood vessels tear, they release blood into areas of the brain in an uncontrolled way. The problem with this is there is no room for this extra blood. The skull does not expand. The blood begins to press on softer tissue, like the brain. Brain tissue is very delicate and will stop working properly or may even die off. With large amounts of bleeding in the brain, the pressure will make areas of the brain stop working.

I have studied the brain so much this past year. Such an amazing "motherboard" that handles the entire human body. I do not have a technical mind so to understand how a three-pound organ can coordinate breathing, heart rate, body temperature, metabolism, thought processing, body movements, personality, behavior, vision, hearing, taste, smell, and touch is way beyond my understanding. The human skull acts as a protective covering for the soft brain. It is estimated to have about 100 billion cells and I've heard it compared to a phone system. If you take the entire phone system in the world and all the wires, the number of connections and the trillions of messages a day would not equal the complexity or activity of a single human brain. I have not fact-checked this information, but it sounds downright amazing to me. All in a little three-pound organ.

SEPTEMBER ARRIVES

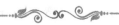

I'm sitting in a recliner with Rusty at my feet. I just got Mom to bed. She had a follow-up appointment today in Monroeville. The nurse in the office took the eight stitches out of the incision by her nose. She still has over sixty stitches in the left side of her head. She came out of her room the other night about one thirty holding the bandages from her head. She was upset because she had blood on her hand, and over her dressing. she didn't know what was happening. I walked her back to bed after putting the dressing back on her head. She required some reassurance and she went back to sleep. Some of her memory is doing really good—other parts I can't seem to find. She is totally exhausted and tires very easily. She takes short naps many times a day and still sleeps all night. Her appetite is still good, and her balance in walking is very compromised. I keep ahold of her when we are walking anywhere other than in the house.

For her own reasons, she just won't use a walker. She truly thinks if she uses a walker, that she's going backward in her recovery. She does enjoy going "shoppin' walkin'" as I started calling it. She pushes the cart and it's all she needs for her balance. She can't handle her money, as she has no clue as to what it may cost. I must prompt her or help her to do most everything. We hope that when they get all this infection cleared up that her memory and mind may improve. When we look back over the year, she has truly been a survivor. She had a bladder infection when she went in the hospital with the large bleed last August. They treated it then. She had the bladder infection again when she went into the hospital with the broken hip in March of this year. They had to treat it then before they did the hip repair.

She then had all her upper teeth removed and they were in very bad condition. And then she developed this infection in her head wound that required this surgery to remove the 4 little plates and screws in her head that were holding the bone in place that they had cut out in the first surgery. My sister Jane went with me today.

I told her Mom would not be with us if she had not lost her memory of everything. I think that's what kept her going, because she didn't remember everything that was happening. Her mind is a real puzzle to us—we can only be hopeful and keep working with her. I'm just so glad she is the most pleasant and cooperative lady I know. She truly needs someone to protect her from herself—cause she just isn't safe. She can't seem to reason what could possibly happen in the end—if she chooses the wrong direction. Jane was with her in her bedroom last evening when Mom put her shoes on the wrong feet. She asked Jane if they were wrong. She didn't know if they were on the wrong feet herself. She is the sweetest most precious little lady. I have her wearing disposable panties, because she's not always holding her urine now. I can't seem to get her to initiate or start anything herself. But then, look at the major surgeries that she's had in one year at the age of eighty-nine?

In the name of God, stop a moment, cease your work, look around you.

The left side of the brain deals more with language and helps to analyze information given to the brain. If you injure the left side of the brain, you're aware that things aren't working but are unable to solve complex problems or do a complex activity. Impaired memory is one of the universal problems of people with head injury.

A Needed Veterinarian Visit

We had taken Mom's favorite dog to her vet. Mickie has been drinking large amounts of water, day and night. She has been diagnosed with diabetes. I needed another opinion, because I couldn't think that it would cost between 350 and 400 a month to treat a pet for diabetes. This first family vet suggested euthanasia. That will be too hard to help Mom deal with. My mom has a compression bandage around her head for a leaking wound—her IV antibiotics have been reordered for 7 more days by the infection control doctor—she is weaker and sleeps more—I was concerned that she had had enough this year and was too tired to continue to fight. Then I see symptoms in her fav dog that were new. My worries came true

Mickie has diabetes. She needs to have insulin injected into her twice a day—and get some regular blood sugar checks at the vets until he gets her stabilized. The blood sugar checks will be done at his office and cost $10. He advised us to buy the insulin and syringes at Walmart because they have their own brand. We bought the vial of insulin and 100 syringes for less than $40. The vet visit was to cost $60—he only charged us $45. I had explained to them yesterday the concern with "letting Mickie go" because of the status of my mother with brain injury and repeat surgery this past year. Jane and I took Mom with us with her bandana around her head. She sat in a chair by the exam table and kept talking to Mickie. What a difference a second opinion makes.

Mom is so relieved and less frightened. She didn't understand—and probably still doesn't—that "keeping Mickie comfortable" wouldn't work. Diabetes is not an easy death, it's a slow killer.

She was so frightened that we would have Mickie put down. She got Mickie about one year after my dad died. Her condition is fragile—and I didn't want it complicated by having her soul mate die and not be with her. She is the only dog that Mom recognizes (most of the time) In fact she calls Annie the "white Mickie." So Mickie had her first insulin injection tonight after her supper—and we will continue twice a day now. I now have two patients to take care of—bless both of their hearts.

LATE SEPTEMBER

I would like to be in Florida for Christmas and New Year's this year, so I'm working on making it happen. We are going to celebrate Christmas early here at Mom's house. I'm thinking about the weekend of December 5 and 6, and no later than the weekend of the twelfth or thirteenth. I'm trying to find out if anyone has company Christmas parties or anything already planned for any of those days.

I don't talk on the phone much anymore. I find that Mom hears some things and then perceives them wrong. When we took her to the doctor last week, she believed we were taking her to a place, getting her a bed, and her head would be shaved again. She didn't realize that she had already had her surgery and hospital admission. I thought if I worked hard with Mom in the beginning, that we could get her recovered better. The hip fracture setback, the infection going on in her decayed teeth, and then the infection that was brewing inside her head was not in the plans. She has finished all the antibiotics, and finally there doesn't seem to be any drainage coming from her head. Maybe we can get some more of her memory back, but as of now, there is no way she can ever be left to live alone. She becomes confused and anxious.

October Arrives

My life is pretty much a constant continuing routine. Mom is a 24-7 watch, monitor and protect from injury. She is mostly confused and trying so hard to sort out her memory and present situation. It varies from minute to minute. She doesn't usually know who I am, but knows that I am always with her. It's evident that she is frightened to be left alone. I can see why when she doesn't know where she is at times, how she got there, how long before she has to leave, and how she's going to go.

She is the sweetest little thing all the time—she has become very helpless in her confusion and disorientation—but her personality remains sweet and cooperative. We had her to the surgeon last week because her head is still draining from the left temporal area. He wants another CT scan next week and wants to see her then. He wants to make sure the wound area is decreasing in size and healing from the inside out.

I made flight plans for Bri. He will fly up and then plan on leaving on Sunday—two days after Christmas. My hope is that Mom and I and five dogs will return to Florida with him. It all depends on the attention this head wound from her last surgery is doing. It scares me to have this open area so close to her brain. She is now having urinary accidents—and Jane and I think she has another urine infection. I'm going to try and get a urine specimen by morning and Jane will run it to the lab. Jane is so extremely helpful to me. She gets our groceries and sends up meals often. She just lives next to Mom, so she can walk back and forth.

Mom has problems doing just about everything. She needs help and prompting and one direction at a time. I have only seen my son and his two little children once since I came up. I only seen my other two grandsons when I took them shopping for school clothes. My whole time is here at the mobile home with my mom and five dogs—one who gets insulin shots twice daily.

Jane stayed with Mom today so I could participate in the event of taking my oldest grandson, Gage, to his college dorm today and getting him settled in. He doesn't plan on coming home till Christmas break. My daughter wanted me to be with them today so bad—so I decided I could do that. I hope so much he can make this schoolwork. He's the one who had brain surgery twice for a tumor removal—and he has some memory issues and brain injury also. He can't drive yet because of that—so he has to rely on others to drive him to and from school.

Start by doing what's necessary, then do what's possible, and suddenly you are doing the impossible.

It's Now Late November

Let's see, it's Sunday night. Bri is trying to hold himself together. The doctor wanted to put my daughter in the hospital on Thursday for shortness of breath and chest congestion. I don't know if it's her chemo wearing her resistance down to everything. She has had breast cancer with radiation and chemotherapy. She still continues to smoke. She still sounds so terrible tonight. She goes back to the doctor in the morning. Tomorrow will be the third day of work she is missing, after being written up once, and suspended for a day already for absenteeism. I'm not seeing her employment status as turning out well. Her son is in tech school with monthly tuition, so I don't know how that can continue.

I have to get my mom up and moving to leave here about 6:00 AM tomorrow, and pick up my sister Jane. When I changed the dressing on her head today, I could actually feel the jagged edge of her skull bone. She gets the CT scan of her brain in the morning and then to see the surgeon. He knows I'm bringing her to Florida at the end of the week, but she still needs medical care. She fell about 5:30 AM a few days ago and has a nasty skin tear on her right hand.

I'm dealing with a heal spur on my left heel, and a damaged right knee.

Bri says he hopes we leave here next Saturday about four or five. Maybe Mom will start to get tired and as it gets dark, we hope she will rest. Often I can't get her to stay in bed here in the house—so I don't have high hopes of easy travel with her. I'm quite sure she's going to drag her feet and refuse to go. Somehow, I just see that happening.

Jane and I took Mom for her scan and doc visit. He says we have to close the wound, or we are going to have infections and worse problems. He tried to call the plastic surgeon, but he was in surgery. We have an appointment at three fifteen today. I broke Brian's heart and spirit—I canceled his flight home tonight. He insisted he wasn't coming up here to Pennsylvania unless he takes Mom and me back with him. He has a really rough day and then he had an appointment with his psychiatrist and totally lost all his composure and patience. I have two days of dinners and Christmas/birthday/thanksgiving celebrations all lined up. I should be going to the airport tonight, and now I won't. Everything is in Limbo now, but I sure don't want to be in Florida with a wound in Mom's head that drains and has openings in her skull that lead right back to her brain. Every bit of my nursing experience is being pulled to the front.

Mother, if you could look through our eyes just once.

It is now about four hours later. The transformer blew in front of Mom's home. They had to get an extra crew of men to get it fixed tonight. I was typing from the computer battery—when it went dead. We now have heat and light and all the comforts of home. My days and nights are pretty much the same, only the visitors change. We had a big successful Thanksgiving/Christmas/December birthdays meal and get together. Then my son Brent and my two little grandchildren came Friday.

I've been busy with Mom's dog Mickie. Another trip to the vet confirmed Lyme disease. I never had a dog with Lyme disease. She went downhill fast, but we already had her on antibiotics and pain meds. The fact that she is diabetic and needs insulin injections twice a day complicated things. I had to carry her off the porch to toilet—and often she couldn't stand up. I was afraid we would lose her—and she is Mom's favorite. She woke up improved this morning. I was so grateful. Mom's surgery is scheduled for December 10. The surgeons plan on doing a skin and muscle graft to close the head wound. This will be the third time, but hopefully it will just be a skin graft—but I have my doubts. I would truly like to know what this drainage is and why it's continuing to drain.

So I've been clipping dogs nails and trimming their coats and then bathing them to keep a check on ticks. Since Mickie has been diagnosed with Lyme disease, I'm on my toes. I found two new ones on Mickie when I did this. I mean no offense when I say this, but Mom is no help at all anymore. As I was clipping JoJo on the counter, Mom said, "She's going to jump off," and then she watched her do it. I've lost the mom that used to react to things. When I clip their nails and they yip or cry—she gets upset—so I have to stop. She feeds them cookies and table food, even though I have asked her so many times to stop. I explain that Mickie has an illness and the treats she gives her will make her sick. She tells me she is sorry and she didn't know that. But she doesn't know who or which one is which anymore. She thinks she has more than one Mickie, just like she has more than one Jane and many Judy's.

She is unable to do much more than toilet independently anymore. She tries—and she wants to help me all the time—and that means the task takes about ten times as long. She doesn't like the seat belt on cause it "chokes her." She doesn't want to drink water because it makes her get up to pee at night. Her skin is super dry and I know she's showing signs of dehydration. I have to run her into Quest in the morning for pre op blood work. Jane came up and stayed with her the other day, so I could go down to Gage's school and bring him home for the weekend. That took a little over three hours round trip. That was because his mother Heather, was so sick with asthmatic bronchitis.

My oldest son, Brent, has invited me to come to his house and stay if I want. I could babysit one of the days. I did that once before and fixed their supper when they came home from work. I got to spend all my time during the day with Samantha and Jeffrey. It was a dream. I tried to explain to him that when I'm not with Mom, she spends her time waiting on me or trying to find me. She doesn't really know who I am most of the time, and she doesn't know where her home is, especially at night—but when she sees me—it gives her a grounded feeling. Therefore, I can't stand to leave her. The girls tell me that she continues to look for me when they stay. My mother doesn't know any of the visitors, until I tell her—and then explain how they are related. Her grandson, Lee, stopped the other day. After he left, she asked me who his father was. When I told her "Ken is his dad," she said she hadn't known that.

- So I'm hoping her surgery is simple and we can leave soon afterward. I broke Bri's heart when I told him we couldn't come home after Thanksgiving.
- She will be ninety in a few weeks. I thank God he's left us enjoy her pleasant personality for as long as we have. She is so lost within herself. She struggles to think and remember and find the right words.
- So as soon after her surgery as we can get clearance—we will hope to return to Florida. Until the surgery on the tenth, and I find out how involved it will be, I won't have any idea what's in our future.

ANOTHER SURGERY DAY

Again, my mother is in surgery on the left side of her head. This is the third time she has had cranial surgery in less than two years. It seems surreal, that the quick decision we made last year—brings us here—we are still signing consents for surgery to our mother. This time the surgeons did a muscle and skin graft to the left temporal areas. The bone was debrided, and she has a surgical drain in place along with a bandage that surrounds her head.

MID-DECEMBER

Mom has been doing really well since this last surgery. She has a drain in and many stitches and a doctor's appointment tomorrow. I expect them to take out the drain, and then probably get the stitches out next week. Her memory seems to be improving and she tires very easily. Bri is flying up next Wednesday, on December 23. He plans on starting to drive to Florida on Saturday, so he can rest and yet be back to work on Monday. Mom says she isn't going, but I tell her she can't be by herself yet. Also, Her dog, Mickie is getting antibiotics twice a day for Lyme's disease from a tick. Mickie also gets insulin twice daily for newly developed diabetes. Sadly, I have no idea what her blood sugar number is, as It's impossible to get a blood sample from her with the glucometer.

So the plan is to drive to Florida the day after Christmas. I'm going to guess that we will be staying at Bri's house for a short time, but I'm not sure. He wants me to brighten up his house with some new paint. He has recently survived an emotional financial life-change. He went to make some toast the other day and realized he no longer owned a toaster. He has no guest beds now in his house, so I'm going to have to buy a mattress and box springs for Mom. I can sleep on the sofa, but she needs a quiet room when she gets tired. I can do a lot if we stay there, because Mom requires a lot more sleep than I—so I can get a lot done while she is with me there. I have to make sure the fencing he has will keep my little guys, especially Rusty, from touring the neighborhood.

How can I help her believe how truly beautiful she is? She asked Brian where the girl found all those stitches. She didn't know they were in her head. She truly doesn't know she had major surgery to her head a number of weeks ago. She knows that something leaks and runs down her face. She knows that she doesn't have much hair. Almost every morning she walks into the bathroom and comes to the kitchen with freshly combed hair—at least as much as she can. She has always tried to keep her hair looking nice. She thinks she looks so bad now. If only she could see herself through my eyes…if even for a short time. If only she can recall at ninety people and events from her past. Some parts of her memory resurface during conversation with all details, but not always. In fact, very seldom.

Things seem to be going haywire. Both the neurosurgeon and the plastic surgeon were with our mother on December 10. They had considered leaving the bone out during the surgery, as it had been a source of infection and had to be debrided. This would leave her head concave, requiring future surgery after a replacement plastic form was made to insert into her opened skull. They were considering closing her skull without the bone—meaning she would need a fourth cranial surgery to place something in her head to replace the infected bone. Enough is enough. I'm drawing the line. God bless this lady who is not making her own decisions. Last year removal of the clot putting pressure on her brain seemed like the best option. Relieve the pressure from her brain, let it heal and see where we were.

Not expected was a fall and a broken hip. Not planned was wound infection that caused her head wound to reopen. Not considered was having her in cranial surgery twice after the initial surgery. Now we are to consider this ninety-year-old lady have a concave head until a form of her skull can be made to replace the bone. And then we are to give consent to have her head opened again—the fourth time in fifteen months. And then what after that? Each time she goes under anesthesia, which has already been five times, she seems to lose more ground.

You can't go back and change the beginning, but you can start where you are and change the ending.

The infection control group from the hospital have ordered further IV antibiotics for our mother. The plan is twice a day for maybe six weeks. It has been one appointment after another since her Dec.

ten surgery. She is to be seen on New Year's Eve for insertion of a central line for the IVs to be administered. Our plans were to leave for Florida the day after Christmas. Our plans have just been changed—again. Mom will have an IV port inserted and we plan on leaving for Florida the first day of the new year. Bri had to stay with us longer than expected, and we don't want to jeopardize his employment. He has flown up to drive us back to Florida.

Dear God, if I have referred to you at all as being my co-pilot in this life adventure, may I ask you now to "trade seats" with me, please.

NEW YEAR'S EVE

The central line is inserted, and the hospital pharmacy has pre-pared us with enough IV solution containing antibiotics for five days. That gives us time to contact infection control in Florida and get her established with home health. I will administer the IV anti-biotics, and home health will keep a check on the level in her blood, adjusting the dose to maintain safe levels in her blood.

It's been said that an optimist is one who does cross-word puzzles with a pen—I am an optimist—but I still use a pencil, and I make sure it has a good eraser.

A Brand-New Year
Has Arrived

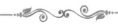

We will be traveling in what I call the "snowbird"—a van that has a third seat that becomes a bed. As Bri drives, our mother will receive her medication just as ordered. To quote a former movie series. Don't you love it when a plan comes together?

The trip to Florida was unremarkable, compared to some of the travel days we have had. Our mother spent most of her trip reclined in the bed. Keeping the dogs from climbing on her was more of a problem, but we managed. I had all the supplies needed to administer her antibiotic until we made contacts at home. I had the referral information and suggested home health agencies in hand. She would be followed by the Infection Control Group under Dr. Cooper. We had a potty chair, a cooler with food and drinks, medical supplies needed to administer her antibiotic, a driver that couldn't wait to have us back in Florida, and all our dogs. We have everything we need within the confines of our "snowbird" van.

As soon as we arrived home and got Mom settled in at Bri's house, I made all the phone calls. Everything went smoothly. Home health admitted her and then kept a check on her blood levels, notifying the infection control group here in Florida. The dose was adjusted to once daily when the levels were too high. The IVs were mixed and delivered to the house.

Every minute with your loved one is precious, because every minute keeps getting smaller.

Let's see if we can add some extra elements to Mom's cauldron of life. I went back to get my mother up for the day. She has been sleeping in Bri's spare bedroom. I don't see a denture in her mouth. I asked her where her "new teeth are." She says she doesn't know. They are not in her mouth, nor in her bed. I look under the bed and find many pieces of what had been an upper denture. Even though there were many chewed up pieces, it was evident that there were many pieces missing. I can only surmise that her dog Annie had a busy night.

So we have added the need for another appointment in my mother's schedule.

I called the dental clinic to update them on her denture. They wanted me to bring in the pieces and it may be repaired. I assured them it wasn't reparable, and many of the pieces were probably inside Mom's little white dog. We will now have to schedule appointments to have another upper denture made. I guess we are back to mashed potatoes and cream soup for a while.

We sometimes consume our tomorrows fretting about our yesterdays.

Another beautiful day. I've ordered another one for tomorrow— How can it not be, when you reside with the most beautiful person that has been in your life every day. We have been very lucky—very lucky.

We are still staying at Bri's house right now.

Mom asked me if Bri's neighbor, Bill, "Had anyone?" He (Bill) was over last night and Bri grilled one of the best meals ever. I told her his parents are gone, and he is an only child. He has one son who lives in California and one who lives in New York. He has no grand-children, so basically he has very little in terms of family.

I said, "Mom, we are very lucky with the family that we have, and the way you have kept us close. We thank you for that."

The lady that looks and sounds like our mother has rhinestone, glittery stickers on her pink manicure. She was so pleased with how pretty they look. I tell her that her mother would never believe her fingernails these days. She agrees and tells me how her mother used to try to stop her from biting her nails.

I've also found a spray-on hair color that adds a lot of body to her hair. She says it "looks like I have hair now." She also has painted toenails after her pedicure the other night. Funny, it was so much easier to paint her toenail than reach my own anymore. She loves to have creams or lotions rubbed on her back and body. Her skin is so dry I try to keep it moisturized. It works better than trying to get her to drink water.

She has a doctor appointment with infection control group tomorrow—I'm trying to get some resolution with her head wound, but I may be out of options. She then has a dentist appointment on Wednesday, when I hope we get her new denture. It's been a challenge to smash, dice, squish, and chop her food to make it easy for her to eat. She loves mashed potatoes with cream of chicken soup over them. She did so well when she first got her denture, before it landed under her bed in so very many pieces. I made the mistake to let her denture in her mouth at night. This will not be a redo.

We also stay very close to the bathroom these days. We have to be able to get there quickly, very quickly. It seems the ability to monitor such situations has declined.

She loves to be pampered, fussed over, dressed up in "pretty dresses." She said she has always hated picking her clothes. She told me she used to hang them on the rack, and just rewear the same ones all the time. Yet when she has something pretty on, she fusses over it and tries to keep it clean. My other mother would not have enjoyed that kind of attention at all.

This lady tries so hard to carry on a conversation. She can answer a few questions and appear that nothing is wrong. But then her ability to add to the conversation has dissolved. I wish you could see her facial expressions and hand motions on this side of the phone line. After every phone call from family, she asks, "Now who was that?" When she talks to Jane, it's the lady that takes care of her banking and lives in part of Dave's house. Jody is the one married to Ken. Jeani is the one married to Mike—the pirate fan. As I write this, I realize the dilemma she has with who I am. There is no man to reference me to. All at once it is so clear. She will tell me that she did something and then ask me if I am her? Brian is my "relief pitcher" for my mother's care, and she doesn't know he is related.

In all honesty, it is the part of her brain that gave birth to four daughters that has disappeared.

She has even said to me, "How can I not remember that I have four daughters?"

Oh, Mother of mine, I wish I knew. But know that I know—and that will be all we need right now.

When we are back at our other life on Sunset Drive she feels we have an "upstairs" This special lady that I spend all my time with "goes upstairs" to bed. It's just a long hall back to her room. She also "goes upstairs" when she takes her dogs and "goes home." The opened can of dog food ended up in the freezer. I took the bread basket with the tea towel out of Bri's cupboard to put bread in. It already had bread in it—kinda green and moldy Italian bread...Apparently someone had put the basket away for me after a meal. She sets the table for me—a few days ago Bri had 3 knives, 3 forks, and a spoon. She could only find one place mat one day—so she spread out a napkin at my place and placed my silverware on it. One special day she "set the table" for me. Bri had his silverware placed on a pair of her clean white socks next to his plate.

I have six dog crates in the family room—three medium-size and three small ones—and when we go somewhere, I have started to crate the dogs. Mom was so upset that I "locked up the dogs." She didn't want to stay very long because the dogs are "locked" up. When we are ready to leave—I ask "who wants a treat?" I don't have to crate one dog—the three bigger ones go in the first medium crate that's empty and waits for their treat—I usually have to take JoJo out of an already occupied crate—but she's right there with the rest. I try to explain to Mom that they are content and they go dormant in their own space. I show her how they lay in their crates during the day when the doors are wide open. I don't seem to be gaining any ground in that respect.

I still get scolded for "yelling" at them.

While we were still staying at Bri's house we had another fall. We came home from being out with Bri. I left the dogs out of their crates and was taking them outside. Mom was trying to get to the dogs and fell off the step that goes into Bri's family room. She hit her head and hip. She denied any injury. She told me today that when she fell, someone fell right on top of her. I had to turn away to smile. That's how fast Bri was trying to get to her and cushion her fall. She actually thought he fell on top of her.

I know everyone misses our mother and Mawmaw. I live with her 24-7 and I miss her so much. She was so compassionate that she would have been a big help taking care of my second mother. I tell everyone that our mother was the easiest going, sensitive, compassionate woman that I ever knew. Our second mother is the same, except that she needs protected and guarded and clued and reminded and cared for in a totally different way. This mother is still the most beloved patient I have ever cared for.

We have been blessed our entire lives, with a father that stood tall in character and morals. He sheltered us in love. We have a gentle spirited mother that Dad knew needed sheltered and taken care of after he had to leave. Mom will tell you that "Homer made sure I was taken care of after he was gone." She may not know how, but I think she knows how he took care of her while he was here and just knows that he had provided for her in his physical absence. In caring for Dad, and then Mom, so much has become obvious. I hope I'm making you proud Dad. I feel like I'm giving all I got in taking care of your wife. When I think I've run out of strength to carry on, something changes, and I'm energized to pick up and keep moving. It makes you wonder how life works.

Don't assume we have tomorrow. Tell those folks how much you love them now, for they may not know who you are tomorrow or understand what you are saying. Grab a life experience today, as someone may not be able to join you in a golf cart or fishing trip or pumpkin carving tomorrow. Make memories, don't bury your talents to keep them safe, for they will just deteriorate anyway. Laugh out loud with someone you love, even if it is at yourself. Smile so your teeth show and your eyes twinkle. Wear your good shoes and your wedge heels while your equilibrium enables you to walk in them, for someday you may be down to wearing one safe pair of tennis shoes.

Wear those good clothes and use those good dishes. Who are you saving them for? Record some family history while it can be conveyed to you, don't assume you will remember or that you "always have tomorrow."

Encourage those little ones, even in defeat, that they are valuable and so very worthwhile, for what they receive as a child from their parents will form their self-worth their entire life. Teach them that they never lose—they either win or learn. Make sure they know that sometimes their behavior is wrong, but it has nothing to do with the amount of love you have for them. And probably my favorite, remember that often the person that needs our support the most, is the one that deserves it the least.

I am forever grateful of the long talks I had with my mother and father years ago and put together an effort of a family history album. I was given pictures from family that I could work with, and stories that I could print. Dad spent time in Italy during the era of World War II. He has many small pictures he sent to Mom. Many of the pictures he explained, but we had more to do. Mom is able to give me some stories even today, of something she remembers from her childhood. It is missing pieces, but sometimes we get it put together.

Our dad's mind stayed with him, so that he was even aware that his body was shutting down on him. He knew when he went into the hospital that last time, that he wouldn't come back to his earthly home. He completed a project we started for every grandchild before he would consent to be hospitalized. Not one was left undone. He worked on Brent's for a few minutes at the kitchen table, then he would have to go and lie down. Soon he was back at the table to finish it. Brent's was the last plaque that he made. He picked a story or poem or verse that he felt fit the personality of each grandchild. He used metal letters and pounded the saying onto a small wooden plaque, then enhanced them with markers. He had asked me to buy frames for them, and also a small frame to put a picture in. I thought he was going to put his picture in the small frame, but he wanted a picture of each grandchild and that's what went into the smaller frame. He so loved his grandchildren.

Dad always said he tried to live his life so he could lay his head on his pillow at night with a clear conscious. He said he didn't have riches to leave his family, but only his good name. He thought out all his actions, and reactions, so he could establish a good name and root base for all of us.

While he was hospitalized, I asked him, "Dad, when are you going to pass out all the plaques you made for all the kids?" He said nothing for a few long seconds, then he pointed to me and as he shook his head in a negative answer he said, "I won't be, you will." Neither of us had to say anything else. As it was, I passed out his gift to each grandchild the afternoon of his funeral. As always, I listened to my father.

I have loved this other mother just as much. I don't want you to think I am keeping her away but I am staying here in Florida for a while longer. It's so convenient living two miles from everything. Bri lives alone so living in his home works for all of us. Even when we go to my Sunset house Mom wants to "come home." I am just trying to protect the image she has kept for eighty-eight years. We live in a world of "fifty first dates" most days. All sewing knowledge, all cooking or baking knowledge is gone. She is more a spectator and wants to watch me do stuff. Sometimes I can pull a memory from many years ago and she can add to the story, but not very often. In her mind, the part that is missing is the part of her daughters. That means she can't remember who their kids are also. She remembers the sons-in-laws' names? I can explain who everyone is and who their kids are but it doesn't stick.

It's a different world she lives in now. I want her to be remembered in the world she lived in for eighty-eight years. She did so much for everyone. She loved her family and loved knowing about them. I don't want family hurting because she has no idea who they are. I live with her and she often struggles with who I am. She knows Bri's demeanor and voice. He is with her every evening and takes her to lunch on the weekend. He takes her back to her bed every night at the same time he goes to bed. I'm afraid that when we come up north and don't have Bri that it will affect her, and also Bri, in a negative way. I'm afraid to uproot her comfort zone right now. She still has a draining wound on her left temporal area, so I don't know how long we can get away with an open wound to her brain. And just like the recent fall, I don't know if we will have tomorrow. All I can say is she has 24-7 gentle attention and all of me.

Do I keep you in touch with the lady we knew and the lady we all love so very much? I keep telling Mom how we are going to be ready for Christmas. She loved Christmas. We are working toward that pleasant memory. She has no concept of time or place. She told me that it was so nice that everything was so green in December. I agreed. (Well, it is green here in Florida in December, so she is basically right.) Keep smilin', family—we do.

MIDYEAR ALREADY

*O*ne *thing about the speed of light—it gets here too early in the morning.*

I poured a margarita tonight—and I'm sitting here eating cheese balls with it. I have country music on the TV—and Mom is in bed. Bri will be here about 4:30 for coffee and to drop off Lucy and pick up his lunch. Mom didn't want to stay in bed tonight, she kept getting up and asking me what time it was. She asked me yesterday if I had a mother. I told her that I certainly did. She then asked me if my mother was still alive. I looked into her pretty face and said "she certainly is." Some days are so much tougher than others.

I try not to get into melancholy. I try to look away with the romantic scenes on TV. My life is scrambled with a handyman at the house, a roommate that requires constant supervision, dogs that bark at everything and anything, and a son that is starting to get his life back on track after a life changing event. Financially, it will be awhile before he regains the ground he lost.

I moved Mom and I and the dogs into Sunset. It is still under construction or I should say reconstruction, but I needed to get Bri's house back into his. I have too much clutter when I get busy and it became overwhelming trying to do things at his house. The dogs barked at any movement so sleep and sanity were very limited

Life with Virginia, Mawmaw, Mom, Aunt Gin, and the sweet lady that I live with.

Life remains interesting in Sanford village. Life has no agenda, and it certainly doesn't have a script or a plan of any type. The sweet little lady that I share living quarters with has been dealing with some problems related to having the diarrhea. I am treating her with medication, and it has helped to some degree. She has started to resist taking pills citing she had "just taken them," (meaning the morning meds) and since "time" seems to be an area of misunderstanding for her, evening pills seem to be repetitious to her. I had to run up to Walgreens tonight when Bri was here for supper to restock some medication. I gave her medication and a glass of water when I returned. She shook her head "no" and informed me she didn't want any more pills. Bri had to remind her how he missed several days of work a few weeks ago, when he had stopped taking his pills. So they have agreed to continue to take their pills, even if it seems like they are not working. Thus the "Cheers" agreement between the two of them was invented. They take their water glass and clink them together. They say, "Cheers!" and both put a pill in their mouth, then take a drink and swallow the pill.

Now my laptop has been giving me a lot of trouble. I hadn't received any emails since May 22 and I had "lost" a few "updates" that I had started to compose. When I dropped it off at the best buy geek squad, it had a lot of viruses on it, including one at the top that I was using to research from. Every time I researched something, I spread it worse. So this virus story gets really cute. As I had just ran to Walgreens for more meds for Mom's condition, I received a phone call from the geek squad informing me my laptop was finished. I was telling Bri about the virus that was at the top of the screen and wondered how I get these viruses when I have the virus protection on. I wondered what I pay for, if my laptop still gets these viruses? Mom got the most puzzled look on her face and asked me if "it had caught what I have?" You know, you just can't make this stuff up. But if you want to test your teaching skills, try explaining to my little roommate what a virus is on a laptop, neither of which she understands very well.

We have moved into our little cottage on sunset drive. Since it is much smaller, it seems to be less confusing for my roommate. I still have to show her where the "restroom" is every time she needs to go. If the door is shut, she figures there is someone in there, and comes out to inform me.

She worries about the dogs being hungry from the time she gets up on the morning. They can be laying all over the floor sleeping, and she is so obsessed with the fact that "they are so hungry." She always asks me how many dogs we have, and she then wants to fix their food. If Lucy is home with Bri, she can't downsize her preparation to 5. I can even remove one of the dishes from her view and she will use one of the dishes from the kitchen shelves. So I don't mess with her system. I propped open the storm door and was working with a chair on the carport, in full view of where she was at. I told her where I would be and what I was doing. I stepped inside to check on her and found that she had put several spoons of "I can't believe it's not butter" into all the dogs" dishes and was mixing it through the dry food. I had to stop her and asked why she was using the butter. She informed me in a rather firm voice, "There was no one around, and I couldn't find the can of food anywhere, so I found the next best thing." I tried to explain that the butter would cause the dogs to poop all over the house, because it would act like a laxative, so we would have to remove it from their dishes. She will not call out to me, or ask for help or assistance of any kind.

I colored her hair this afternoon and set it. She asked me not to cut it too short. I explained that I was coloring it the soft brown color she liked, and I was not cutting it. She nodded and asked me again to please not cut it too short. I reassured her that I wouldn't do that, so she could relax. I then changed the dressing on the left side of her head, where there are still two open areas. She doesn't feel any discomfort in the area, except when I remove the tape.

She has fallen several times recently. She had two small cuts on the back of her head, and the most recent fall gave her a badly bruised right shoulder. She had full range of motion and minimal discomfort so I didn't take her to the hospital. It's a golden yellow color now, so it's healed quite well. I'll keep giving her the multiple vitamins, osteo biflex, fish oil, along with her ordered meds. Something is protecting her from more injury, or someone, or possibly a whole squadron of guardian angels. Her appetite is improved, especially if she is eating with Bri. It seems he can put it on her plate, overriding her resistance, and she will clean up her plate. She especially does this if we go out to eat. She truly does enjoy eating out. She never picks her choice of meal, she never even has a suggestion, so her and I almost always "share" a meal. She has discovered that she loves a western omelet, eggplant parm, and almost everything I prepare except for RICE. Bri teases her that her worse fear would be eating rice in his boat. She adamantly refuses any invite he extends to her to go for a ride in his boat. She tells him to "go ahead and go" and she will stay right here with the dogs.

Bri has removed the big pool from his back yard. The upkeep was overwhelming when he lives by himself and doesn't even use the pool.

My roommate is not discontent, nor is she unhappy. She usually understands sarcasm and humor quite well. She is extremely protective of the dogs, even though they only have the name "mickey." She sets the table with adequate silverware, in fact, it is usually an interesting display. The handyman has joined mom and me for lunch several times. He has said a prayer before eating with us at times, and it is not a standard prayer. At the end, we all say AMEN. The other day, Mom must have been a little hungrier than usual. After the first sentence in his prayer, she announced "AMEN." I guess she was ready to eat.

Mom sleeps on a single bed, with safety bars on both sides that she can use to pull and turn herself with. Her room is her "home," so when she says she needs to get her kids and her dogs and go home, we know the way.

This awesome lady that I reside with came through the first cranial surgery well, as we remember. The second one, where they removed all the hardware left her with a little less memory and a little more damage. The third, the muscle and skin graft (which totally failed) played a toll. Too much invasion within too little time. Our mother had always told us she would never let herself become a burden to any of her daughters. This has not occurred. I am apparently someone who comes in and helps her, so her daughters are not so directly involved? She knows she has four daughters—because we tell her she has them—not because she remembers. Considering the care and supervision and protection this awesome little lady requires, dementia has almost been a blessing. This little lady is usually very cooperative and unlike our first mother, she loves to be pampered and fussed with. She gets foot soaks and massages, manicures with rhinestones to embellish, her toenails are presently a pretty pink. Body rubs with lotions and creams, hair coloring and sets that last for the week are done regularly. She loves looking pretty and wearing nice things.

She doesn't usually like to go to bed and "leave me alone" so she says she will sit up with me. But when Bri comes for supper, and then they have ice cream and watch "their shows," she lets him escort her "home" every time without any objection. Of course, she appears quite tired by then, because she refuses to nap during the day. Sometimes I do require Bri's "suggestive encouragement" to reach a certain goal, because some nights she just firmly states that she's not taking any more pills.

I want you to know that this awesome little roommate of mine is doing the very best that she can. She makes me smile every morning when she combs her hair, not even realizing that there is no hair on the left side of her head. She is predictable, in that she has frosted flakes every single morning.

COMMUNICATING WITH
THE HANDYMAN

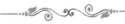

Mom was looking at one of the hanging hand towels that she made for us, one for each of the main seasons. This happened to be the one for the red/white/and blue holidays. She pointed out to me how pretty it was, because it had a strip of the patriotic material across the blue towel, and then the top part was the same material. She looked it over and commented on it often today. It seemed to have caught her attention. I think pointing out to this dear lady that she made it, along with hundreds more, only brings more attention to the memory loss. This time I agree with her and allow her to point out all the details.

She was on a nonsleep marathon this day, starting with last evening. She didn't appear tired. She was almost hyper. I, on the other hand, felt the lack of sleep that she was having. Since the handyman was here working, I laid down on the sofa, knowing I would fall asleep. I had the three little dogs on the sofa with me, and since the sofa was by the door, I thought I had all bases covered.

I guess knowledge does not always automatically come with old age. I startled awake with her talking to the handyman, and him trying to relate to her problem. She was at the kitchen island and had been working on the 6 dishes of dog food. She was holding an unopened can of dog food in her hands, and the carpenter was trying to understand what she wanted. I don't like to "assume" things, but it was a pretty sure bet to assume that he didn't follow her train of thought, let alone relate it to the situation she was talking about.

It seems she was telling him about how "they" were sleeping over there and the dogs were sleeping too. "They" were all sleeping and she didn't know if she was doing this right. Meanwhile, she has an unopened can of dog food in her hand. I asked her if she wanted him to open the can and I got an adamant "No." As I sorted out the items involved in her communication attempts she was more upset that "they" were sleeping and so were the dogs. She had already opened two other cans of dog food and mixed it with the dry food in six dog dishes. This group of canines is really having moist dog food tonight.

We talk about any and all things throughout the day. She had talked about "doing something different, and going somewhere else, because "they" need to get on with what they want to do." Of course, we are dealing with "they" again. I reassured her that we were all right where we are supposed to be, and we are doing exactly what we are supposed to be doing. I asked her who she would go to, if she made a change.

She said, "I don't know, but I have daughters up north."

I agreed with her and said, "Mom, I am your daughter."

She looked at me without saying anything. I said, "I am your oldest daughter, Judy, and I have been with you for a couple years now." That's where the conversation stopped.

Today I had all the dogs outside and was doing a little weeding. She appeared at the carport door and came down the steps. I walked over and she asked me, "Who is feeding my chickens when I'm not there? I remembered them and I don't know who is feeding them." I walked her back in the house and assured her that "Jane" is handling everything up north and Jamey and Mark are helping with the chickens. She was satisfied and the subject was closed. I understand their son Luke is in charge of the chickens, but I needed to keep information simple tonight.

I took her shopping today. It gets harder and harder to do that because she refuses to use any assistive devices. She pushes the cart, but it also requires me being in front of it and pulling and directing it in the right direction. And there are always those spurts of energy she gets which runs the cart right into my feet.

I got the special sports package from direct TV so we could watch the Pirate baseball games. I am sitting here watching it by myself. I am recording it, so I can use it for entertainment as needed in the future. Hopefully they will keep winning, so Mom can watch a good game. It will be fun, because she will tell everyone they won regardless. They better hold up their end and maintain their lead tonight. Game is 6-8 right now, so go, Buccos.

Mom wants to go without a dressing on her head wound. I was washing her hair and setting it when she wanted to let the dressing off, and she wants me to comb the hair down over it instead. I try to take her requests into serious consideration. I reminded her that there will be drainage from that area. But she was ahead of me:

"It docsn't have any, unless it gets wet in the rain." Mom's wound is open to the air at this time. I may have to put a covering over the wound if it starts raining inside the house.

She was watching a tape of the pirate game the other evening. I commented about the one player being described as a "no hitter" and said that I felt that wouldn't be a nice thing to be said about a baseball player. Again, my mom was ahead of me. Her response was, "Why would you want him to get hit?'"

Yesterday she told me she has three daughters and a son. I wasn't sure I wanted to explore this comment any further, but as always, I do.

I asked Mom if she knew their names. She said, "Yes, they are Tom and Franny—and Jody—no, not Jody. There was Fern? And OH YES, THERE WAS ME." Tom, Franny, and Fern are her three siblings, and of course, she does make number four.

We were talking about the Pirates coming home to their own field on Friday and it being "Free T shirt Day." She informed me that Mike Rattay had taken her to the new ball field. She told me that there was another lady there with them, Mike, his wife, and Herself. She said they did a lot of walking, and they were by the first base. She was trying to remember who was on first base. She said she was "racking her brain." And I thought that sounded dangerous in her situation, so I texted Mike and asked him. He named a few of the first basemen during that time, but she said that was not the name.

He then named Willie Stargell. She immediately told me that was him. When I said that he wasn't the first baseman during that game, she assured me he was. Who am I to argue, because I wasn't there so I informed Michael that Willie was on base that day. He jumped right on my hay wagon and agreed. I told Mike that I'll bet he never thought, on the day he took his mom and his mother-in-law to a ball game, along with "his wife" (no name Jean) that it would mean so much to her at this time in her life. Thank you, Michael, for allowing that memory to be so good for this lady today.

She fixes the dog dishes daily, and always does six. She always asks if that is right. She feeds Bri's dog, "the brown dog" along with our five. A few times Lucy wasn't here and I tried to assure Mom that she only needed to fix five bowls that day. That didn't work. Somehow she is fixated on six bowls, and that's how it will be. Welcome to our dinner time, Lucy.

Yesterday we invited the handyman to stay for supper. We set the table for four, but Bri wasn't here yet. Mom went in the living area and sat on the sofa. She stayed there and when Bri came in, he invited her out to the table. She said she wasn't eating, and that there wasn't room because other people were here and coming. He assured her that her seat was at the table, and he had to work at getting her off the sofa and out to the table. When she got there, he was helping her into her chair but she wouldn't sit. She kept asking where he was sitting, and he said he was in the same place as always. She wouldn't sit down, and was asking me where my seat was. I showed her my seat and started fixing her plate. She said she wasn't hungry and didn't want anything. I made her a half hotdog in a bun, baked beans, and half baked potato. We put lots of butter on the potato and she ate every bite. Even though the handyman was here several times, she got anxious with 4 at the table. The conversation at the table was between the worker and Bri, so it was not something she was included in. It's interesting to watch how she perceives things, because she doesn't talk unless the conversation is addressed directly to her—and one on one. Fortunately Bri does this on a regular basis—so she was made to be part of the conversation at times—on her level—with her interests. He always asks her if she sewed today.

She usually says she does. She irons his work shirts, and I leave them on the hanger as she puts them. The sleeves are often totally inside out. He told me there was one sleeve inside the other when he went to put it on. He said it makes him smile in the mornings. We have a keeper here. Ironing makes her feel useful, and Bri smiles at 4:15 AM.

She is always doing the dishes, or putting hot water in the dishpan and putting them to soak. The other day she was frustrated and trying to do something with the drain. I walked over when she told me she couldn't get it to stop leaking. Now, I have a plastic dishpan in a large enamel sink. She was running the water into the sink, not the dishpan. She was upset because she couldn't get the water to stay in the dishpan, even though she was running the water outside of the dishpan. Of course, it was running down the drain and she couldn't get it to stop.

I asked her to peel an onion, and we would have it for our hotdogs for supper. I watched and observed as she worked at peeling the onion, and peeling—and peeling—and still peeling. I remembered the day I had her frying the bacon. She fried it—and fried it, and turned it—and continued to fry—until I had to intervene and remove the basically burnt charcoaled bacon from the pan. There doesn't seem to be an ending—a finish line—to her tasks. I took the onion and thanked her so much. We are now down to about half onion, which I diced for our meal. She will help with any task, but she doesn't know when the task is complete.

It's like she doesn't know the ramifications that some things could bring concerning her balance, feeding the dogs her cookies, not drinking enough liquids, letting her head wound open to the air, refusing to use the walker with the seat—although I did ride her back to bed last night on the seated walker—after she watched Bri wheeling himself around and through the living area—telling her how neat it was, cause his legs were tired. He breaks through to her more often than you know. He calls her his grandma and tells her he is her grandson but he knows she only knows him as "familiar." That's the label I carry also, because I often get told how "they wanted things done" or how "they put that there" or I guess the other night someone came in and folded all our material. Mom didn't know who "it" was, but they did a nice job. Indirect compliment, unknown acknowledgement, wondering if someday it will occur to her how many of those people I am? It doesn't matter. I know who she is. She is comfortable with me unless I fall asleep on the sofa, then she becomes anxious.

I can live for two months on one good compliment.

She's watching the Pirate game now. She doesn't know which team is ours, but I continue to narrate them. I will ask her questions during the game, and she repeats some of the things that the commentator says. Or she repeats a portion of the statement. She still doesn't understand why they make them so long now, because "they were never this long before." "Time" is difficult for her.

She was sewing this afternoon. I sat at the table with her. Nothing comes easy to her anymore, nor does it get more familiar as she does repeated tasks

I asked her if she was "okay"? She was touching her head. She said the noises were getting to her. I explained that she can hear the noises because there is no airtight dressing over her wound. I told her she was hearing noises because it was the air moving in and out. She sat down and I cleaned the wound and replaced the dressing. There were no more noises. She told me that she had asked the other girl to curl the hair down over it but it's not long enough. That other girl sure does set the bar high for my caretaker tasks.

At supper, Bri and her took a few of their pills. He is going to bring over all his vitamins and supplements so they can take their pills together. They take them one at a time, at the same time. She doesn't hesitate to "play" that game. Tonight she wrapped four of them up in a napkin and laid them under the little saucer on the table. She said she was "saving them for later." Tomorrow Bri and her will have the same amount at the supper table. Thank you Bri. They take a pill, click their water glass, and say "cheers." It works wonders with Mom.

Some things I hear that I don't have an answer for. She had a bed pillow under one arm, one blue top and a pair of slipper socks in her hand. She said, "I'm going across the street to my mother's house."

"Where did your father-in-law go?"

"He was standing right there in that aisle."

"Where did that man go?"

"He was dressed in a suit. He was right there, and then he was gone."

While eating half Klondyke with Bri, "This is really good. I don't think I ever had this before."

"I don't have a car. I don't have a phone. Would you call someone to help me get these kids together so I can get them out of here?"

"I need to find a place for me and my dogs for the night."

I assure her that she is staying with me tonight, along with all the dogs. She is so grateful and continues to thank me.

"I am so tired of them doing the same things over and over. They throw the ball, then they run, then they throw it again, and they run again. The same thing over and over." She is talking about her formerly beloved Pirates. "They changed the rules again. The game never used to be this long. They keep making it longer and longer." My only guess is at one time, the ballgames must have been shorter than nine innings?

"Is this all that's on? Is there anything better on?" She has no interest in TV shows anymore.

"Have you seen Judy? Where did she go?"

And the day she got so upset with the person taking care of her in the house. "Why are you doing this to me? Why do you have me locked in and I can't get out? I have heard of this happening to other people, but I never thought you would do it to me. Call someone so I can get out of here." Meanwhile she is addressing a storm door that is propped open and the outside door left wide open.

It was about time for Bri to arrive home after work when she went down the three steps onto the carport and was standing by the gate. I left her go but kept constant watch of her activity. Bri pulled in and got out of his truck. He addressed Mom and said "Hi Mawmaw…How was your day?"

She looked at him and said "I want to go home."

Bri said, "Okay, come on, Mawmaw." She almost ran to him and he put her in the truck and they left. He never misses a beat when it comes to Mom. They were gone a short while. He pulled into the same place he had just been and helped Mom out of the truck. She asked him how he got her here—and when she saw the dining room table—she was so glad to "be back home."

Bri had taken her down a few blocks, then they went through a drive through car wash. This distracted her thoughts. She was returned to the exact same space she had just left—yet she was so glad to "be back." Fortunately, I was there when she returned—and not the other person who had locked her in.

Apparently, her own world isn't a place that she can find her way through these days. I welcome her into everything I do. I'm just too tired trying to keep in touch with a lady that has lost touch with herself and everyone she knows. I still can't "give back" as much as she has given in the first eighty-eight years that we were blessed with her presence.

Any time I talk on the phone, Mom hears one half the conversation and it gets misunderstood. She always listens, and if I walk outside, she asks me if I'm going to talk about her. She has problems carrying on a conversation and is always looking to me to lead the conversation. She wants to be able to carry on a conversation, but when she attempts that, it doesn't happen. We talk all day long, as I try to encourage her to use her brain. Sometimes she can pull from her memory.

Other times, like tonight as she sat on the sofa close to her bedtime, she looked at me and asked, "Do you know where I am to be now, 'cause I need to go somewhere?"

I told her she was right where she needed to be—that her, her kids, her dogs, and me would be sleeping here tonight, and she has her own room in her house right here. She always seems so very relieved when she hears that. Tonight she answered me that she was ready to go there now. Before I tuck her in, we wash her face and put her favorite cream on her face. I kiss her forehead and tell her that she is "so loved by so many." Then I reassure her that I will be here all night. And I remind her that I am right outside her room. And tell her tomorrow will be a brand-new day. She thanks me. She doesn't want the door shut tight, and there are nightlights in her room, and lights in the hall that throw light under her door. Things are so different than they were before her injury and her surgeries.

EYE EXAM

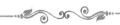

Bri took today (Friday) off. It was a safety day that they had to take before the end of the month, or they lose it. So I made Mom and me an appointment to have our eyes examined. I wanted to make sure she was seeing as well as she could, since she's had two more craniotomies since her last script. The eye doctor was great. She had been updated on Mom's status, and I wasn't sure how they would be able to assess her. She used some tactics that are used for kids, and she took her time with our mother. As it was, she could only improve her script ever so slightly. When I checked with her insurance, new frames were covered up to $100, the exam was covered, and the only charge for new glasses would be $59. We picked out two frames, since she didn't want the little plastic and metal nose pieces. She wanted the solid plastic nose piece. We picked two pair that looked good on her and she liked. One was exactly what she had, so we picked the other pair. This way she will have two pair of pretty much the same script. Bri was there with her the whole time, and then sat with her while I got my eyes examined. I wasn't as fortunate, because my eyes have been burning and tired, and I haven't enjoyed reading or computer time for some time now. I have dry eyes and some clogged tear ducts, so I am to use artificial tears, and warm compresses to my eyes. She also increased my script 3 levels. We shall get them in a few days. I also got an expanded eye visual field in my lenses, which the doctor recommended.

Mom kept wanting to leave and come back another time. I'm not sure why. We then took her out to eat and came home afterward. She eats so very well when we are out, it's amazing. She drank a large Carmel iced coffee and loved it.

She was to help Bri mow tonight but she kept wanting me to walk her and her dogs home because they needed to eat. She fixed the dog food here and we fed the dogs. She still needed to get home because her dogs hadn't eaten yet. When this happens, I know the evening is going to be difficult. I pointed out her two dogs while they were eating. I told her this was her home and those were her dogs, and they were eating. She said "stop it, and just walk me home so I can feed my own dogs." I told her we would get her where she needed to go after the dogs all finished.

Bri came over on the mower, but she didn't want to get on. She stood on the carport and watched him mow the front yard. He stopped and asked her if she wanted to help him mow several more times, but she declined again. We are in a negative type frame of mind tonight.

Her half-moon night light shines in her room over her bed. I told her she sleeps under the "moon over Miami." It casts just enough light for her to see well enough to use the potty chair. So she goes to bed with her "nonslippy socks" on her feet and the "moon over Miami." I'm watching the monitor right now and can hear her snoring. I think when I hear that sound, she is truly at peace. How confusing it must be to wander around in her world. Sometimes she calls me Judy but is always telling me that "she" or "they" or "those other people" were here also. I try not to correct her, knowing it doesn't change anything anyway.

But today, I asked her who those other people were and were they here today.

She said, "Yes, where did your sisters go? They were here."

So girls, my dear sisters, all three of you, if you are reading this, when you come to visit, you could at least let me know and spend a few moments with me. I think it's rude that you just show up in Mom's world and not mine.

God put me on earth to accomplish a certain number of tasks. As of today, I am so far behind I need to live forever.

We would bring her home in a minute if I thought it would work in her favor. She is so anxious with anyone in her home space. She is content in her house with all six dogs. She is upset when we are away from home and don't have the dogs. I don't really know if she would know anyone, but I know she doesn't now. I know she can't carry on a conversation without much help. I know that sometimes she tried to converse, but it's not easy to follow. She struggles and struggles with word finding. I deliberately keep Jody's soap operas on and tell her we have to watch them so we can find out what's going on every day. I question her throughout the show—as to "what are they trying to do now, Mom?" or "did they tell him about the baby yet?" or "is that women telling him the truth?" She loves giving me her version of the answers— and she loves feeling that she's explaining something to me. I've found this is a good activity for us. She repeats some of the things that were said, mixed in with her idea of what's going on. This is often her time to shine, and I let her shine. Does it follow the story line? Oh hell no, but whose keeping score? I'm relishing how good she feels at these times.

I know that a lot of her actions are not those of our other mother. The last two surgeries were not so kind to her. There is zero chance of getting her head wound to heal up at this point. I use flesh colored bandages and pull her longer curls down over the top of the dressing for her. We try to keep the bandage side out of most of her pictures, to maintain her image. I do not make fun of our mother in any way, but I do hold onto my humor with every breath. Sometimes I can share it with her and pull her right in. Other times I shield her from it so she doesn't misread its" intent. Sometimes her questions are priceless, other times they make you wonder how she came up with that thought.

Bri always sides with her against me and that makes her laugh.

She doesn't refuse her pills anymore. She takes them with Bri, as they both say "cheers. He has shown her how to take the pill in her hand, click the glass, then take the pill and then a drink of water. We have had a time where she takes the pill in her hand, clicks the glass with Bri's, puts the pill in the water glass, then takes a drink.

We will probably sew tomorrow as she likes being at the machine. I will no longer try to get straight lines from her. I will just help guide the fabric, so I don't have to thread the needle or fix the bobbin' many, many times. When that happens, she gets frustrated and I don't want that. Another piece of our Sanford life so you don" t miss a beat of "life with Mawmaw."

MID-JULY

Jumping around with my note takin.

Tonight, after supper, Mom helped to clear the table. She puts things wherever she can find a spot for them. Sometimes the half can of moist dog food ends up in the freezer. Sometimes the condiments or jelly end up in the cupboard. Sometimes things end up in the dish with a napkin stuffed onto the top to keep it covered. It's always a great effort on her behalf—and it lends me another period of scavenger hunting. Her sincere efforts and the need to feel "useful" far exceeds any of the end results. Tonight, she was going to help with the dishes. I was trying to pay some bills online, when she came in and sat down in the TV room. I turned around and watched the water running full blast into the sink. I waited, what seemed minutes, and then asked, "Do you know the water is running?"

She said, "Yes, I'm filling up the sink with water so the dishes soak." And she never moved a muscle.

I waited another long second and said, "It appears the dishpan is full and running over."

She never took her gaze from the TV and responded with, "Okay."

Another long second and I asked if she wanted me to turn the water off. Her tasks don't seem to have an ending, unless I am monitoring what she does and help her make closure. It's like the thought involving that task just dropped off the end of the neuron and died from lack of oxygen.

I tell her about a daughter's golden anniversary. I tell her of a granddaughter's graduation from nursing school. I tell her about a relative dying at the young age of 50, and how he was related to grandma Clarks brother's family. I tell her about people that ask about her at church and at the funeral home. Her face shows no acknowledgment of who they might be. She wants to sew at the sewing machine, but the machine "isn't working"—just as the paring knives are so dull…and the scissors don't cut like they did at first. I help her sew from corner to corner on a square patch. I sit right beside her, as she needs close supervision. She resews over the very same stitch line that she just did.

She will prepare six bowls of food for the dogs, and always wants to know what she can add to the dry food. We either use some canned dogfood, or cut up some table scraps to make their food look good—for our mother's sake.

The dogs are all fed before our supper is ready, and Mom constantly moves the bowls around on the floor. As a dog walks away, she picks up the bowl and follows them around, trying to get them to eat more. She is so very preoccupied with feeding the dogs and giving them treats. We are eating supper, and she tells the dogs that she needs to get them something to eat, because she knows they are hungry. I tell Mom to look around at all the bowls on the floor, and remind her that they were just all fed. I remind her that they were so happy with the way she fixed their food that they ate till they were full. My heart follows her as she looks at the white Mickie, who has her paws on her knee, and tells her that she just ate. I know that she only repeats what I said to compromise. If I give her access to a bag of treats—it totally disappears. She doesn't know when she gave them treats, just that they don't have a treat this very minute. White Mickie will take treats or eat food until she throws up—gagging and gagging. This our mother also forgets as soon as the episode is over. I find half cookies on the floor between her paws as often as the cookie jar is handy.

I am trying very hard to get Mom to drink two liters of water a day. I work from her arising until I walk her back to bed—and we can't make the goal. If she gets one liter in, it's been a good day. I know she needs more fluids, so I tell her if she just drinks all day and does nothing else I will be so very happy.

Yesterday I sat three plates at the table and she asked if we needed silverware. I said, "Yes, we do." I had to show her which drawer the silverware was in…when I sat down to eat there were two spoons in the middle of the table…we each had a fork…no knife…and we each had about three spoons. There must have been a sale on spoons today—but the look of amusement and acceptance on Brian's face as he decides which tool to use is beautiful. She does nothing wrong in this house, and he will vouch for her without question.

You have to be available to the invisible voices that are swirling around you.

I'm in sunny Florida—so let me tell you a little about my day. It starts early, because I am used to Bri stopping every morning at four thirty to have coffee, drop off Lucy, and pick up a fully packed lunch before he heads to his job. We have coffee for an hour and watch the news to see who was shot in the last twenty-four hours. So living with five dogs—we have all settled into this routine. Now Bri is battling with bipolar every minute of his life—and he tells me that this "hour" is the best part of his day. He calls from work several times to check on me and Mawmaw. Then he comes for supper every night about five or so. Mom sets the table so we may have nine forks between us, three knives and no spoons. The next night it may be different but it is seldom the right amount. She helps clear the table after we eat. She has put the peanuts in the fridge and the canned—and opened—dog food into the cupboard. Now when I find that can—it has become quite odorous. I keep harmful chemicals or products out of her reach since she put the Clorox into the fridge one day—and tried to give the dogs a treat—which was a dishwasher pod. She made herself a sandwich with peanut butter and my strawberry scented shampoo one day—after I had washed my hair at the kitchen sink and left the shampoo set there. Back to my day—Bri came over for coffee and then had breakfast with Mawmaw. He then had errands to do and the need to repair his hot tub, so he left. I assisted Mawmaw at the sewing machine, which she loves. The problem is, she needs constant supervision and guidance. She doesn't remember how to use the foot pedal.

July Ends

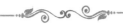

I am so tired these days. She lives my life, so if I sit down, she watches me. If I fall asleep on the sofa, she moves to the chair at the dining room table and waits for me to wake up. She stays very quiet and then tells me about the ones who were sleeping "over there." Last night she told me she had a problem. I had helped her to the table to have a cookie before bed. I asked her what her problem was. She told me that the one who dropped her off here, never came back to pick her up—so she didn't know where she would sleep tonight. I asked her where the one would take her to if she came back and picked her up. She said it was up to Elderton. I have no idea how Elderton came from her memory, but she sundowns every night not knowing where she could stay. She is so relieved when I tell her she will stay with me and all the dogs—and I have a room that's all hers. A few nights ago she came out at midnight, thinking it was morning. I put her back to bed, and I woke up to water running in the kitchen sink. She was up again and told me she was going to help. Again I put her back to bed. She has no concept of time or place, and talks of her sister "Franney" more than her present family. She calls Bri "the boy" when she asks about him—even though he tells her she is his grandmother. Lucy is the "brown dog." She never knows or calls Annie by her name. She is sometimes "white Mickie." I feed Rickie up on the kitchen island so the other dogs let him alone. She knows a dog goes up there, but never knows which one. She wondered why he wouldn't stay one day—after she put Rusty up there. Her life—on her own—involves feeding the dogs. That's the only thing she can almost complete on her own—almost.

291

How our world—as we knew it—changed with her. She would be so upset if she knew what her condition is. We protect her former image with everything when we can. Bri only posts pictures and events that make her look good. It makes her sound like she is doing so well. That's the facade that Facebook lets people partake in.

What do we live for; if not to make life less difficult for one another?

COME ON IN AUGUST

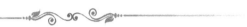

I've been using emails to tell my story, but I haven't been on this sight for a while. Today, Mom worked at getting the dishes washed and putting the clean dishes away. I watched for a while and then asked her if she needed some help.

She said, "No, I'm just finding empty spots to put these."

Oh, let the games begin again.

The other night Bri's red skinned peanuts that he uses on their ice cream nights was safely placed in the refrigerator. We had two bags of peeled apples in the fridge from a few days ago. I asked her if she could get them out of the fridge. She turned around a few times, and then asked me "which one of these is it in?" I pointed to the big white thing right beside her, and she thanked me. I watched as she opened the fridge and found the one bag of apples quite quickly and then watched her search for the second bag. It looked exactly like the first bag. She picked up the butter container, she picked up the cold cut container…and several other plastic items in the fridge. I watched her for what seemed like forever. I walked out to the kitchen and said "let me help you." I reached in and picked up the second bag of apples and handed it to my mother. She told me she had looked, but couldn't find it. I just explained that it was hidden behind the egg carton.

This explanation satisfied her as she carried both bags to the counter. She then asked me what she was to do with them. I demonstrated how to slice the apples and lay them in the pie dish, so we could tell when we had enough for a nice full pie. This is how my mother used to estimate enough apples for her very full pie, but this memory has lost its way. I left Mom to slice the apples. When I rejoined her, all the apples were back in the bags. She had an explanation, but she wasn't finding the proper words. So we just picked up the few steps to get ready for the pie crust. Mom doesn't have her recipes and tells me she doesn't know how to add the needed things to the apples. When we were ready to put the top crust on, I told her to cut a few slits in the top. She didn't know what I meant, so I handed her the butter knife and told her to just cut a few little vents. She was unsure how to make them, or where to place them. So much is gone.

Later when I was helping her sew, she forgot how to use the foot pedal. She thought maybe her shoes were too big. Then she thought the machine was not turned on. I finally picked up the foot pedal and showed her how it works, only she was to use her foot to make it go. I was using my hand. She sewed a few inches and then stopped because she said it wasn't sewing. I checked out the machine, and told her she was doing a good job. I finally had to show her the seam line, along with the fact that the needle was threaded. Today was not our best day. I've tried to tell her how important drinking water is—but she feels she is drinking too much…and it makes her go to the bathroom. She has now decided that she needs to cut back on eating because she is "full." Not to mention the fact that she no longer thinks the pills make any difference, so she doesn't need to take them anymore.

My only saving grace—I tell her that if she goes in the hospital…and she will if I quit pushing her to drink water—that the dogs will have to be in their crates while she is hospitalized—because I will be with her. She hates this; she doesn't like the dogs to be in their crates, even if they go into them on their own and sleep. She has been worried that Mickie is just laying around and sleeping all the time. Where did this concern come from? Most of the time she keeps her hands entwined into Mickie's harness while she sits beside our Mom. I often wish Mickie could verbalize her concerns to me.

Tonight she was not going to sit at the table—she said she wasn't going to "join our party." Fortunately Brian can always get her to come to the table and "join the party."

A REVIEW OF THE LAST SEVERAL YEARS

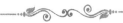

I'm going to write up an email tonight, to keep family informed. Those are the people that were such an important part of a certain lady's life. She will turn ninety-one in a few months—that would be quite a status marker in other circumstances. This lady had a severe cerebral bleed, followed with surgery on Labor Day two years ago, Monday. It's been two years plus that we had noticed that things just weren't "right" with this special lady. She did some remarkable recovery following this surgery, and even traveled to Florida so we could keep her active during the very dormant cold months up north. Sans the broken right hip incident in March of the following year, and the upper teeth removal—We were pleased. Even during her post op period of her hip repair, she didn't "remember" that she had broken her hip, so she didn't "remember" that she had a large incision and it was supposed to be difficult to keep moving and stay active—so she did it anyway. I constantly was reminding her, "Watch your hip, Mom," and her usual response was, "Why, what's wrong with my hip?" Some things you just can't make up. She continued to progress fairly well. She even had a "smile" that she would have cherished—in another time. She was always self-conscious of her teeth, therefore her smile. After her dental removal and placement of an upper denture—she flashes a smile that is beautiful. Now we have already had a second denture made, after she lost it one night, and we found it in a million pieces. It came out of her mouth and Annie chewed on it all night. I remember calling the dental clinic and explaining that her denture was ruined. They told me to bring in the pieces and they could fix it. I smiled as I explained, "I don't think so, not this time. I'm sure part of it is in her dog Annie, and I'm not about to follow her around for several days."

The wound on her temporal area had started to drain. On assessment, the surgeon felt she must have been rejecting the metal plates and screws used to replace the bone of her cranium that was removed to excise the clotted material putting pressure on her brain. Surgery was scheduled for August—and the incision was even larger that the initial surgical line. This is the third major surgery with anesthesia in less than a year. This would be tough on a young person, but this lady was about to turn ninety. The wound on her temporal area still didn't close and she required a dressing over the sight. Months of observation resulted in a plan to do a muscle graft followed by a skin graft to cover the wound. This was scheduled for December. She tolerated the surgery but the wound continued to drain. IV antibiotics were ordered through the next six weeks, at which time we left the northern state to head to Florida. It would be much easier to keep her active while healing when we are not closed in during the winter months. She received IV antibiotics for six weeks and was followed by infection control clinic here in Florida. This plan sounded good, in the planning state. Mom's head wound did not heal. Both the muscle and the skin graft failed. An area of cranial bone is exposed, with two areas at the edge of the bone that remain open—and continue to drain. She has a dressing in place over this area at all times. FAST-FORWARD TO TODAY. AND LIFE AS IT IS IN HER WORLD NOW. She is weaker. She is probably dehydrated, as she barely sips water. Her appetite is decreasing. She weighed 129 a few days ago. Her tolerance for walking has decreased drastically. When I take her "shoppin' walkin,'" she holds on to the cart, but I pull both her and the cart. This gets difficult when there is anything heavy in the cart. There is no "push" coming from her anymore. I put an elevated seat with arm rests over the toilet, as she can't get up and down independently anymore. I elevated the legs on the potty chair at her bedside. I guide her or assist her or do things for herself at all times. She wouldn't brush her teeth, if I didn't push the issue and prepare things and take her into the bathroom. I bath her and change her clothing. She wears depends at all times. There is a handrail on both sides of her bed, to assist her in getting in and out and turning while in the bed. I also added a lifting pad under her hips to help in turning her and positioning her. Her lower back hurts at times, following her most recent fall in her bedroom. She had a small bruise on her upper arm, but still tells me her right rib/lower back area hurts at times.

I often sit her on the seated walker to take her back to bed at night. She doesn't want to go to bed until she knows that I am also going to bed. Occasionally she goes on "all-nighter marathons," where she is up every hour thinking it is time to get up, then she is wide awake all day. She is very unstable in ambulation, and often tries to pick things up off the floor, and continues to topple over. It seems she always lands on her head—you figure? We've already had to have her new glasses refitted because of one of her falls. Bri ordered a bed alarm which gives me more warning that she is getting out of bed— if I've fallen asleep. I have a baby monitor on her bed at all times. Sometimes, no matter what we do, we can't protect her from her own actions. She is obsessed with "feeding the dogs." They must tell her that they are hungry—all the time. She has no concept of time or place. So she is always wanting to feed the dogs, even though we just did less than one hour ago. This goes on throughout her entire day. Annie puts her feet up on Mom's chair all the time—and this is when she tells Mom that she is hungry. Every action of the dogs is interpreted as being hungry. If they are laying all over the room and sleeping, she tells me they are worn out because they haven't been fed. Now that Mickie is diabetic, she can't be fed all the time. There is no comprehension of this in Mom's world. I have explained that she needs a shot when she eats, and that's only once or twice a day. She just explains it back to me, "But she is hungry. Some of the other dogs got to eat, but she didn't."

Mom is never thirsty, and she figures if she doesn't eat or drink, she won't have to go to the "restroom" as often. I can't explain this concept away. The only battle I can win is—"if you have to go into the hospital Mom, because she aren't drinking or eating—the dogs will have to go into their boxes while you are at the hospital, and I

297

know you don't like the dogs locked in their boxes." We were in the van today about 4:00 PM—and Bri said to me "she's getting really upset and anxious. You are taking too long. We are going to need to take her home." It happens every day about the same time, whether we are out or we are at home. It is called "sundowning."—and she does it every single day. Bri thought it was because we weren't home, but it happens at home every day. I explained that it happens shortly before he gets home from work every day. Sometimes I just have to throw him under the bus and let Mom know that he will be home in a few minutes to help her fix things—things that I apparently refuse to fix. He picks up the ball and carries it like a pro—and she succumbs to his presence, his calming voice, and the fact that he takes her side and always makes things right. We bounce off of one another—and it seems to work for this little lost lady.

No, she doesn't know us. But she knows us as being familiar—and that is comforting to her. She never knows where her home is—until I open her bedroom door, and then she knows she's home. We are discussing the holidays, but it puts a lot onto Bri as far as driving us back and forth. He is thinking about changing his job from Disney over to Cape Canaveral in a month or so—so if he starts a new job, it may be six day weeks with ten hour days. Right now we have no plans. Each time I hear Mom fall, I wonder whether we will be heading to the hospital "this time." So we are working on Christmas ideas and gifts—Mom watches everything I do. Sometimes she will wash the dishes, but mostly she just watches anymore.

Mom is our 24-7 activity, sometimes entertaining, sometimes interesting, sometimes challenging, sometimes frustrating, sometimes exhausting—but never can we match the care she gave us all as kids and as adults—or the care and attention she gave our kids during their lifetimes, she set an example that puts the bar pretty high.

She doesn't remember this—she doesn't remember having four daughters—but we do. I just try to imagine what it's like inside her head, even for a short time. I watch her struggle with word finding or trying to think—and I realize how easy my job is, compared to the one she's living in. Bri does so well with her, because he says he knows what it's like when your brain doesn't work the right way.

A Message to My Mother

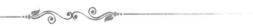

I watch you open the door and walk down the three steps to the carport. I watch you stand at the bottom, holding onto the railing and look all around. You wait a few minutes, then turn and come back up. You walk over to the sofa and sit down...without a word. No words are needed Mom. I can tell by the look on your face. You started somewhere, but you didn't know where. You came back in before you forgot how to do that. You feel safe and comfortable inside our Sunset home. You sometimes seem a little frightened outside—you don't move away from the bottom step or let go of the railing, maybe the world is too big out there. You have said to me so often, "Don't forget me." I won't, Mom—I know where you are every minute of your days—and your nights.

You are seated at the table while I lift the food from the stove. There is a container of diced onions and the soft butter already on the table. The silverware and plates and napkins are in place. You spread some diced onions on your plate, and then start buttering them. These you lift onto the red napkin, which you then roll up. You take your butter knife and try to slice the napkin with its contents. Brian says to you, "We'll save this till later, Mawmaw, 'cause Mom has other stuff for us to eat now. Mom, put this in the fridge for later, okay?"

You have fallen several times. We are so lucky. Your guardian angel's safety net has cushioned the landing. You are usually bending over to pick something up, or attempt a task—so you are already close to the floor. You always land on your head, but you have had some sore ribs, sore lower back, and also hips. We purchased a memory foam pad for your bed, and you seem more comfortable. You aren't as restless with finding a comfy position.

You also have fallen asleep the last few nights to the sound of crickets and summer night sounds. It's as if we are sitting on the back porch of the farmhouse, swinging on the swing, and listening to the sounds of the evening. I may even hear some of the frogs from the pond in the night. Maybe this gives you the feeling of just where home might be. It's in your heart and mind Mom—but since some of those parts aren't connecting as they should—we will put them in a white noise box and make them available to you. If they help your busy mind relax and rest—goal accomplished.

You stand and watch me cut out a "butterfly" dress for my granddaughter. I suggest you walk around the kitchen island for exercise. You take me up on the suggestion and begin circling the island. You are concerned that you might get dizzy. I don't think you will be going that fast Mom, so give it a try. For a few rounds, you count the "laps"—but after about three, I ask, "What lap are you on Mom?"

By then, you have forgot that you are counting and answer, "I don't know, I will just go till I'm tired."

I answer, "Good idea, let me know when you get tired." Immediate response, "I'm tired now." You are so precious, Mom. You are so innocent. You are so helpless, one of the things that was never in your vocabulary.

You know your dog's name is "Mickie." You have two dogs, sometimes you think you have three. Only one name stays with you, so we have white Mickie and black Mickie. Brian's dog is "the brown dog." My three dogs are lost somewhere in the midst. None of them have names. Mickie and Annie have always been protective and loyal to our mother. They still are, but you can tell they are a bit confused. It's been over two years now. You have had to leave them four times to be hospitalized. Each time you have come home confused and lost. They don't understand, but they are adjusting. They see our mother surface at times, and then they are climbing into her lap. You are always worried about getting their leashes, and taking them home late afternoon. It happens every day. I call it "sun downing." Brian goggled it, trying to understand it better. We are still working at ways to make this transformation less traumatic for your world.

You have been coming outside and sitting more frequently lately. You will watch me mow or water plants for a short period, and then you are done. I pace my activities around your attention span. I'm usually out of energy about the time you have moved on anyway. It's like my battery powered weed eater. When the battery pack dies down and needs recharged—so do I.

Brian is about to change jobs, and his hours will change also. Often you are awake when he stops in the morning on his way to work. He goes back to your room and tells you he will be leaving for work, but you get to go back to sleep. When he tells you it is 4:30 in the morning, you are amazed that he is up so early. You do fall back asleep, usually.

Your nightstand is now positioned against your potty chair, which is pinned between the nightstand and the bed. Your bed has a railing on both sides, which helps you with changing positions. Hopefully there will be no more potty chair and Mawmaw landings across the bedroom floor at 2:30 am. By the way, the large skin tear you collected on that landing is knitting together well. If only we could have gotten your head wound to knit together. I don't see that happening. I think we will be dressing the open wound on the left side of your head for the rest of your life.

We had the three neighbor ladies in for supper on labor day. I wasn't sure how that would work out, but they all offered to leave if you became upset. Bri sat with you most of the afternoon, along with some medication—and it was a nice time. You listened and watched, but because multiple people were in the conversation, you withdrew. Bri sat beside you and maintained the one-on-one that you can take part in. You smiled and looked comfortable for the meal and dessert, but then you were done. Bri excused both you and he, and knew you needed to be distanced from conversation that you couldn't follow.

When Bri comes home from work, I take a back seat. I know that you work best with One-on-one—that is the only way your mind can follow. He has other things to talk to you about, from our events of the day. You relate well to his voice, his presence, and his calming demeanor. (those words, calming demeanor, and the name Brian in the same sentence will go questioned by the rest of the world—but when he is with you Mom—that is exactly how he is). If his day is too rough, he excuses himself and recharges in his own space. He tells me he knows what it is like when your brain don't work like everyone else's. He has to stay with a routine to function well. He has to use medication and environmental aides to stop his mind enough to sleep at night. He knows when he awakens each morning, he will have to fight his own mind to get through the happenings of his work day. I watch him deal with his own battles, and I watch you wrestle with yours—and I realize that of the three of us—my days are the easiest.

Today I fixed the dogs food. I also fixed our plates for supper. As you started to eat, I sat the dogs' dishes on the floor, and they all started to eat. As you took a bite of food, you looked around at the dogs eating. You said, "Now this is nice. We are eating and so are the dogs. I like that." Now it sounds like we don't do this same thing every night. It sounds like this is the first time we have fed the dogs and ourselves at the same time. It's really sad to think that our mother doesn't know that we feed the dogs every day at supper time. But then, she never knows where she is going to stay at night. She never knows how she is going to get her dogs "gathered" and transported. I try to imagine what it would be like to not know where I was going to lay my head at night. Not just tonight, but every night.

In search of my mother's garden, I found my own.

Mom has finished eating. She says, "May I be excused."

I turn and look at her face to see if she is being serious, or sarcastic. She is serious.

I say, "Yes, you may."

She thanks me.

Tonight I offered our mother half Klondike before bed. She looked at me with a puzzled look. I said it's white ice cream with a chocolate coating. She agreed to just have a small one. I cut a Klondike in half, then cut her half into bite size pieces. She took a few bites and informed me that it was really good. I ask if she remembered having them before. She didn't think she had—After she finished it she told me how good it was, so I told her we would have to have them more often. (Mom used to have half Klondike every night before bed before the changes of the last two years.)

I was sewing a Christmas gift with Mom watching closely. I showed her that I had used a "double seam" to keep the stiff material from irritating Samantha's arms. I told her that she had taught me how to make a double seam many years ago. She studied it, and then told me that I would have to show her how to do it now.

I put a small table covering on the table outside this morning and Mom ate breakfast out in the carport. I showed her the crocheted edges and the appliques on all the corners and asked her if she remembered doing it. She said she didn't remember, but she used to do that edging. She studied the crochet and tried to explain to me how the stitch is done—but couldn't put it into words. You could see that she knew she used to do it—but had no idea how to begin now. I told her that I watched her and her mother crochet years ago, but it never became comfortable to me, it was always hard work. Then I told her I would rather sew, and it changed her focus.

Today she was watching Mickie chew a bone in front of the sofa. She asked me what I was going to do with him. I sat down and asked her what she wanted me to do with him. She said she didn't know, but she wanted someone to take care of him. I informed her "he" wasn't going anywhere—that we were keeping him, and all the dogs will be staying here at our home with us. The relief on her face made me feel so sad—I told her that we will take care of our dogs just like we do every day, and nobody will be getting our dogs. I told her we are keeping them here, where they can go in and out and play in the fenced yard whenever they want. She thanks me again. The other night she was telling Brian of her concern with what to do with the dogs. He informed her that we would feed them and keep them right here at the house. She was concerned that she didn't have money to pay for them right now, because she didn't have her wallet. Brian just informed her that we will take care of it "tomorrow." Thank God our "tomorrows" are always a brand-new day on a brand-new page with no notes scribbled from the day before.

I have her monitor on, and I'm sitting here with the Pirate game one. I can hear the crickets from the summer nights setting on her sleep therapy machine. It made me think, I don't hear crickets down here in Florida. We have a ton of little lizard like creatures—lots of squirrels running about, and too many barking dogs. But our summer nights don't sound the same as they do, or did, up north. Funny how things surface when a memory is stimulated. Mom has lost that ability. Maybe the machine will help supplement the connection that's been altered in her own memory—and she can just enjoy and relax to the sounds.

ANOTHER DAY IN OUR NEIGHBORHOOD

Mom's bedroom door is left partially open, with a wooden child gate across the doorway to keep the dogs from running in and out. She woke up this morning, put on her shoes and opened her door the full way. Four dogs were sitting by the gate watching her every move, quietly. I took the gate down and wished her a "good morning." "another beautiful day in the neighborhood." She looked at me and said, "I must have been in here all night."

I said, "Yes, you were, this is your room."

She said, "Oh, that must be why I was here then."

I said, "Yep, that would be why."

She asked me what should she do now.

I said, "Why don't you come out to the kitchen for frosted flakes with a banana, and some coffee?"

She said, "Okay." She looked down at her pajamas and under-shirt and said, "I have on these, and these pants, and this shirt. I have on so many clothes."

I said, "You are a rich woman, with so many clothes. Do you want to change them?"

I received an adamant "No."

I then helped her to the table, trying not to focus on her shoes—which were on the wrong feet. Of course, in her slightly altered world, they were the only feet she had—Two shoes, two feet...how could a person possibly get this wrong? God blessed us with another day—a day with no script...no plan—no schedule—and most of all…no memory of the day that preceded this one. We start with a brand-new slate. Not everybody has that opportunity. Most people have to pick up where they left off yesterday. That doesn't happen in our world. We are reborn every day. We will redo what we did yesterday, and all the days before—as if it is the first time ever. Maybe we will even try a Klondike later, knowing that it will be something she hasn't tasted before. I bet I know the outcome on that one—just sayin'.

A Snowbird Trip

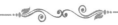

We counted sheep to aid in relaxing so she could go to sleep. I would count a few sheep, then pause, and she would name the next number. When we got to the fourth sheep…I asked her if she could tell what color he was. She informed me that he was gold. We continued to count a few more sheep until we got to sheep number 11.

I said, "I think this one is black."

She quickly answered, "He's black, but he has brown on him."

I was quite impressed. I continued to count sheep with her, and when to number 16; I asked her what she could tell me about it.

She didn't hesitate to tell me, "Oh, they smell so good."

I have now climbed onto the fence that holds her in the lost world she has resided in for two years. She is so into counting the sheep, describing their color, and now the smells—It seems to be keeping her awake, rather than relaxing her into a comfortable sleep. Also, I have now realized that we could count for a long time, and she would stay right with me.

She has fussed with her seatbelt and continues to try to get it off. She has sat straight up and told me she needed to get the chains off the kids. She has asked me if the driver is my husband. During a gas stop, as Bri got back into the van, she asked me why we were changing drivers? She has asked why it was taking so long. She was watching the trees as we drove, and said "we're not going to see them." Apparently she was remarking on the hunt for the colored leaves. Almost all the trees up and down the hills were still green. She doesn't handle "time" well, whether it's a trip or a wait in the doctor office, or patiently waiting for a certain time during the day when there is an event or appointment at a certain time. I've learned that one minute can mean ten months—or vice versa—in her recalibrated mind.

We made a quick impromptu visit up north to see if something familiar would bring a reaction to my Mom. Some things she would recall, like the building in North Vandergrift that stood through the flood of 1936. The home was just as confusing as her days are here in my home. She never knew where the "restroom" was, and always had to be directed. She was ready to leave a few minutes after we arrived.

We are back up in her own home.

LATE SEPTEMBER

S ome things spark a memory with my mom. The trailer is not familiar. Some of the surroundings here at the farm are. She does not know the family, but she fakes it well for a short period of time. My sister Jody and her husband was over the other day. She talked to ken for a short period of time, but then became a spectator.

After they left, she asked me, "What was his wife's name?"

It seems that the memory of all her daughters has disappeared. While we are here, my niece gave birth to what would be Mom's great-grandson. I'm not sure what number this would be, but I'll have to count it up for her. Mom had her doctor's appointment, and the only thing off is that she needs to drink a lot more water. Yesterday we took all six dogs to the vets and got their three-year rabies vaccine and flea medicine, and I had help doing that. Now I can send for their dog license when we return to Florida. Bri also had a doctor's appointment and had blood work done. He needs some adjustment made in his medication regime when we get back.

My days with Mom are much the same for me. My sister has sent several meals up to us, which is such a prize for me. We have had a lot of company, all family. I haven't seen any recognition. She will ask questions about Bri…and want to know if he is feeling better. She still don't know where the "restroom" is in this house. I have been passing out Christmas gifts—Christmas in September. Family know we won't be back up for a while. Bri is still waiting on his starting time for his new job. I am still tired. There is no fenced in yard for the dogs. Family is anxious to see Mom—but they need conversation and information, so that comes from Bri and I. I have seen my daughter and two older grandsons. She works at Kmart here in Leechburg, and just got a second job at Sprankles grocery store. That may be a good start and help keep her busy. I have not seen my two youngest grandchildren.

We returned to Florida, noting that the "snowbird" sure does meet all our needs. Mom does not get out of the van during the entire trip. She can walk around, lay down, eat, use the potty chair and cuddle with her dogs the entire time. She can see out all the windows.

We had beef pot pie from the turkey farm today and it was so good. Mom actually requested a second helping, and Bri really fussed about it.

I also made Taco soup and took over a serving to my neighbor. Jane had purchased the pot pie for us to take on our trip back to Florida. She also sent all the ingredients for the Taco Soup. What you do is so appreciated sister.

I hear from some people that they don't have the patience to do what I do. I simply explain that it is those times that I seem to be blessed with even more patience. I told them all I have to do is look into our mothers" eyes and accept how lost she is. I said that has to be the most frightening feeling, just like how she has to always know where I am so she can see me. I can't imagine feeling that alone.

MID-OCTOBER IN FLORIDA

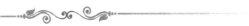

Let's see if I can document some of the happenings of the last few days. I did leave her alone in her room yesterday morning. She got up and was moving about without opening the door. She came out of her room dressed in a different set of pj's—from what she wore during the night. She had put shoes on, the wrong feet, but she was dressed. She went into the bathroom, put in her teeth, and combed her hair. She presented herself at the breakfast table ready for a new day.

I had some apples in the crisper, so I told Mom we would peel them and make an apple crisp for dessert. I put several knives on the table, along with two bowls, and all the apples. I was doing some other things, when she began "chopping" the skin off the apples. I left her work at them, for she is always wanting to help. I walked over when she told me the knives were "terrible," and she had to "chop" at the apples. She had five apples, intact, with the skins removed. I told her I would finish removing the skins, and she could slice them in the baking dish. I put quarters of apples in front of her when she asked what she was supposed to do. I showed her how to slice the apples and layer them in the dish. I went back to peeling and left her continue. She had picked up one of her peeled apples and started slicing it in the dish. I had to remove the core pieces from the slices, and explained to her that she could just slice the ones in the baking dish. We finished the apples and I told her we needed to make the covering for the top. She said, "I'll just watch." And that she did.

We have been having some issues with Mickie. She has become more irritable and aggressive. I probably would too with such diminished eyesight. Yesterday, mom filled up a little dish with water and chased all the dogs around in the kitchen, sitting the water down in front of them. Some would drink, others did not. She did this for about half hour.

When I fixed our lunch, she took half slice of bread from the bag and brought it over to the table where we were sitting. She broke it up and fed it to the dogs. She then started taking her sandwich apart, when she got back up and brought another half slice bread back to the table. This she fed to the dogs, mostly Annie, rather than eat herself. This happened the third time, by then I had finished eating. Rather than offend or embarrass her, I left her alone to "treat" the dogs.

Brian was here for supper when she looked at him and asked where the other girl had gone. He looked at me, and then mentioned that I was right there. She said, "no, the other girl." Bri said she had left and he saw her leaving when he came home. She was content with that answer. Bri was just as quick with his response.

She doesn't want to go outside. She has gone out with me while I was doing something, but she usually brings herself back in after a short time.

I have bought boxes of dog biscuits, puperoni, etc., but it doesn't seem to matter. They can be sitting on the counter or the island, and she still gives the dogs cookies or bread or some of her food. I try not to intervene, but with Mickie being diabetic, I have to watch her consumption. It's hard, because Mom's life is the dogs, and she wants to feed them all the time. She gets upset when the dogs are sleeping, just as she does with me. She tends to pick at the dogs while they try to sleep. When Mickie goes outside, she goes to the door and keeps calling her to come in. Even when she does come in, she can't seem to see her. She is most content with one of her dogs on her lap.

I have an appointment with a new doctor on Tuesday. I hate the idea of starting over with history and diagnosis. I will be taking Mom with me, and I will not let her sit in the waiting room as I did several years ago. In those days, she carried a purse with cash in it. I exited the doctor's exam room and she told me she had been counting her money. Her cash was in bunches in her one hand...and as I know her ability to count paper bills, this may have been going on during my entire appointment. I watch her count six dog dishes over and over again on a daily basis, and often come up with different numbers. She also does this with the dogs, but in her defense, it is hard to count moving objects.

October Winds Down

We had a two week trip up north, and nothing was familiar to Mom. It was something I needed to find out, because if she was kept from being happy by living with me in Sanford, I would have changed something. We had her up to the farmhouse we lived in our entire life, and she couldn't wait to get out of there. The mobile home wasn't familiar. The family wasn't recognized, even though she could fool most of them part of the time. At one time, Bri thought she was recognizing people and enjoying herself more. It would be then that she would come off with one of her infamous lines like… "I need to find a place to stay tonight, for me and the kids…and I have dogs." Reality check again

She wouldn't sleep on the way back down. She fought the medication. She was anxious I'm sure, not knowing the driver or myself most of the time and not knowing where we were taking her…and then make it dark outside—it's even more scary.

Since we've been home, there is no mention of our trip or the time spent up north. I had a Christmas tree up and decorated the house with lights. No mention of that. We passed out all the Christmas gifts for everyone, but she wasn't really a participant. She would just quietly watch. It's like she was in a room with strangers.

Since coming home and getting settled, I needed to do some maintenance.

I cleaned the carport floor with cleaner and etching. I then primed it and then painted it with floor paint. I've also painted the railing. Now I can get the furniture out of Bri's screen room and bring it over.

I'm trying to fix up my house—even though I need the activity and exercise, the paint and stain sure didn't hold up. I pressure washed the front porch today. I need to get it treated. Paint is peeling off my house, and many other places it's discolored and dark. The stained wood looks terrible, and the front door is rotted out at the bottom. I'm painting the stained trim white. So I'm putting a sealer/primer coat of paint over the dark stain. Then I will paint it with white. I'm going to get paint to paint the house also. The eves were never finished, as was the trim in several places. I can't do much about the back deck, but I can try and fix or finish some of the other stuff. I'm going to check with Lowes and see if they have someone that would install the two storm doors and replace the front door. Meanwhile I can paint and trim the outside. If I could figure out how to sand the hump off in the middle of the room, I will then finish the floor myself also. At least I'm going to try. I've painted the plywood, so I can keep up to the accidents a few of the dogs have. It will be much easier with the vinyl floor laid.

The handyman that was working here, is under treatment for Hepatitis C. He's really fatigued and weak It's been so many workers now—and still unfinished. The door didn't hold up on my shed, so I've kept one of the solid doors. I don't know if it can be cut to fit.

They haven't picked up all the lawn debris yet, so I've been trying to get the limbs and branches to the street. We had some severe weather that brought down a lot of tree branches and limbs.

I mow my back yard, and I'm falling behind. I didn't even weed eat it the last time I mowed.

Bri contracted the front and side yard to be mowed when he calls them.

I worked with Mom for a long time yesterday, trying to get her interested in solitaire—It didn't work. She never seems to know whether cards are to be face up or face down. She used to play solitaire in all her free time.

The best and most beautiful things in the world cannot be seen, not touched…but are felt in the heart.

I'd like to share another bit of time with family. The determining factor of my success will be if I find myself "waking up" at a later hour. It happens often—right in the middle of whatever I was doing. I watch my roommate on the monitor. When I hear her snoring, I feel myself relax. It has become one of my most appreciated sounds.

You see, I talk almost nonstop all day. From the time I greet her in the morning and ask if she is ready for a brand-new day—Until I hear the successful sound of a sleeping lady emit from her room. If I don't talk, there is no conversation. Sometimes there is no conversation anyway…just answers. Sometimes there aren't any answers—because she can't seem to make any decisions or choices. She wants to converse, but it is such hard work. It takes explanations and direction and word finding, and sometimes that isn't enough either. I will leave the subject and quietly refocus her efforts to a more simple subject—that may only need a "yes" or "no." And even then, I am sometimes left with the general answer of "whatever is easiest for you."

It's been said that you truly don't understand something unless you can explain it to your grandmother. You are a grandmother to many—but you don't know that—and I can't even explain that.

I am fortunate. My roommate is pleasant, nonconfrontational (most of the time), appreciative, loves and praises my cooking (most of the time), hasn't had any bad nightmares in over a year, loves and lives for her dogs (she doesn't know their names—except Mickie—and she doesn't always know the number of dogs we have, but she loves to feed and treat them).

Just yesterday, she lost the little gray dog. She told me he hadn't come in from outside. All six dogs were accounted for, as I showed them to her one by one. The six we had in our house did not include the little gray one she was hunting. She looked everywhere, so I told her we would prop the door open so he could come inside when he was ready. She stood at the door and called for him. No name, just telling him to "come on—come on." She even told Bri when he came home that she couldn't find the one dog. It bothered her until she became drowsy in the evening. I knew that tomorrow would be a clean slate, "a brand-new day." I knew all the pups would be accounted for, and present for roll call.

The dogs always go to her bedroom door when she gets up. They know she is moving about in her room, and they wait at her door.

When I open the door, they rush inside and she fusses over them all. She walked out to the table this morning. She saw her frosted flakes sitting in the bowl, a pitcher of milk, the spoon, and a glass of water.

She said, "Look, it's waiting for me."

Every day she enlivens our life by just trying her best with what she has. Bri and I cannot fathom what it must be like to function with her brain. It works differently than his or mine. It works differently from minute to minute. When she gets frustrated or scared, she seems to run like the Eveready bunny. I think that's why she resists any medication on our trips back and forth from Pa. She doesn't really know Bri or I and we both change into other individuals during the trip. For example, Bri was "the boy" and then "the driver," and then we switched drivers so I don't know who he was then. She never really knows where she can sleep at night with her "kids" and she also has dogs. She tells me not to forget her, for she tells me she could never find her way home. So when she is riding for a long period of time with strangers who keep switching with other people she must be so frightened that she is being taken somewhere and won't be able to get back home. Home is "the house with the dogs" and that works for her. Where her dogs are there be her heart also. When we pull in front of the house, she wants to know why we are stopping here. Seldom is anything familiar. Does she say anything about being up north? Does she say anything about her long ride to get south? Does she say anything about Christmas decorations or passing out blankets? I told her the other day that we actually made forty-eight rag quilts…we still had one left over.

She said, "We did?"

I said, "Yes, we made them for everyone for Christmas gifts."

She said, "Did anyone get them yet?"

I said, "Yes, we passed them all out."

She simply answered with "good."

She watches me, and waits for me. She is uncomfortable if I take a power nap on the sofa, even if we are watching TV. She doesn't like when the dogs are "all lying around" either. I can only guess that she is more frightened if I am not talking and my eyes are not open.

I did nap the other day—I tried to get her to lay down and gave up at 2:10 PM. The next thing I knew was I heard her say, "Will you please wake up." I rose off the sofa, I think I even levitated off the cushions and asked her what was wrong. I was trying to orient myself while concerned with the tone in her voice. I did see that it was ten till 3:00 PM.

I said, "What is wrong, Mom?"

Her answer: "I don't know what to do—you are sleeping and they are all sleeping—look—they are laying around everywhere—they are just sleeping everywhere (pointing to the dogs sleeping and dormant all over the living area). I don't know what to do." By now I realize that I don't need to use CPR or direct pressure and calculate that I had about thirty-five minutes of sleep. As I look at the face of the lady I live with, I realize the importance of my presence in her environment. She is frightened with myself and the dogs sleeping. She is not comfortable. She doesn't know what to do. Bless her heart.

Life isn't a matter of milestones or mileage—but a matter of moments.

I am now awake, with adrenalin kicking. I asked her if she was ready to make the dogs food. She said she was, so I set out six bowls and put dry dog food in them all. Mom tends to keep adding dry food and stirring and adding. I have now put everything out of mind and started Mom with the canned dog food. I am now starting supper.

I did come back in and lay out on the sofa for a few minutes—regaining my mental stability (don't laugh). She told me she was done with the dog food, so I got up and was about to help her lay them down. Laying on top of the food in three dishes was a piece of white cardboard. I was going to ask, then I decided to just use my imagination instead.

I watched Mom put water in a dog dish and go from dog to dog, putting it under their head asking them if they were thirsty. She made the rounds several times when the dogs actually would get up and move. I showed Mom where the big white bowl was that always had water in for the dogs. She has even added water to the bowl. I guess she felt they needed "room service" at this time. I let her go, for the dogs are her whole reason for living. She has called Mickie her "ole faithful" several times. I put her reflective harness on her so she could be seen by Mom. When she lays on the dark floor, she disappears. Mom has gone through a large box of dog biscuits in less than a week and she wonders why no one wants to eat when they are fed. And the dogs still get cookies, whole ones sometimes, and I have abandoned that issue. I need to paint the house. I will have accomplished something when I'm done.

ELECTION NIGHT

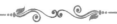

It's election night. All of the people have been watching the final campaigning of both sides. Supporters of both sides are firm in their choices. People all over the United States are going to the polls. This is the general news. It's all that's on TV.

But here in happy valley, life is different. My roommate is concerned with the "kitten" that has the pink thing on. JoJo has a pink harness on, and Mom is carrying her around. She has informed me that "this kitten" was in the basement yesterday, but it didn't come out. She told me that the kitten just came out of the basement a little while ago, but there is nobody in the basement now. She wants to know who it belongs to. She has informed me that there is no name on it. She wants to know what she is supposed to do with it.

Now just to keep you all informed…as we don't have an "upstairs" in Florida, neither do we have a basement.

I told her she didn't need to carry it around, that she could put it down. JoJo is going to be the obsessing receiver of the day. Often it is Mickie, but not today. JoJo is very timid. Her eyes tell me that she is confused, but she shows no objection.

I bring Mom into the kitchen and ask her if she wants to make the dog food. She puts great love into the way she mixes the canned food with the dry pellets. She makes sure that she gets an even amount into each dish. She then stirs and stirs, mixing it throughout the dry food. Sometimes she has to take a teaspoon of food from one dish, and adds it to a different dish, making them exactly the same.

Once she has finished and is pleased with how the dog food has turned out, we sit it down on the floor for the dogs. JoJo runs around

320

in her circles, and then starts to eat out of one of the dishes. Mom is concerned. She points out to me that the kitten is eating from one of the dishes. I tell her, "It's okay. She must be hungry, and we have enough food." I can tell she isn't quite convinced. Again she tells me that she doesn't know who the kitten belongs to. I simply tell her that it's okay—she can stay here until we find out who she belongs to. She watches as JoJo eats, and just shakes her head. Mom has now decided that one of my little dogs has become an abandoned kitten.

I sit the daily pill container at her breakfast cereal every day. She takes the morning pills without any incident. She doesn't fuss. She hasn't been drinking coffee, as the lady that used to wear her title had done. She requests water. It has improved since her UTI and her trip to the doctor during our trip up north. She has to be reminded, but she will drink a small glass of water at each meal.

The nation is concerned as to who our president will be for the next four years. I have Fox news on and I'm watching the news between duties. Mom is sitting on the rocking chair, and she wants to know where her dogs are. She is relieved that I want her to stay with me tonight. She reminds me that she has dogs. I tell her, "It's okay. I have dogs too, and they all get along."

Again she thanks me. She asks me if she can go to her bed.

I tell her, "You sure can, I will walk you back."

She is concerned that her dogs won't go with her.

I say, "Annie, let's take Mom to bed. Rusty get your bunny. Mickie, let's go to bed."

Immediately we have many dogs leading the way to her room. It makes her smile.

She is tucked in. I assure her I will be here all night. She is relieved and thanks me. I tell her we will wake up to a brand-new day. She is tired. She works her way into bed, and lies on her right side. She is covered up with her purple fuzzy blanket. She tells me goodnight.

I tell her, "I love you."

She says, "I love you too."

The sound of summer nights and crickets is softly filling her room. The yellow moon nightlight is shining on her wall. The monitor is positioned to show any activity or movement that she makes in her bed. The dogs all follow me out of her room. Again I tell her that I will be right here with her all night. Again she thanks me. I close her door. My day has wound down.

Bri comes home from work about fifteen minutes after she goes to bed. He is working late hours this week. He feels so bad that he missed her. I tell him to go see her. He checks on her and talks with her for a few minutes, helps her with her blanket, hugs her and kisses her goodnight. She is tucked in twice. She is loved, safe, and content.

Outside her room, the nation continues to wonder who our president will be for the next four years. Inside her room, the world is much smaller. The needs are much simpler, but they are much more important. The lady that resides there is "the world" to so many people, this I know. There may be just a few people working in her world right now, but the love and concern and support from the others that hold her in their hearts is well known. I know how her family loves her, and I also know that another person resides within her that is not familiar with those in the first eighty-eight years of her life. That's okay, because we remember. It's something that she can't fix, and it's definitely something she wouldn't have wanted, given a choice.

But all I have to do is look into her eyes and hear what she can't quite say. I see what she can't find words for. She enjoys meals so much. She likes to look good, and feels good when her nails are polished and her hair is fixed. She wants to help me, and often washes the dishes. She tells me what "the other girl had done or said," how "she" changed her bandage yesterday, how she spent a lot of time fixing lunch. She never recognizes me as "the other girl."

Yesterday I was painting and cleaning and trimming outside. She came in and out, watching me. Finally, she asked me where all the other ones were? I asked, "what other ones." She said "all the people that are coming to our party. No one came, and you spent all that time getting ready. How come nobody came?" I told her it was early, but we are here, and that's all that matters. It bothered her.

When Brian came home, I said, "Tell Bri about the other people."

She told him that nobody came to the party.

He said, "We were having a party?"

Mom said, "Yes, she worked all day getting ready, and nobody came."

Bri told her that was terrible—and they discussed the sadness of nobody coming to our party. Brian is her "go to man" at the end of each day—after spending all day with me and the other workers here at the house. She lights up when he greets her at supper time. He greets her in the mornings if she is awake, and she always tells him to "be careful."

Outside our world, the nation is deciding who our president will be. Inside our world, all needs were met and the lady is resting quietly. Our day is complete. Tomorrow will be a brand-new day—regardless of the choices the voters will make. Our day will be the same—only different.

Great moments occur from time to time in life. At the end of the day, if you have done all you can do to enable another to have a great moment—you will be blessed with some matchless moments yourself.

THE BEAN STORY

We had baby lima beans for supper. I knew Mom loved them in her previous role in life, so I put a nice pile on her plate. She asked what they were, and I told her they were baby lima beans. She asked me the second time, "What are they called?"

I said, "They are baby lima beans. You must tell me if you like them?"

She tasted them and marveled at how good they were. She commented on their good taste several times while eating, and I thought, *Some of my other mother is in there—somewhere.* Occasionally she makes herself known, and it feels good.

Brian came home about three hours after we had eaten. I sat the dish of baby lima beans on the table, and mentioned to Mom, "Tell Bri about these, Mom" (deliberately not mentioning the name).

She said, "They are so good."

Bri asked what they were, and Mom answered, "I don't know what they are called, but they are shaped like a bean…and they are so good." He asked her what they tasted like? She answered that "they taste like a bean." Bri responded without hesitation, "Mawmaw, if they are shaped like a bean, and they taste like a bean, maybe they are a bean." She looked at him and paused for a moment.

She then said, "They could be."

Later Bri asked Mom is she wanted to talk to Sadie, which he had decided to FaceTime. She said "yes" and got up and started walking. She then bent over and addressed one of the dogs with "Hello Sadie." The eye contact between Bri and I was spontaneous.

Again…we have to remain available to the invisible voices that are swirling around us.

Jane noted to me that Mom talked about the "kitten" being on the sofa. She told me that Mom never used the word "sofa," that she always used the word *couch*. This is something that I didn't pick up on, as I always use the word *sofa*.

Mom still thinks that JoJo is a cat, that nobody has claimed. She told Bri that it was tame and that it lay on the sofa and slept. She carried it around most of an afternoon one day, telling me that it was in the basement yesterday, but today it came up. She said it has a pink thing on, but she doesn't know who it belongs to. She has wondered if anybody is out there looking for her. She wonders if it belonged to "one of the people that were here, and they just left it here" Or maybe someone dropped it off, and they just haven't come back for it." Somedays she just makes me smile and smile and smile. She is so complaisant, avoiding confrontation at any times. She loves giving the dogs treats, and has already finished a box and a half of those we keep on the counter by the fridge. She will not eat a meal with the dogs at her side, and not have something to feed them. She talks to them about getting them something, and will use her cookies if she can't find the dog treats. We keep them in full view now, since Oreo's laying around on the floor just doesn't seem right.

ALMOST THANKSGIVING

I left Mom's head open to the air all day. Tonight I cleaned it with sterile saline and put salve and a dressing on. I put one of her little stretchy hats on, 'cause I needed to try and hold it in place. The whole section of the incisional line had opened up this morning. No symptoms. no headache. no temp…no nausea or loss of appetite—nothing.

Maybe it was just a pocket in Mom's incisional line. I'll probably call and talk to them, but I know that means another appointment… and what will they have to culture. I just don't want to put her through any more procedures. She was frightened last night when she went to bed. She doesn't quite know why; she just knows something is different. After all, she felt a lot of pain in that area of her head. Bri sat with her and held her hand. I then brought her out to the TV room and gave her a little more anxiety medication. She relaxed and then I could take her back to bed. I can see her trying to figure out what was wrong with her shoes. Her focus changes so quickly. We have to be able to jump subjects quickly with her. She couldn't problem solve it at all. I tell her every night that I am here all night, and she will not be alone.

Bri stayed with her while I did a hundred errands today—I went to Lowes and paid to have two storm doors put on the house. I had to pay for the air conditioner repair guy this month—so that's it for this month. I did find a pair of sandals with a slight heel with foam heel areas. I needed to find something to wear a little dressier if I needed to or had the opportunity. I go to Rosses or home goods or Marshalls. They have the best deals, maybe not as much to choose from but then the smaller choices are easier for me.

There is some changes in Mom's memory. She does recall some things from the day before. She has been upset the last few days because of all the things I do and nobody shows up. I don't have a clue where she got that idea. I've reviewed things, and the only thing I can think of is the day the man came to measure the storm door places. I explained to her that he would be coming back another day to hang the doors, and we would have to put the dogs in their crates. I told her that workers are not permitted to be in the house if the dogs are not confined.

Mom referred to the dogs as the kids again tonight. She worries about the kids. Today when I went to the stores I bought a bunch of dog treats for her to dispense. After her head opening last night, I just wanted her to have fun. When I buy pee pads and supplies and dog food, it adds up. Do you know Rusty's license cost me $25 because he's not neutered?

I see pictures of my niece, Jeani's daughter, Audrey, in Costa Rica. I wonder if she'll be moving there?

I'm dealing with the satellite company. It's the only way I can get the pirates. Bri said, "But, Mom, she doesn't watch them anymore," and I had to admit that I follow them now, when I don't fall asleep. It's so good to be able to get them on TV when I'm not interested in most of what's on TV the rest of the year.

*****

It's 4:30 AM. I just talked with our mother and explained that it's really the middle of the night, and she should try and go back to sleep. We are all on Bri's work schedule of getting up before 4:00 AM. Dogs have been out several times already. It did get cooler last night, which is a change for us. I had the weather channel on yesterday, and left Mom watch the snow storms going on out west. She will be watching for the snow to come here, I'm sure. As I plant some flowers, she reminds me that they will be gone when the frost comes.

As I sip my coffee, I think of the last few days. I reported that there has been some improvement in Mom's memory, and that is true. She recalls some events that hold over until the next day. She was waiting for "that thing to go up," and it did last night. The rocket went up from the cape. Funny thing is, I had it on TV and she really couldn't have cared less. She was watching it as it went through several five- and ten-minute delays, but when it went up, she didn't seem to be able to relate it to the "thing going up" that she had been waiting for. It's how her brain is working, and it puts me in awe so many times.

I've been laying out her clothes and giving her sometime in the mornings to independently dress herself. She came out with her purple slippers over her nonslippy socks over her regular socks, which she does often. She said she needed to put her shoes on because "these aren't mine. I don't know who they belong to, but they aren't mine."

She went back to her room and brought out her shoes. Seated at the table, she had the shoes on her lap. One shoe had the toe pointing forward, and the other shoe had the toe pointing the opposite direction. She held the shoes, she lifted one and sat it back down, she looked so puzzled as she studied the shoes. I waited for what seemed like hours and walked over. I picked the one shoe up and faced them both in the same direction, as they would go on her feet. The relief that she showed and how many times she thanked me—could break a strong person's heart. She then was able to put her shoes on. There is no problem solving ability whatsoever—none. Things are as they are, and sometimes it's like a major roadblock to anything she was attempting. I saw the same thing with sewing, or helping with cooking, or even breaking some eggs. I emptied Bri's lunch box the other night and set the containers on the sink. She went over and started washing the dishes, as she is usually able to. She washed four plastic containers with the lids on. That's how I set them on the sink, so that's how they were washed. She tries so hard, and generally doesn't even know when something isn't right.

She fussed with her head, and I realized the bandage had irritated her forehead, so I left the dressing off during the day for several days. The other morning, she was still fussing, and I told her to put her finger where it was hurting. She placed her finger on the oldest incisional line, well above and further back on her head from the three areas draining from the open wound. I separated the hair and it was hurting her. Then the incisional line opened up, about two inches in length and drained purulent drainage. There was no swelling, no evidence of a problem, because I had just colored and set her hair two days before. Now for the weak of heart, I'm sorry, but I expressed about a tablespoon of purulent drainage. I dressed it and the pain had left that area of her head. I was somewhat confused as to how she felt it, when it was under the surface of the incisional line, but she did. The next day, there was only a speck of drainage.

The night that it opened, she knew something was wrong and different. Bri was here for supper, and he sat with her and held her hand when she went to bed. She was frightened, without understanding. It's truly heartbreaking when you see that type of look in her eyes. She worries that I will forget her, or that she doesn't know where I am…even though I tell her and let the door open when I go outside. The storm door is propped open, but when I am out of sight—I am not there. I can't imagine how insecure she must feel at that time.

So I went to town and bought a bunch of dog treats and snacks. I had been trying to explain to her that the reason the dogs won't eat when she sits their food down, if because she has fed them so many snacks. She will go through a half box in a day. She then follows the dogs around, holding their bowl of food in front of their face, when they walk away. I try to explain that an eight pound dog can only hold so many treats and he will be full. She will then put water in one of the bowls and go from dog to dog, putting the dish of water under their face, wanting them to drink.

So I threw caution to the wind. I don't care how many treats she feeds these neglected dogs right now. It's the only thing she seems to get happiness from. She smiled from ear to ear, and carried all the treats over to the corner of the countertop, where we had placed the other box. It took her two trips. They are in full view and under her total control. I think that is what will be under the tree for her. It made her so happy to have so many dog treats available. I'm sure Annie is smiling also, except she is white Mickie to this lady.

We also have a white cat that was left here one day. For some reason, JoJo has become a white cat that was in the basement but came up one day. She couldn't understand why no one came to claim it, because it was so tame. She carried it around one day, wanting to know who it belonged to. She says it just lies on the sofa and sleeps all day. Bri suggested that we call it JoJo, but she said there was already a dog here with that name. And life goes on.

I'm watching her head…I don't know what's going on under the surface. I know the bone was deteriorating the last several surgeries. I will probably call the infection control doctor down here on Monday—and explain the situation. Whether there will be anything to culture, I don't know. Whether he will order oral antibiotics, or order a cat scan, or IV, or nothing—I don't know. Meanwhile, I will try and get the incisional line approximated and see if it will heal. The two wounds, the one I have been dressing and the new one, are not connected.

This wonderful lady that I live with has a good appetite, loves anything I prepare in the kitchen, eats a good breakfast, lunch and supper, along with coffee and cookie breaks midmorning and midafternoon, and ice cream with strawberry jelly every night. She has no symptoms of an infection, and she has no pain except when I pull her hair removing her head dressings. She loves her manicure, which she is sporting blue nail polish right now. She combs her hair every morning, so when the color and set is good, she is proud.

She feels good when she is dressed and often says, "This is too good to wear for every day."

I just tell her that every day is a good day to wear something good. She still layers to keep warm, and I turn on the furnace every morning to take the chill off for her (certainly not for me. Seventy feels so good to me, but not her). She has no interest in TV unless we narrate about everything that is going on to keep her attention. Most of her day involves her sitting in a chair watching me, or standing where I am—watching me. The dogs are the center of her universe.

She doesn't know who they are, and often doesn't even know Mickie.

Today will be a brand-new day.

FACEBOOK POSTINGS

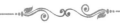

I don't put much stuff on Facebook. That is all Bri. He puts nothing negative on it, and keeps a good image of Mom for the outside world to see. I checked with him, and then invited Doris up. I told her to bring her little dog Gracy and stay overnight. I have Bri's two bedrooms cleaned and decorated with a full bed in one room and a queen in the other bedroom. Doris stayed in the end corner room and raved about the soft blanket I had on the bed. I also have two white noise machines in his house. I then have three different lite up stone lamps, which he put on timers. We are trying to let him fall in love with his house again, for it has depressed him for a year now. He is always handing me his phone to record time with Mom. He is her hero, and he maintains the most "up" spirits when he sees her, his voice it always the same happy tone, and he walks directly to her each time he enters the house. He says all his energy comes from being in our house, and the minute he goes home, he feels drained.

She had that area on her incisional line open up about a week ago and drained the worse looking drainage. It drained for about two days, and now it's drying up. The other first wound is still draining as always. She didn't want me to call the doctor She kept telling me it didn't hurt anymore. I've held off, because I know they will schedule an MRI or a CT scan or something. How else would they know what's going on. I personally feel the bone is continually deteriorating. Meanwhile, we see an improvement in her memory, except for her daughters. She retains some things over into the next day. I've been copying the family album for Brent, and she's been looking and studying the pages. I've updated some info that we have been able to pull from her mind. I can't get her interested in anything, but she does keep up to the washing of the dishes. It makes her feel like she's helping me.

I pulled some of the sayings from the notebook Jody gave me and put them in Bri's lunch box. That book must have cost her a fortune in printer ink, because I know what I've put in printer ink.

Our mother's physical condition just keeps going, like the energizer bunny. The other night she looked at me, about 6:00 PM, and asked, "Where is the custodian of this place?"

She is forging a path through her mind every single day. Bri battles depression and "I don't care" every minute of his life. I keep my life preserver on and dance as fast as I can. I don't have any music on, but I can hear the song, so I just keep dancing.

IT'S ALMOST CHRISTMAS

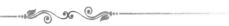

I asked myself, "Hey, Judy, why don't we write a Christmas Letter this year?" Okay, so I checked the internet to get some pointers. There are eight tips to writing a good letter:

1. Start on a positive note (that's a given).
2. Keep it short and sweet (now we may have a problem here).
3. Use your own words (I always do).
4. Write to the specific audience (that would be my family).
5. Don't embellish (oh darn! Stopped at the starting gate).
6. Make it personal (it is personal; it revolves around our Mawmaw).
7. Use photos selectively and sparingly (maybe, or maybe not).
8. Write down a family recipe, write an award you received, a trip or a class you took (that paragraph won't exist, unless they want me to push Marie Callender's, Swanson, Mrs. Paul's, Sara Lee's, or Tai pai). So here goes!

Hello family: It's hard to start on a positive note, when I'm saying we won't be seeing you this Christmas. So I will say it this way: It was great spending "Christmas in September" with all our loved ones. We have been told we have a wonderful family all our lives, and that we are so lucky to have stayed so close. It is very true… and we certainly are…and in spite of the miles between us…we will continue to stay close.

Keep things short and sweet. I won't be using any 50 cent words, just good ole country conversation. Our house is all decorated and colorfully lite. There is a large snow laden tree in the corner. I had to put it up on a table. There is one glass jar tree, one tinsel tree, two medium trees, and 6 small ones in the living area. Santa is climbing up a rope ladder on the tree. There is Rudolph, Mr. and Mrs. Clause, snowmen, angels, and the canine stockings are hung high on the windows with care…for lack of a better place. There is garland on the fences and lights on the garland. There are two lite trees on the carport, 3 wooden ones by the gate, and another one on the front porch. The pathway is lite with candle sticks so Santa doesn't miss our house and fly over. All the lights will be reflecting off Florida's neon sky.

There are snowmen and angels, Santa and Mrs. Clause, Rudolph, Christmas placemats and Napkins. Mom watches me and I try to keep the action close to her so she feels she's a part of everything. She tells me everything looks good.

There are no black skies at night here—not like in Pennsylvania.

Keeping it personal, Mawmaw has a little improvement in her memory at times. I went to the airport yesterday, and she thought it was the Pittsburgh airport (some things are better left unexplained). She thinks all you guys live right down the road (except Angie-on-the-hill, she lives up on the hill) and thinks you stop in at times. In fact, in her world, you apparently stop in often. We have started to look at her head wound as "a minor inconvenience" and a badge of honor from having four major surgeries within the span of two years. I made her an appointment on Monday with the infection control office with Dr. Cooper. I'm concerned that there might be something I should be doing. On the other hand, I'm leery of what is going on inside). Her life revolves around the six dogs. She makes their feed, and gives them treats from breakfast through supper. If she doesn't have dog treats close, there will be Oreos lying on the floor. Of course, we also have the new cat that nobody has claimed. (the one that came up from the basement a few weeks ago) Mawmaw calls her "the baby doll in the pink thing." Bri and I call her "JoJo." Funny that Mom hasn't missed the little dog that came missing when the kitten came up from the basement.

Bri took a friend to the airport the other night, she was visiting with her uncle in Kepple Hill. Mawmaw struggled with that for a while, and finally asked, "Why did she have to get an airplane to just go to Kepple Hill?"

Every night she asks if it is okay if she stays "here"—and then she reminds me that she has dogs. She asks me where she is to sleep. I walk her back to her bedroom, and as soon as we open the door, she says, "There's my bed." I have a purple fuzzy blanket on her bed. She now identifies its presence on her bed, as her room.

Bri is working for a different boss on the Cape now, and he took his buddy Jason with him. Ironworkers need to have each other's back, and Jason is over 400# and 6 ft 8 inches. His boss said he brought his own crane with him. Bri says if he can't fit in it to do the job, Jason will move it. He teases Jason that he has Toyotas for shoes. He says this boss plans on shutting down the job between Christmas and New Year, so since Christmas is on a Sunday. He will have a nice holiday.

The "cook" will be working overtime, it appears, but she won't have to pack a lunch. I'm sure Santa will be putting more dog treats in the dog's stockings, so Mawmaw will have lots more treats to pass out. She won't eat in front of them without giving them treats.

Our wishes for the new year would be good health and happiness to all. Mawmaw seems content here in Florida, but spends most of her time inside the house. There are so many of me. Mawmaw will be outside with me, and go in the house to see what "she" is doing in there. No matter where I am, she looks for "her" somewhere else. I have the opportunity to be outside and busy with painting and planting and mowing and trimming and looking after the neighbors. She has little interest in TV unless it is narrated as we watch it with her. Her attention span is very, very short. She doesn't want me to do the dishes, because she feels it is the only thing she can do to help. So hard as it is, I bite the bullet and leave the dishes alone so she can help me.

She doesn't want me to make any doctor's appointments because her head "doesn't hurt anymore." She makes the food in the dog dishes almost every day. One day she put a spoon in all 6 bowls because, "how else are they going to eat?" Amazing how this lady thinks of everything. How inconsiderate I have been. All these years I have fed the dogs without any way to get their food from the dish to their mouth.

All hearts go home for Christmas, as will ours. But more than that, please know that our Mawmaw gets a lot of attention. She will have festive nail polish on and she will be enjoying many meals that she loves. I have purchased more baby lima beans, the rolls that you heat in the oven, and lots of mashed potatoes. There is a peach cobbler and a key lime pie in the freezer. We keep lots of double stuff Oreo cookies available. She drinks half cup coffee twice a day, because she says "they say I need to drink more water, so I'll have water." Today I gave her half glass of orange juice, and she liked it.

She kept asking me, "What is this again?"

So many new discoveries in her world, so many new foods that she hasn't tried yet, and beans that she didn't know they made, and so many people who come into the house and help out with all the tasks at hand. I just hope the cook shows up, 'cause she needs to fix at least three meals a day, plus a bedtime snack. If you see her up the street at your house, please send her back down to Sunset Drive.

I spent an entire day helping Mawmaw sign the Christmas cards...I walked outside once, and when I came back in...Mawmaw had signed an envelope. So know that she truly signed your card. I may have stated that wrong when I said "an entire day"—it took entire "days"—which is the plural version of just one day. It definitely took the plural version.

No Sassafras Tea This Month

Every day is the same—but yet they are different. Everything involved in her day can change in an instant—and with unknown reasons. Like the last few days, she has been ironing, because she can do that. Ironing and washing dishes are her two gifts to society these days. So the ironing board is set up in the living room, dining room area. It has been there for two days.

She has done a lot of ironing material pieces. Ironing, along with hand washing the dishes, are both activities that she can do. It gives her a feeling of worth, and she feels she is doing something to help. Some days she goes to the kitchen sink every few minutes, looking to see if there are dishes to wash. She did the same with ironing the past few days. She would get tired and take a break. Soon she would be asking if something else needed ironed. Yet tonight, she was hunting for the iron on the kitchen island. It was right beside her on the ironing board—yet she didn't know where it was at this moment.

No matter what you face in life…don't let go of God's hand.
Every blessing assigned to you will come. Just trust Him

For the past year, she has just existed. She was here, and she functioned, but there was no life in her actions. Now recently, she has regained some quality to her life. She remembers from one day to the next. She recalls things that were discussed at another time, and re introduces them into the conversation. Millie, the neighbor, gets her hair done weekly. When we took her to her appointment last Thursday, she made the statement, "I thought she already went there." That kind of observations are big steps in the way her life has been the past year.

Her life changes quickly. An outside person may see her ironing and feel that she has regained this ability. They could watch her preparing six bowls of dog food and feel she knows what she is doing. They may watch her washing dishes in the kitchen sink and feel like she is functioning within the household as an independent person. They may see her serving herself something at the dinner table, or adding a condiment, and not realize she may have a mental injury. What they don't see: The dishwater is cold and there is no detergent added, instead she has added hand lotion that is on the sink. She has washed a plastic container used in Bri's lunch, with the lid still on. They don't see how many times she has counted the dog dishes, and they don't know that she puts the opened cans of dog food in other places than the fridge. She has put spoons in the dishes to enable the dogs to eat. She has added cottage cheese to the dogs' food dishes, after she had put some in dishes for our supper.

For her to iron, I need to keep the water level in the iron, and help her with what to iron. She had ironed several pieces of material and laid them on the dining room table. She turns away from the unironed material, and started reironing the pieces she had already done. She asks how to turn off the iron every time, and must be instructed in how to unplug it. She has started telling me if it quits steaming, so I can add more water. They don't see her when, all at once, she can't find the iron. I truly believe she forgets what it looks like, while she's hunting for it. There is so much to see behind the scenes in my mother's daily life. I love it when I am trying to find something in the kitchen, and she helps me look for it. She admits she has no idea what she is looking for but says she will help me look. Things that a person may not be aware of, because she has learned how to cover her actions so well.

At the dining table, she may put butter on her potato up to three times. She may do the same to her bread. She may put mac and cheese on her hotdog, or cottage cheese on her potato. I tease her that she is writing new recipes every day when she fixes her plate. She counts the dogs off and on all day long. She wants to make sure they are all in the house, yet a week ago, when she answered Bri's front door, two dogs ran out and she wasn't even aware. She still believes that we now have a kitty, and has never questioned what happened to our dog Jojo, that apparently disappeared the same day that the new kitty appeared. She explained to Jane the other day that the kitty is growing (Jojo is probably twelve- or thirteen-years-plus old), and she has a little pink dress on.

I cleaned and skinned a few sassafras sticks the other day. I then cut them up and cooked them in water for quite a while. I then semi strained it and removed the sticks. I poured it in a pitcher on the sink so I could restrain it with a coffee filter. As Mom finished washing the dishes, I noticed that the pitcher was washed and draining in the rack. She had emptied a whole pitcher of dark fluid and never questioned as to what it was. There goes a day or two of work "down the drain." Sorry Bri, but you won't be trying Sassafras tea today.

Today she had her shoes on the wrong feet. She wiped her nose on her pajama jacket top at the lunch table. I asked her if she needed a Kleenex, and she informed me that she had some in her pocket. I have chocolate Oreo cookies with chocolate icing in the cookie box. She has told us that they don't look good at all, so she doesn't think they taste good. She describes the chocolate Oreos as "they just aren't right."

She needs monitored, with her every step or action. She doesn't seem to be able to explain herself to me. She often sits and looks pensive. She cannot tell me what she is thinking about. Her whole reason for being—seems to be taking care of the dogs.

Her memory is showing some amazing improvements, but her head wound is regressing.

SCATTERED THOUGHTS

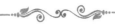

Mom kept going out and staying on the carport this afternoon. I was on the sofa and Bri had gone back to my bedroom to sleep a little before work. The car's tires were dangerously bad, so the car is also at the shop. The snowbird has been there, and we dropped off Bri's truck a day ago, because it wouldn't start easily. All three of our vehicles are presently at Tire City. I was to wait for the phone call that the car was done, so I stayed close to Bri's phone, which was charging. I couldn't get Mom interested in any TV for the past week or so. When I put a game show on, she tells me the same show was just on yesterday. She tells me the same thing when I put on one of the half hour comedy shows. Even when I record her favorite show, keeping up appearances, she tells me she has seen it before. I should have seen this coming when she started to become disinterested in the Pirate games. I remember her telling me, "They keep doing the same things, they hit the ball and then they run, then they hit the ball again, and do it all over." She's also told me they made the games longer than they used to be, showing her interest levels are shortening.

Back to this day, I thought she was enjoying the outside, and maybe wanting to be away from me for a short period of time. I walked outside and she was holding onto two of the dogs. She told me she couldn't find any rope. I asked why she was looking for rope? She told me there was only four dogs right here, and she had to get them all together. I again, asked why? She looked at me and asked if all the people had come, that's why she was trying to keep the dogs together. I told her that Bri was still sleeping, and he was the only one here, except for me and the dogs.

HOWEVER LONG IT TAKES

She looked at me and said, "So it happened again, nobody came just like the other times."

I am confused as to why she always thinks there are other people who are supposed to come, and they never seem to show up. I sat down and explained that Bri would be getting up and going to work. Her and I and all the dogs would be staying here for the rest of the day and also the night. She seemed relieved, but still upset, that nobody showed up again. Maybe all those people that used to help out here at the house have stopped coming to help?

The last few days she has had no interest, except involving the dogs. She has informed me that I don't have to entertain her all the time. I try not to challenge Mom, or correct her, but her feeding cookies and pancakes and her meals to the dogs is totally out of hand. She will feed them whatever she has, and trying to explain the need of insulin for Mickie when she eats, comes on blind ears. I do know that Mickie spends more and more time at the water bowl, day and night. Annie's belly is taunt and large. Feeding the dogs is her only interest. She does it from morning until bedtime. When she sets the dog dishes down on the floor, the dogs will walk away. She will pick up the dishes and follow the dogs, sitting the dish right under their face, and encouraging them to eat. The food dishes will still be on the floor, and Mom will ask me if the dogs were fed yet. They sit and beg at her chair, whether she is at the table or in the other room. She lowers food to the dogs while she eats. If the dogs are laying or sleeping in their crates, it seems to upset her. She thinks they are hungry and need to eat. When they are laying about and quietly sleeping, she gets concerned. I have watched her pull a dog out of the crate, while they slept, because she felt they were "stuck" in there.

Last night I had tucked her in bed. I watched the monitor and about fifteen minutes later, I see her sitting up at the bedside. I walked back and asked what she was doing. She said she didn't know. It seemed like she was getting ready to get up for the day. I explained that I had just brought her back to bed about twenty minutes ago, and she hadn't even fallen asleep yet. She said she didn't know that, so she will go back to bed.

A few days ago, I had three dogs up at the grooming center at Petco. I helped Mom prepare to make six bowls of dog food, telling her that we will feed the dogs after I go pick them up. Needless to say, I left to go pick up the three dogs. When I walked into the house after returning with the other three dogs. I noticed that all the dog dishes had been placed onto the floor, all six dishes. I asked Mom if she had fed the dogs. Her answer was "yes, they all ate." (To say my days don't hold any mystery or surprises, would be an understatement.)

Valentine's Day

M om received a delivery from UPS. It is a Vermont Bear, dressed in a red Valentine dress and with a red bow on its head. I sat it on the table in front of her and sat the opened box on the floor. She looked at it, and would touch it, while she ate her sandwich. After we finished eating, she got up and put the box on the table. She started putting the bear into the box. I asked her to leave the bear out, since it was so pretty, so we could all look at it. She sat the bear on the table. Two more times within the early evening, she started putting the bear into the box. She didn't give a reason. It just seemed that she wanted the bear put away in the box he came in.

March 26

This is Mom and Dad's anniversary date. I'm wondering if the date will spark anything in my roommate's memory bank. The doors on the bank seem to be getting less assessable. Last night, Bri walked her back to bed. She was tucked in for about eight minutes when I watched her get up on the monitor. She appeared to be standing by the potty chair. But then she disappeared from view. I knew she was headed for the door, so I got there just as she was opening it. She was having trouble finding the words, but by watching her lead, she apparently needed to use the pot. The problem was the lid was down, and she didn't seem to know what to do. I put the lid up, but confusion has already reared its stressful face, and it usually snow-balls after that. Next issue was waiting for her to get on the pot. She forgot what to do next. I helped her by having her turn around and getting pants in position. But it still wasn't easy for her. I had to give one slow instruction at a time—then help her physically to get to that goal. Then we took another step—going very slowly tonight. Mission accomplished and assisted her back to bed. For how long? We shall wait and see.

I was cleaning on the carport today and had Mom sitting in the area so she could see me. I walked over and sat down beside her. I initiated a simple conversation.

"What do you think about when you are sitting here?"

"I was just watching"

"Is it hard for you to think?"

"Yes, it is."

"Do you see Homer sometimes?"

"No, cause I haven't seen him for quite a while."

"Why haven't you seen him?"

"because he has a car, and he has wheels. So he doesn't stay here very much."

"You mean when someone has a car, they go other places."

"Yes."

"Do you remember very much about him?"

"yes, somethings. But I haven't seen him for a while."

"Do you know what relation he is to you?"

"yes, he is my husband."

"do you remember how you met?"

"we were in school together. We graduated at the same time."

"did you date when you were in school together."

(Noted very confused look on face). "I think, I don't know."

"Do you remember how he asked you on your first date?"

"No..." (Long pause.) "But he had a car, and we would go places."

She has a sense of humor, and she "gets" sarcasm. Her memory shows improvement. After the phone call from her granddaughter Sara the other night, she looked at me and said, "She's a teacher, isn't she?"

I had two grapefruits laying on the counter. She asked me the other day, "I've been wanting to know what these are, so I'm just going to ask, what are these?" I told her they were grapefruit that I picked off the tree in the yard. She looked confused, and asked what you do with them. I explained that you eat them, and followed up by cutting one in half. She watched my every move, so I loosened a bite and told her it might be sour, but to taste it. She made a face and spit it in the sink, agreeing that it was sour. I then sprinkled sugar on a bite and offered it to her. She ate that bite, and then told me it was really good. I asked her when was the last time she ate grapefruit. She stated that she didn't think she ever had.

I put chocolate Oreo cookies out, which had chocolate icing between the cookies. She said, "they just don't look good. They don't look right." When Bri would ask her about the specific cookie in the cookie box, she would refuse. When he asked her why she didn't want it, she said, "they are black."

MY SISTERS ONLY VISIT MY MOM

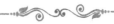

Oops, let's just put this glass back into the dishwater. I admit, getting a milk ring out of the bottom can be a little difficult. In fact, let me wash this glass and therefore eliminate this problem before it recycles again through my dishwashing roommate.

This remarkable lady exits her bedroom in the morning and she has put on her own shoes, her glasses and her denture. She is wearing a brightly colored yellow nonslip sock on one foot, and a conventional white cotton diabetic sock on the other. She is also quite bipedal, as her shoes apparently work on either feet.

She did question, "The hole in my head, is this getting better?" She was palpating one of the residual healed scars from one of her previous surgeries. It is a very evident indentation right at her hairline. I took her hand and placed it over the bandaged area, explaining that the "holes in her head" are under the bandage. I've ceased to use the word, "dressing" for rather obvious reasons related to dual meaning. She flinched as her hand pressed over the wound area, as it is tender to touch. She said nothing more. She had no more questions.

I'm still slightly offended that my sisters do drop in, and then leave without saying goodbye. I have had to hide stuff, in "case one of the kids drop in." Often this lady starts getting her stuff together and gathering up her kids and the dogs, so she can get home.

I like to spend time outside, so I leave the door propped open so the dogs can come and go. She has walked to the doorway and told me "you need to come in here, because I have things to do—and you need to tell me what they are." I truly love some of her questions.

"Is this a step down?"

"Which way do I go to go to my bed?"

"Where did those other people go that were here?"

"Where did your dad go?"

"Where is my husband, he was just here?"

"Where are those long things with the lines that your mother brought and put on the table?"

"Why aren't those boys coming in to eat?"

Brian told her he doesn't have a boat anymore, so she can't go riding with him on the boat. He does have a bike, if she wants to go riding with him on the motorcycle. She looked at him and said, "well, they won't let me drive a car, maybe I will drive that."

She has no concept of time, none whatsoever. Some nights she gets up, puts on her shoes and eyeglasses, picks up her denture cup, and heads to the bathroom. I walk her back to her bed, remove her shoes, and explain that it is the middle of the night. I advise her to try and stay in bed-at least until the sun comes up. She says she is still tired, so she says she will do that. She admits she looked outside and saw it was still dark. A digital clock sits in her room. She pays no attention to it. When I try to point out the time, she just agrees. She often gets up four times, thinking she has slept all night.

She prides herself on keeping up with the dishes. We used to let them air-dry, and then I would put them away. She has started drying them and putting them away. Maybe a better way or better wording for her efforts would be "and placing them someplace." Occasionally we "misplace" something, at which time I will ask her if she knows where it is. She joins me in the hunt. She hunts and looks everywhere. I know she has no clue what we are looking for, but I wouldn't call her bluff. She opens the fridge, lifts out the mayo jar and asks; "is this it?" I answer "no," so she resumes her search. She pulls a can of dog food from the pantry and asks again, "is this it?" I decline again. I know she wants to help. I let her ask once more, and then I tell her that I found it. I hold up "something" and tell her where I found it. She is glad that our search was successful. Not knowing what we were searching for, allows us to "find" it without question.

She will tell me a story about "something" but the words are either lost midsentence, or inappropriate. I try to follow her thought process, so I can respond properly. Often, it's a story she heard on TV, but some of the parts are missing. She likes the "judge shows" and often picks up on a partial reason why they are "fighting and yelling" at each other. Often, she will tell me they are "fighting over a baby." She watches *Ice Road Truckers* with keen interest.

She is attracted to the drama and action of *Dog the Bounty Hunter*. As we all know, the Pirates have changed their way of playing and she doesn't enjoy watching them anymore. She tells me they have made the games longer, that they never used to be this long. She tells me they keep doing the same things over and over, like one guy hits the ball and they run. Then another guy hits the ball and they run. Then they do it all over again. No matter what game show I put on, she has already seen it. She doesn't like the talk shows and lets me know when she doesn't like one of the speakers on the show. I will ask if she wants to watch a cooking show, or the "fightin' channel," which is one of the court channels where they fight and scream during the whole show. She always picks the "fightin channel."

Brian and I took her to a doctor's appointment, I needed the doctor to see the change in her head wound and it's drainage. When Jane talked to her later that evening, she asked if Brian went with her to the doctor Mom said "No, he didn't," and then adds that "the other boys went." Jane also asked if Judy was here. Mom looked at me holding the phone and told Jane she hadn't seen Judy all day.

Sometimes she leaves me speechless.

Someone once asked me, "Why do you always insist on taking the hard road?" This person must assume that I see two roads?

She's not walking as well as she had. She finished one week of an antibiotic for her head wound, but the culture showed two other bugs, so she will be starting two new antibiotics tomorrow, since it is raining and getting late.

She said, "Well, maybe Homer will pick them up." Sometimes she leaves me speechless.

We had pizza for lunch and after watching her try to eat it, even though Bri had cut it into small pieces. I asked her if she wanted to trade her pizza for a half sandwich? She readily agreed. I made her a sandwich and removed the pizza from her place at the table. She looked at the sandwich and then tried to use her fork to eat it.

I said, "Mom, it's a sandwich. You pick it up and eat it from your hand."

She looked at me, and I placed it in her hand. She then continued to eat the entire sandwich.

I gave her a dish of ice cream with topping on and was watching her eat it. I watched her give a spoonful of ice cream to Annie, letting her eat from her spoon. Then I watched her wipe her sticky mouth on her pajama top. I have watched her lay her napkin aside and wipe her mouth on the placemat when eating.

She fell again tonight. She was moving the rocking chair but couldn't give me the reason why. As she tried to slide it forward, she leaned backward and just kept going. I was able to grab her sweatshirt and hold her back to slow the fall. She doesn't use any self-protective moves when she falls. She shows no sign of self-defense to protect her head when she falls. She ended up with a small bruise on her shoulder, another on her head, and denies any other injury.

April Showers Bring Sister Jody to Visit

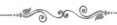

My sister Jody flew down last Wednesday to spend about ten days with Mom and me and Brian. We have spent a lot of quality time—with a few runs to the Goodwill Store, Joann Fabrics, and Walmart. We sewed, shopped, cooked, baked, drank coffee, and drank wine. I could say that visitors seem to upset her almost solitary routine. She doesn't know enough about her children to enable her to ask questions relating to their lives or family. I have been with her for almost three years now, and I do not have a stable identity in her mind. She can call me "Judy," and in the next breath tell me she has a daughter named Judy.

We took Millie to her hair appointment on Thursday, so we left an hour early so we could allow Millie to shop at Walmart and I could do a little shopping myself. I put Mom in the wheelchair, because I couldn't pull her and the cart through the store safely anymore. There are no more signs of Mom pushing the cart on her own power. She drags her feet and walks with a shuffle gait. When we are out, I keep my hand under her arm to enable her balance and keep the forward movement. This is impossible to do-along with pushing—or pulling—the grocery cart. Therefore, I used the wheelchair for her. She was angry. She wanted to walk. She wanted to push the wheelchair and not sit in it. I insisted she stay seated. I left Millie go on her own so she could get her shopping done. Mom called out to her, asking for her help.

As I pushed her past other customers, she would reach out to grab hold of them. She would talk to them, but it was hard to make sense out of her statements. If I stopped the wheelchair, she would immediately attempt to get out. If I pushed the chair, she would take her feet off the footrests and attempt to stop me. She constantly kept telling me to "stop this." At one time she informed me that if I didn't let her walk, she would scream really loud. I knelt in front of her and firmly stated, "You go ahead and scream. They will come and arrest me, and they will take you to the hospital. If they take you to the hospital, the dogs have to go into their boxes. Now, do you want to scream, go ahead. That threat was gone for the time being.

We brought supper home from Wendy's. She put spoonsful of vanilla frosty on her baked potato. She poured her coffee into the small pitcher of milk, and then drank from the tiny milk pitcher.

Mom's legs are not as strong as they had been, and she seems to be shuffling her feet rather than picking them up. I took the wheelchair today...and she was not happy with us. I felt it was better than having her stumble in one of the stores. She just finished three different antibiotics for infection in her head wound. I'm hoping she can get stronger with longer endurance for walking—like she used to. I realize she's ninety-one, and she has quite a memory issue, but I try to maintain as much strength as possible.

If you can't fly, then run. If you can't run, then walk. If you can't walk, then crawl, but whatever you do—you have to keep moving forward.

MORE RANDOM HAPPENINGS

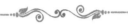

This lady removed the scissors from the dog grooming box and cut Rusty's harness into several pieces. She walked out of the bathroom with her disposable brief down around one ankle, and her pajama bottoms on backward.

While eating her Frosted Flakes Easter morning, she picked up the cloth table covering and wiped her mouth and face with it.

Black Mickie jumped up on her lap, and she hugged him and called him Buster.

I have to keep the butter dish away from her reach, as she butters her bread, the food on her plate, and then rebutters everything several times.

She opened the kitchen pantry door, looking for the restroom

She washed the dishes and put them in the dish drainer. She sat down for a rest, then got up and washed the dishes from the drainer and placed them on the other side of the sink. She sat down again, got up, and then started putting them all on the kitchen island, silverware inside water glasses, plates wet with water, piled on top of pans and cups. She tends to keep moving things from place to place, like she's putting things in their place.

She wished my brother would come by, so he could make the heat work. She told me the dogs were cold, and I needed to put more clothes on them. She kept walking around feeling the dogs to see if they were getting warm yet. She tried to cover them up with the throws from the sofa, but the dogs wouldn't stay still.

She is talking and laughing, but she is the only one privy to what is being said. She joins the conversation, then sees something on television that joins her sentences, then she sees something in her environment that now takes over the main talk. She finds it very funny, so Bri and I join in on the laughter. It's so good to see her happy, regardless of what we are—or are not—talking about. It doesn't matter, she is truly laughing. I hope we will have this conversation again tomorrow...for obvious reasons.

Tonight may the angels kiss away your sadness.
If only for tonight—laugh mother—and let us laugh with you.

Brian was sitting beside her for dinner. He fixes her plate. As she is eating, I asked if she was hungry? She said she was really hungry and everything tastes so good. I asked her if Brian was hungry? She told me she hadn't seen him yet today.

She's outside, then she's inside. She walks fairly well, then she can't stand up by herself.

She answers a question appropriately, then the conversation completely flies out to left field.

She can't find the "restroom."

She is always asking me where I want her to go now.

She takes off her shoes and walks about in her socks. This is normal behavior for me, but very strange for my roommate.

Her condition is changing. Is it the head wound that hasn't healed? Maybe what is going on behind the bandage? Is it too many falls? Maybe falls are causing "shaking baby syndrome? Maybe seizure activity from the brain injury? Mini strokes? Dementia? Old age or senility? Whatever it is, we won't know. I won't put her through any more testing. No more hospitalizations if I can avoid it. We are blessed by the fact that she isn't aware of what we see. Every day is a brand-new day for her, starting with frosted flakes with mini marshmallows and sliced bananas. I have many colorful headbands that we now use to keep the bandage in place on her head.

The cookie box is always filled with her white double stuffed Oreos, which she hits very hard all day long. She has her ice cream every night at bedtime. She basically toilets herself and feeds herself. She needs supervision or assistance in almost everything else anymore. But she is not unhappy. She doesn't know what to do but declines any suggestions. The Pirates are back playing on "Extra Innings," but she doesn't watch them. She feels she has already seen whatever we have on TV. Sometimes the TV works adversely on her, as she seems to think that the shows are the news and it is really happening. This is so true with the weather on the shows, or shootings or wrecks. She is confused with single verbal commands now, and usually requires assistance. When given a choice, it is always, "whatever you want." I don't think she can remember what the choices were. She hears the first choice, and when she hears the second choice, by then the first choice has already left. Her quality of life is questionable, but her physical condition is rather good.

I do have to tell this story. After our altercations with the wheelchair and Walmart a few days ago, my mother looked at me and said, "your sister almost ruined things yesterday." I asked if she meant our trip to the Walmart and she said yes. I asked "how did my sister almost ruin things?" She said, "by the way she treated me." So I got a "get out of jail free card" sisters…but one of you have to take the fall for the treatment of our mother in Walmart. Sorry about that.

Sometimes I get wordy, but things have changed so much and I want to keep everyone informed. My roommate is very restless tonight. She is now sleeping in the TV room on a roll away bed by my sofa. It's lower, so she can't fall far now. She is now upside down and has her blanket on the floor covering the dogs, and her pillow on top of "the kitten" who was sitting quietly on the sofa. Now she is messing with the blinds on the window. It's gonna be an interesting evening.

Brian now has one of the guys that he works with, residing with him in his home. Since that occurred, I have another dog at my doggy day care. My cousin Bill would come visit and be surrounded by the dogs. It has been said that he doesn't truly care for dogs, yet they won't stay away from him. Maybe they are trying to convert him to a canine lover. There are more dogs for you to meet. You haven't met the four-year-old 110# blue-nosed pit bull. He makes #7 under my leadership about fourteen hours a day—I'm not sure if Brian's dog Lucy was here when you visited—but she is #6.

Jody and I are sewing new kitchen curtains for her home, hemming three long dresses to a shorter length, finishing an appliqued and embroidered tablecloth, and made a table runner for her antique kitchen table. She plans on painting her kitchen with the two girls she is raising when she returns to Pa. Mom watches us while we are busy, but she doesn't join in. She is showing more agitation with the presence of a house guest, but she does that when she has a doctor's appointment, a visitor, or even when the neighbor stops over to chat. Anything that upsets her normal routine causes her anxiety these days. That certainly isn't the mother that I remember, but it is the traits of this sweet lady I live with—I kinda refer to her as my "second mother." Even her tastes are different from her first eighty-eight years, as she was eating potato chips and cheese curls with Jody the last few evenings. One night I had packed Doritos into Brian's lunch and had a few left in the bag. She finished them and then said—"what are we gonna eat now?" I don't ever remember her eating cheese curls or chips of any kind.

We finally got a good rain today…one day I don't have to manually water my plants.

Bri will be stopping to pick up his and his roommates dogs after work. They are working eight-hour days this week so he will be here about 2:30 AM.

When I tell Mom about the snow and ice you guys have up north, she starts watching for it "to come our way." Bri wanted to go buy a snow machine and run it out the window where she sits. She will just have to keep "watching" for it—cause I don't miss the chilling weather that affects my muscles and bones in a negative way—not because I am getting older, but because of the change in her familiar routine. (That's my story, and I'm sticking to it.)

Into the Second Quarter
of the New Year

God is surely on the job…Mom was just up trying to walk around. I said, "Mom, what are you doing?"

She never knows; I asked if she had to pee. She said yes. So I helped her to the pot.

She looked at it and said, "How do I work this?"

I said, "You have to pick up the lid."

When I did, she said, "Oh, there it is."

Her innocence is so very priceless.

HELLO, MAY

I just ran back to mother's room—she could barely walk back to bed half hour ago—requiring much help from me. now I find her standing at the foot of her bed. She has pulled the bedrail out from between the mattress and box springs. And she's going to "go over there and do that." Of course, this is just the ending of a day where she was very talkative during the entire baseball game. Talkative—to say the least. She said that one guy kept moving his hat, because he was cold—that girl just ran over that, and it was a girl—they just gave that one a hat—and her informative chatter continued throughout the game, leaving Bri with a strange look on his face when he stopped over. On the way back to her bed, she said to me, "Did you and Judy decide to switch out?" I just ran back again—this time stepping in a puddle of pee in the hallway—(damn) in time to catch her getting up to "get the corn fixed in the corner and to move them over." Her eyes aren't even open. Do you think I will get to watch the special on Princess Diana?

I Set Up a Hospice Evaluation

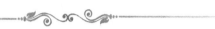

Good morning, sisters and family.
As you already know, I set up a hospice evaluation. I picked a facility in Altamonte Springs. They all know that the entire remainder of family is up north. Altamonte Springs is the neighboring town where I had taken our mother to see the infection-control doctor when we came down to Florida with IV Vancomycin, a year and a half ago.

On Friday, the "intake nurse" spent about two-plus hours here to evaluate whether our mother was a candidate for hospice. They have guidelines that life expectancy is six months or less, and their own hospice physicians decide if they will be able to accept a patient into their program. If they do accept our mother, their doctor will be her doctor and she won't be seeing any others. He will perform as her family doctor also. Meds will be reviewed and ordered through their pharmacy…the medicine Shopee…and we will no longer use express scripts. They will not do cultures, use IV medication, or admit to hospital, unless there is a change in her condition. They have a social worker, nurses, aides, volunteers, a pastor, and physicians on their staff.

The Intake Nurse explained the head wound and the three-year history and the hospice team chose to accept Mom. If she holds her own with no dramatic decline, in six months they can transfer her "out" of hospice and then use Home Health. Meanwhile all health care etc. will be done in our home. She said they even have doctors that make house calls when needed. This area's team color is yellow—which suited me super fine.

As she has been seen by five different staff in the last four days, they understand her status. They know she has a head wound, basically of two-plus years that has no prospects of healing. They know she ambulates independently in the home, is continent, feeds herself, does some dressing of herself, but basically needs assistance or supervision for about everything else. They know she washes dishes as her "way" to help in the home. They know she lives for the dogs, and makes up the seven dog dishes of food almost daily. They know she treats the dogs from morning to night and feeds them from her own food—and that is her only real enjoyment at this time. I told them of the time she fed JoJo pancakes with syrup from her plate with her fork. Then for the next hour or more, Rusty licked and cleaned JoJo's face of all the syrup. I told them she will not eat in front of the dogs, without giving them something. I explained that Mom's favorite cookie is vanilla Oreos…and because I walk away—she thinks she's treating them behind my back. She actually thinks she sneaks them her cookies, and does it very quietly. I do walk away, as this act gives Mom so much satisfaction. As six dogs were in their crates beside the kitchen table where they all sat to interview Mom, and the large guy was in the hallway on the roll away bed with a child gate between us—they all were so perfectly behaved. I explained that they could see everything—so they don't mind their crates. I told them the real problem when they are in their crates was Mom—but since she could see all them…she was okay too. The dogs have become Mom's reason for life—and now hospice is in awe of this. The pastor wanted to know how I possibly toilet seven dogs, as he has great difficulty with one.

Bri was here for three out of five of their visits. He removed Mom when some of the conversation turned in the direction that she could misunderstand. They all know that Bri and I use our own language and have made notations to be more aware of things they say, and that she can't really answer questions. He explained that trying to answer questions increases her anxiety and frustration. I guess they felt with her confusion, that they could discuss things of a final nature in her presence. They must use a lot of discretion in their hiring process, because the staff is fabulous. After two hours plus with everyone, and explaining and answering questions—I was very, very tired. I also know that involving "hospice" played a number on me also—as it puts a finality or ending on things.

I have refused aides to help with personal care at this time. I explained that if a stranger comes in to undress her—we will have a real problem. I am going to start using Walmart on-line shopping, where you get a time, and drive up and they load the car. I need to make a dentist appointment, so I will talk with the volunteer coordinator and then go from there.

I was trying to get Mom to join in conversations, so we discussed "the baby lima bean" story and the fact that Millie "has never seen snow." She found out the social worker has never seen snow either. Mom's reaction to that was so honest—her show of total disbelief that she knows two people that have never seen snow.

All the staff were complimentary with what they saw. Many compliments as they watched Bri's intervention on her behalf—I called him my "relief pitcher." I told them of her life for the first eighty-eight years and how lucky I was. She is naive, she is innocent, she is not angry, she is appreciative, she is fragile and yet she is so very lost in time. I told them that I could never give back in a few years what she has given family, friends, church, meals on wheels, kids in the cafeteria, etc., in those eighty-eight years.

Her BP was high when first checked. Bri explained how she gets anxious when someone comes into the home, because she doesn't really know anybody. When they checked it yesterday it was perfect. We did have to keep reassuring her that nobody was here to take her anywhere—but until Bri would tell her "I won't let anyone take you—cause they have to go through me"—she was at ease. I just keep telling her that she's not going anywhere and leave me with these seven dogs. She looks over at the dogs and just smiles.

Their pharmacy sends out a "comfort Pac" that has several medications to use if needed. They told me it will have "Haldol" in it, if I needed to try it at bedtime to see if it helps her sleep. I thanked them, but told them we are trying to use less medication as more.

She often forgets she can't "flush" the potty chair, but forgets how to flush the toilet. She got up to the "restroom" during the night because the potty chair "was full." (I have no idea where that idea came from.)

She brought out the Poo-Pourri spray (that I use in her potty chair) with her toothbrush and asked, "Is this what I use." So I have now removed it from her sight. (by the way, that is the first time she picked up her toothbrush on her own, in three years.)

Slippers are almost always on the wrong feet

When the staff asked if she knew what was going on with her head. I left her explain—"tell her what is different about your head, Mom?"

She said, "I have a hole in my head."

When Jane asks about the kitten and how it is doing, she says, "It's growing."

She seldom walks outside anymore. I have furniture set up in the house that she can hold onto something wherever she walks.

Her bedframe is removed, and her mattress and box spring sits on the floor. We haven't had a fall in months. I turned her bed into a "low" bed, so she doesn't fall from it.

This is the update—when I know more, I will let you know. Basically, the interviewing and paperwork should be mostly done.

ONE HALF YEAR OVER

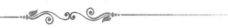

Hi, all, good morning.
I'm going to sit down and write down a few happenings in "happy valley" here in Sanford. Things that happen that amaze me. Things that allow me to wonder into the makings of our precious Mawmaw's brain function. Things that we take for granted. Things we don't really think about because it is so easy for us. Things that are not as easy for some others.

Yesterday our mother was clearing the table of the dishes. She picked up a plate with the silverware and walked toward the kitchen sink. She rounded the kitchen island slowly and walked right past the kitchen sink. The very same sink she checks every ten minutes to see if there are dishes to be washed. She walks to the far end of the island and leans against the corner, placing the plate on the countertop. She looked over to me, with a confused look on her face. She pointed to the storm door to the carport and asked; "I go that way to wash the dishes, don't I?"

I walked over and placed my arms around her shoulders and picked up the plate with the silverware—walked her to the sink, and showed her the dishpan, where she could wash the dishes. She seemed so relieved, and thanked me several times.

A few days ago, I tried to get her interested in helping me make meatloaf. She sat and watched, telling me that I do it better. As I mixed the meat and all the ingredients, she got up and walked over to the island. She loves to watch me do things—she is no longer a participant, but rather a spectator. I formed two meatloaves and placed them in the baking dishes. I took some bacon out of the fridge and cut them in very small pieces. I started placing them on top of one of the meatloaves, and ask Mom to finish. She saw how I started, so she picked up one of the pieces and placed it on top—and then asked me if that was what I meant. I assured her it was perfect, and would she do it to the top of both loaves. I went about doing something else. She finished and called me over. She said she didn't have enough to finish the second one. She had placed all the bacon on top, covering a full meatloaf, and also exactly half of the other one. I look at the loaves and told her it was perfect, because we are going to eat it anyway. A normal functioning brain would have dispersed the bacon pieces, making it cover both loaves. My other mother's brain doesn't work that way. Funny, was our brain trained to work that way—or does it require reasoning and preplanning capabilities? Did she use the bacon as I would have? No, but then it doesn't mean that it wasn't the right way.

It's fascinating...to wonder if I am watching basic instincts that we are born with? Watching our second mother get through a day... and often a night...is not easy. I wonder why she wants to get out of bed in the morning. I wonder why she wants to face one more day, or even half of a day. She has nothing that truly has her interest, unless it is something that I am painting, sewing, baking or cooking, crafting or changing. She watches as I take down drapes, and hang others. She compliments me on how it "brightens things up"—or how hard I am working and she wishes she could do something.

The little rack with the Keurig cups—she now fills it up. We have found another helpful task for her to do. She puts on her slippers or shoes every morning. It doesn't bother me that they are on the wrong feet, if it doesn't bother her. She combs her hair every morning before coming out for breakfast. She fusses when I trim it, that I cut too much off—but when it holds the set and almost looks even, she is pleased. I have explained that she doesn't want long hair on one side of her head, when the bandage needs to be on the other side.

The hospice nurse came today and spent two hours with us. She will come once a week and wants me to document any changes. I told her my emails to my family up north would act like a diary on her behaviors. Our mother told the nurse about all the visitors we get, "And there are lots." She can't name them, doesn't talk to them in my presence, won't go to bed while they are here, and gets upset when they leave without saying anything. The nurse did confirm what we already knew, that some patients do see people that have passed, and get visits from deceased family when they are reaching the end of their life. I told her that her visitors don't have names or identities, but then neither do I. The nurse asked her first name, her middle name, and she answered them right. She could not tell her birthday, and when she asked who I was—she answered "my nurse."

She weighed 135 today, her BP, pulse, temp, lungs—all were perfect. She did tell the nurse "no" when she asked if she ever smoked. She noted how her balance is off, and the furniture is all placed so she can use it to walk around. She offered a sleeping pill, but I told her if Mom is going to get up during the night...I would rather it would be without medication. We haven't had a fall in a very long time. Our mother gets up many times, comes to the door and opens it, and often thinks it is time to get up for the day. When she is told that it is the middle of the night and still dark outside, she goes back to bed. But she does get up—and I don't want her medicated when she does because that's when she'll fall.

As you know, Heather has some surgeries coming up. I'm truly afraid if I bring Mom home, I'll disrupt her stability. She doesn't remember which way the "restroom" is, still worries that the potty chair is full, and she can't flush it, knows where the breakfast table is, washes dishes and moves from chair to chair to loveseat. We watch the baseball game each evening—(thank God for DVR)...if a game isn't on. They are always too long...and she asks where she can sleep. The dogs and her eat double stuff vanilla Oreos every day between meals—and she is really trying to drink more water. She has half cup coffee about three times a day and frosted flakes with "those little white things" every single morning (frosted flakes with marshmallows). We have those little green lima beans often—and they are always "so good."

Six dogs lie in their crates when hospice comes, and the big guy is in the hall with the child gate across. Nobody can believe how well behaved they are while they are here (do you believe that? I was told these dogs are well behaved); they actually lie, often upside down, and sleep while hospice staff is here. Millie was here for supper, and she is afraid of the big dog. So why is it that the large dog Diesel, wants to be right beside her at the table. Of course, his head is above the level of the table. She kinda freezes in her seat.

Mom got up and came out for breakfast and looked so amazed. She said, "Did you do this all yourself when I was in bed? It looks beautiful. You did all this yourself?"

I asked, what are you referring to, Mom?"

As innocent as always, she said, "All this furniture. You put all this furniture in here and it looks beautiful...I can't believe you move this all yourself" (what can I say, every day is a brand-new day in our mother's world. I knew it often came with visitors that I don't see, and sisters that come and go without saying goodbye...I just didn't know every day came with new furniture—life is good).

As a finale, the thunder just stopped so I took the dogs outside. Our mother said, "I have to go to the pot...do I come out too." And she laughed.

I told her she had to go the other direction...and relished her sarcasm and sense of humor. She laughs more often than she has in a long time. It is usually when Bri is here.

As I explained to hospice nurse...we have had a few really good weeks. She's walking better, remembering some things, and happy. She is happy, and I truly believe that. She's holding Mickie on the loveseat right now...she had just consoled Ricky during the thunder storm, and she keeps reaching down to the floor and petting Annie and Rusty's head. There lies her reason for life.

Love to all family up north...from the southern three. Please keep a prayer in your hearts for Heather's upcoming surgeries and keep a check on her in her mother's place. She knows I would be there for her...if things weren't so stable here with her grandmother and brother. Like I tell people, my daughter is a bullfighter, and Cancer is the bull. She's not going to sit and wait on the bull—she's going after it first...on her terms...in her own time. And she's going in for the kill. That's how she rolls these days.

THE HOSPICE DOCTOR

Let me see if I can convey the results of the visit from Dr. Michael Brown here at home to see Mawmaw. He is one of the hospice doctors, and I've been told he has a neuro background.

He showed up with his little gray doctor's bag. I met him on the carport and told him it would be a few minutes. I explained that I had the largest dog blocked in the hallway, when my mother decided she needed to go to the bathroom. I explained that the gate is down till my mother comes out of the restroom. We stood in the carport and talked for a bit. When I ask if he was allergic to dogs, he assured me he wasn't. He told me he had dogs and they have just rescued a dog, since they had just lost a few dogs from old age. He commenced to describe the dog as part dash hound with feet that turn outward, but with some terrier mix also, that he was truly a mutt. Its name is Gusstaff—with a nickname of Gus. I commended him for rescuing, instead of shopping. He said he should have done it that way before. I agreed, and said I felt the animals know when they are rescued and become great pets. He also knew that and felt they were grateful. I said some of these dogs were rescued, a few were shopped for…and a few are staying with us while their owners work during the day.

Oh, so you wanted to know how his visit went with Mom? (Smiling.) Well, that's how it started.

I brought him in and introduced him to Mom…while seven dogs were all saying Hello at the same time. I left them say Hello for a minute—and then I settled them down. There was 6 in their crates, and one in the hallway. The doctor sat down and removed a small yellow pad and pencil from his bag. He didn't bring out a laptop as all the other staff had done, except the Pastor. He didn't have a cell phone making any noises the entire hour he was here. He had a manual BP cuff and a small flashlight he used to check Mom's eyes and throat. He took notes on his yellow notepad.

He explained Mom's type of cerebral bleed and drew a small picture to explain it by. Some bleeds occur inside the brain, and cause brain injury. Her bleed occurred outside the brain, and put the pressure and injury from the outside of the covering of the brain.

He asked Mom her age—she thought maybe eighty-four—and kept looking at me. I told her I wasn't allowed to give her the answers this time. He asked Mom her birthday, or when she was born. She didn't know. He asked her what year this is——she didn't know. He asked her who the president is right now—she didn't know. He asked her where she was born, and she answered Kepple Hill. I explained that the answer was correct. He then asked her if she was born in the hospital. She looked at him with a very strange look on her face and answered, "No, at home."

He said, "Most were born at home back then, weren't they?"

She agreed.

He watched her walk a few steps, then had her shut her eyes and hold her hands out straight; they kept going together. He repositioned her arms and hands and told her to keep them out straight. Again the hands went together.

He explained that hospice is palliative care…and there really wasn't any care to give Mom at this time. They offer comfort measures, pain control, treatment of any symptoms, bowel or bladder management—and she didn't need any of them. He said he will probably see her again in a few weeks.

He wanted to know how I manage toileting for the seven dogs…and how about poop patrol? He apparently had his sons two boxers, plus three other dogs in his big back yard at one time—and the grandkids didn't like to come because there was poop in the yard. He said he welcomed any of them to come and do poop patrol if they wanted to. He said he had to clean up the yard every three or more days, and I laughed. I said I never let it go beyond a day, sometimes several times a day I also explained that I have a fenced in yard, and often just prop the storm door open. It means I'm air conditioning the outside—but it works for the dogs.

As I walked him out, he commended me for what it must take to care for the dogs—let alone taking care of my mom.

I told him she was better than she's been in a year…remembering where the restroom is, knows where the dishes get washed, often recalls something from the day before, or that happened earlier in the day. I also explained that the memory that included the entire family seems to be missing, along with any ability to cook, bake, sew, quilt, can…etc. He just explained that memory is affected in different ways, but not to rule out dementia, Alzheimer's, along with the injury from the clot. I told him I worried about taking her out of her familiar place…and going backward. I remember what happened when Jo came to visit for the week—and how she felt she was the one that needed to go home, when Millie came to visit.

The doctor explained that keeping a routine is very important, and disrupting that routine would be very confusing for her. He explained what happens when they put someone in a different place than they are used to—and how you can't get back to where you were initially…after such a change. I point blank ask—if I took her home to Pa. …could I lose the place we are at now? He answered with an adamant "Yes." I know she doesn't know anyone enough to even miss anyone—so bringing this other mother "home" may cause such confusion that I won't be able to get her back to where we are now. He just said several times: keeping her routine the same is very important to her.

I want everyone to know there is an open invitation to come and stay with us—I have several beds that are not used—and lots of blankets for "sleepovers" in the great room. If I know I get some company, I will purchase some air beds—so know that my door is always open—(that's the truth, propped open for the dogs to toilet).

FUNNY THOUGHTS

When I asked Mom how many dogs we feed every day, she didn't know.

When I asked her how many dishes of food she makes for the dogs every day, she answered, "Seven."

The doctor told me to continue using clues, prompts, directions—and keep her routine steady. He wasn't interested in seeing her wound, stating, "I don't need to."

Now my thoughts on all these visits—seven nurse visits, one pastor, one social worker, one doctor—they are not coming to see Mom. They heard there are seven dogs under one roof, and they come to see how the dog house works. I just explain that thus far...I maintain the alpha dog position—or I get out the squirt guns, the flyswatter, or the puperoni for reward.

The hospice nurse, should be here tomorrow. She was going to save us for her last visit, because she wanted to meet Brian.

So Mom and I are working on some small Christmas crafts; she continues to keep all the dishes washed and now the Keurig tree filled. She fixes seven dishes of dog food...and still feels she is alone when I am outside. Even when I tell her where I am going, I have the mower running, the door is propped open, and I check on her often. If I am not in her visual field, she is alone. If I take a nap on the sofa, "that one was sleeping over there."

So tomorrow we will spin the wheel again and start a brand-new day.

MOM FORGOT MICKIE

Our mother walked back the hall and into the bathroom last night. Mickie went back and laid by the door, as she often does. Mom came out of the bathroom and life resumed in the living area. As I walked back the hall and stepped over a sleeping Mickie, I saw that the bathroom door was closed. I came out and told Mom that Mickie must have followed her into the bathroom. She listened as I explained that Mickie was asleep back the hall. I explained that she follows her everywhere and probably fell asleep before she came out of the bathroom. Mom still listened. She was listening—but not able to comprehend what the meaning was.

I said, "Mom, walk back the hall and talk to Mickie. She thinks you are still in the bathroom." Mom walked halfway back the hall, and said, "This way?"

I said, "Keep going—you will see black Mickie laying back there. She is looking for you."

She walked back, hall lights are lit and immediately starts fusing over Mickie, telling her to "come with me," "come on, honey," "you are such a good dog," as Mickie walked out, following Mom's voice, and lay in front of her when Mom sat in the chair. Mom leaned over and praised her, rubbed her head, petted her back and continued to fuss over her for being such a good dog.

Prayer sent to heaven: "Please let us keep black Mickie as long as necessary. The other dogs are usually just a number from one to six—but Mickie is not. She continues to get an insulin shot every afternoon, and I have no clue what her blood sugar is. I just monitor how much and how often she drinks water. She is basically blind,

370

only seeing movements and responds to voice. She has walked into things, including another dog. I watch closely when she is outside. I call her and she follows my voice to come in. I have tripped over her, she has walked over dogs that were asleep—she actually walked over Diesel's legs as he slept in the doorway. She puts her paws up on our mother, and our mother picks her up and holds her for hours. I haven't told Mom the family and friends that have died in the recent past. She won't miss them, so she doesn't know they are gone. Mickie is not in the category."

She said, "Morning or evening?" (Does it even matter, dear Mother?) She kinda bases bedtime by darkness, and getting up with daylight.

We were watching the baseball game last night. She seldom looks at the TV screen unless I'm narrating. Michael, I'm explaining baseball to my mother. Her questions aren't the same as the ones I call and ask you, but they are questions just the same.

I tell her, "Oops, the other team got a homerun, so they are winning. We are still losing, Mom, but your Cutch is doing a fine job. Mom, watch that guy run and catch the ball...he slides, but he has the ball—watch, Mom...they will show it again. That used to be your favorite player, Mom."

"Who?"

"Andrew Mccutcheon...you called him Cutch."

"It still is...how much more is there."

"Who is your favorite player, Mom?"

"That same one—when does this stop?"

"It has a long way to go yet, Mom...and they are losing."

"Well, I'm going to lay down here."

"No, Mom, let's go back to your bed. You've already fell asleep a few times, and it's hard to walk you when you've been asleep."

"Okay, where do I go?"

"In your room, you have a bed with the purple blanket—oh look, we are winning now."

"Well, I'm going to stay here then...I have to see this."

"Okay, it's fun to watch the game when we are winning, isn't it?"

(Are you ready for her next question...family?) "Oh, are we winning?"

God blesses this lady every day—and blesses me by keeping me entertained at the same time. The world where her mind resides is a place where only angels dare to walk.

Bri burned up a lot of brush and dead tree stuff in my back yard Friday night. I brought Mom out on a chair. She doesn't really like being outside. We kept right beside her—but she wanted to go "back." I think she's afraid she won't find her way back to the familiar interior of the house. I'm so glad the kitchen, dining and TV room is all one big open area—because she can see them all—and she moves from chair to chair to sofa in that area.

She loses her way to the "restroom," and never finds her bedroom. Her world is the big room and the restroom. She opens the storm door and leans out...but doesn't really like to go out. She tries to keep the dogs within her area also—but she doesn't like it when they are all laying down and sleeping. She thinks they have gone somewhere ...and often doesn't see them until they start moving. She still pulls dogs out of the crates...thinking they don't know "how to get out." I think she's telling me a lot about herself when she does that. How many time she has said to me "don't forget me"—and when I'm outside, she is "all alone...and there wasn't anybody around."

We have a lot of afternoon thunder storms this time of year. I've kinda bridged the fear she has of them...by the need for her to sit on the loveseat and calm "the little black dog down" I tell her how afraid he is, and he tried to hide under our legs and feet. She now knows that he needs her to cuddle him against her legs and make him feel safe. She keeps reassuring him. She did that often through this Fourth of July fireworks in the neighbor's yard—every night for over a week. Last night there were many big loud bangs—somebody must have had leftover fireworks.

The nurse canceled on Friday...she had several new admissions and I told her we were fine. She was so grateful...She made sure I didn't need anything...I told her we can handle anything on Monday.

Bri starts ten-hour days on Monday—in this hundred-degree heat—seven floors up on the edge of a building—so she will not get

HOWEVER LONG IT TAKES

to meet him. They all bring their laptops in...except the doctor—he brought his pen and little yellow notepad. It's so nice to meet someone else who is "old school."

WHAT TIME IS IT?

I tucked her in bed tonight.

She said, "I'll try not to bother you so many times for the number tonight."

I kissed her cheek and told her, "You ask me as often as you want, anytime you want to know what time it is. When I hear your door open, I know that's what you want to know...and I will tell you." She smiled, and her eyes even twinkled—when she said "okay."

She just can't read a clock, neither digital or with hands. I've even tried to show her the digital clock, and if she just looks at the first number, it will give her an idea of what time it is.

SOME QUESTIONS FOR MY MOTHER

I'm gonna ask my mother some questions while she eats her break-fast this morning. Mornings seem to be her most livid times—so we will see how it goes.

"Now you know you have some memory problems—do you know why?"

"No...I don't know why."

"Do you know that you've had surgery on your head?"

She nodded yes.

"Do you know why?"

"I don't know—if I fell or what?"

"Do you know if you were married?"

"Yes—"

"Do you know to who?

"I think I was married twice."

"Do you know if you have any grandchildren?"

"Yeah, I think I do."

"Do you know any of them?"

"No."

"Do you know if you have any children?"

"Yes, I have children."

"Do you know what you have?"

(She was struggling for an answer.) "I know I had them, but...?"

"What about brothers or sisters?"

"Yes—Tom—Frances and Fern—I think I had another one—it's in some books somewhere."

"Does it hurt your head to try and think or remember?"

"It doesn't hurt my head, I just feel bad that I can't remember."

"This isn't to make you feel bad—I just want to see how much you can remember."

"Is there any names in your family that you can remember…or names that come to mind?"

"Can you think of the last time in your life…that you can remember things? Like you remembered Tom, Frances, and Fern's name."

"Can you remember the last place you lived—before here?"

"Well, I lived in Riverview—I lived there a good while…with my mother and dad."

"Yes, you did."

"I went to school in Kepple Hill, I graduated from there, and then from Vandergrift."

"What about after that?"

"I went to work in the mill. With my dad."

"What about after you worked in the mill?"

"We had a farm…somewhere."

"What do you remember about the farm?"

"How did you go from the mill—to the farm?"

"The boy that bought the farm. Just made a mansion out of it…it was beautiful."

"Who do you mean by 'the boy'?"

"My son—as far as I know he still has it. I haven't been back to see it for a long time."

"How long has it been?"

"A long time, but I remember all the people that were around there. Like I said…he worked hard on the farm—he deserved it."

"Homer got it…and he deserved it. I think his name was Homer. He worked hard—I think it was his son—he helped Homer…and then one built a house way up on the hill—and we all worked hard… and hauled hay."

So one built a house way up on the hill? Do you know who that was? "yes, that was the one we gave it to—"

"You gave the farm to someone?"

"Yeah, he was our son."

"Did you just have the one son?"

"Yeah, I think, but I'm not sure. We all worked hard."

"Someone turned it into a mansion?"

"Yes—"

"Who was that?"

"Homer."

"Were you related to Homer?"

"My son."

"And you haven't been back to the farm for a while?"

"No, not for a long time."

"What are you thinking about now?"

"Just about all those involved in it—babies, and kids…and all…I haven't been back for a long while."

"Whose babies and kids?"

"My grandchildren."

"So you do have grandchildren?"

"Yes."

"Do you know who they are?"

"Yes…I knew them all, but I can't come up with them now. It would be in books somewhere—I don't know where," but you need the books to remember more about it? "yea…there was a lot of those on the farm. A lot of good times."

"How 'bout a lot of hard work?"

"Yes…a lot of that…mowing and making hay…canning and all that …that goes with it."

"Do you want to go visit there again?"

"No…I don't know."

"Are you content where we are right now?"

"Yes, at this time I am."

"Why don't you want to go back?"

"I wouldn't mind going back…but not to stay…but I'm not sure."

"So you would rather not do any of that right now?"

"Right."

"Is there anybody you miss that you want to see?"

"I'm sure there is…I'm sure there is more babies born—"

"But you are okay…with where we are right now?"
She nodded. "Yes."
"Is there anywhere you want to go…or do?"
"No, not right now."
"Just here with all our dogs."
"Right."

LATE JULY

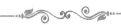

She's struggling to remember, but it's hard for her to understand that she did live an active life before things changed. She only knows that she doesn't remember any of it

How we remember; and what we remember; and why we remember form the most personal map of our individuality. It seems like mother is free-falling, never knowing where she actually is.

I spent a lot of time today trying to get my wireless printer connected to the new carrier, and then getting my laptop to communicate with the printer. Finally, I contacted Tech support and they did remote access and finally got it working properly. Meanwhile they would keep calling me back and then all the dogs would start barking loudly, so I smacked Mickie on her nose to stop barking. A little later I asked Mom what she wanted to do.

Her answer was, "I'll just stay with the dogs and keep them from getting "knocked around." Somedays there just isn't enough chocolate.

Some situations may break your heart or damage your pride—but never give these events the power to break your spirit.

Mom is obsessed with doing the dishes. I knew that—I also know she is most comfortable in the large room where she can see all of her surroundings. She always sits in the chair in the far corner, even to watch TV. It's like she has nothing behind her then. It's also why she likes the back seat in the snowbird—she can see who is in the car with her.

Since I just changed networks and cable companies—it's been hard to get the wireless printer functioning properly and learn the new channels—I forgot how different they are. I don't have as many TV channels as before—but I also don't know just how many I do have or what shows are available. I also am saving over $100 a month—in the contract I was in for over two years. I've spent more time working on the laptop and TV than usual—but I thought it was okay since the TV was on and I was in full view. I brought in peppers out of the garden and had Mom cutting them into chunks so I could chop them and freeze them in little snack bags for cooking. She told me she would cut them up, but she wouldn't use "that thing"—meaning the little chopper. I started bagging up the chopped peppers—she got a little upset when I started cleaning up.

She said, "I don't know where she went. She was getting more of these, so she probably went outside to get more. You better wait till she comes back…because she was looking for more."

Again, dearest mother, I have nothing.

She was acting a little different as the evening went on, wanting to know where everyone went. She didn't understand why some of the family left without offering to drop her off somewhere. When I asked her where she wanted dropped off—she would get anxious and say, "I don't know, but they will know. I just need to go somewhere and take these kids and go home." "Where are those stairs that go to that place?" She looked at the TV, but never seemed to see what she what was going on. She didn't want to do anything other than do the dishes and wipe the dining table. She would dry the dishes and try so hard to put them away. The cupboards they go in has no doors on them…and they are right above the dishrack. She brought in a handful of silverware and started looking around the TV and my little laptop desk. She said she couldn't find the place where "these went." So I directed her back out to the kitchen and showed her the drawer where they go. She is always so very thankful. She knows she should know—and also knows she can't remember. I tried to get her interested in making some sugar cookies. She didn't want to help, but washed up the dishes as I used them.

Hospice couldn't even find a way to hold her under Medicare for the time allotted. You know how well she can appear—and how she can carry on a general conversation without any specifics that require her to remember. When she got so adamant last night about "getting on her shoes and going somewhere" "and nobody knows where I am and they will be hunting me," I called Bri against her will—she was upset that I bothered him and "now he will be upset and call all the rest-and then everyone gets involved." She kept shaking her head "no" while she talked with him; he offered to come over and she declined. Then when Jane called back—she wasn't talking very much. She didn't want me to call Jane—because—are you ready? She just met her, and even though she was her daughter; she didn't know her as a child or while she was growing up…and then she will get upset and upset all the others.

She wasn't going to be "locked in that room"—when someone would be hunting for her. She went in her room and came back out—saying she needed to go home…and someone needed to come and get her. She told me she was messing up my plans…and that I needed to do what I have to do and let her go to that other place where she does the dishes. I turned her chair around so she could see the sink and dishpan—sat her by the dining table…but she only seemed to see what was in her head—not what she was seeing.

She finally sat on the loveseat where she could hold the dogs… but her face was tense. I told her we needed to stay here because we have so many dogs and they are happy here. The baseball game came on…and she watched the TV screen.

I got up this morning and stepped in diarrhea. The four new pee pads had spots all over them, along with the areas on the floor that were difficult to see. I go through pee pads like air—and I try to keep clean ones down because Mom just walks all over them. Mickie drinks and pees all waking moments. Mom feeds Annie on the sly, anything she has access to. She says she just "gave her a bite" and yet half Oreo cookie is laying between her paws. The Oreo cookies she is always getting out of the box—cannot be all ate by her. No matter how many dog biscuits I put in her view—it doesn't work. It's like she wants to feed the dogs her own food—even ice cream off the spoon. We are always changing her shirts…and the placemats get washed constantly. I need to keep a constant check on her personal care and hands. She is trying so hard—like playing solitaire with only

51 cards. The neurons aren't connecting to the right receptors in her brain, but more and more of them are connecting to something.

It's all improvement—and isn't that what we were working toward. I watch her struggle and I wonder—did I do her any favors by working to get her back? I work with her 24-7 to keep her content and happy…but am I?

I just watched her toilet herself…and get back in bed. I am very fortunate and grateful for the simple acts of self-care she does. She feels remorse for not raising Jane—and carries guilt into the next day because of that. She remembers that she didn't know her until a little while ago. She continues to remember, and it upsets her. She knows I am here all the time—but there is more than one of me. I'm not sure who she thinks I am and I don't challenge her or ask. I just make excuses for the one that hasn't come back in with more peppers, or the ones who left without saying goodbye.

I don't entertain. I don't invite people into the home, it's too hard with the dogs. And besides—it just makes more work. I've just left my little workshop in the corner of the living area where I pay bills—do computer and printer things—and Facebook.

I went to Walmart one day, as Bri came to sit with Mom. Often they would both take a nap, while he held her hand. This day he called me at Walmart to tell me I may have to come home, as he just took Mom into the bathroom and shut the door. He didn't know what kind of help she would need and he wanted me to be available. I headed toward the checkout.

Before I was even in line, he called me back to tell me not to hurry. After calling her name and knocking on the door, He opened the door to check on Mom. He found her totally dressed, sitting on the commode with the lid closed. He didn't realize she didn't know what to do for herself. As I finished shopping, all I could think of is Mom wondering why Bri put her in that small room and then shut the door.

The dogs have started peeing in the house when I'm outside, even if the storm door is propped open. And Mom doesn't see any of this. I take the dogs outside with me and shut the door…she opens it and lets them back in. Mickie's eyesight has gotten worse. I have to watch her on the steps…and also make sure she finds her way back in the house when she goes outside. Sometimes I just see her wondering around aimlessly—but just like Mom, she just keeps trying—she takes the hand she was dealt and lies by Mom's feet constantly. The sad part is…Mom doesn't often see her because she does it quietly…Annie is the attention demander…and so she gets the attention Mom loves to give—food and more food. I am seeing that is a good thing. Mom isn't content when the dogs are sleeping—I'm not sure why—but when Annie is always demanding attention—she likes to fuss over her and talk to her. I've thought about kenneling annie during moms meals—but I get lax, and Mom finds things to feed her, anyways—anytime—anything.

DAD'S BIRTHDAY

Dad's birthday came and went quietly. I didn't bring it up. It probably wouldn't have mattered to my mother, so I thought back-quietly-on life with my father. His last number of years was such a struggle. When you struggle to get enough air to breath—I think that you fight the ultimate battle. That's how he lived the last number of years, often developing pneumonia. Each time he dealt with pneumonia, it took a little more time from his life, and left a little more damage to his lungs.

My dad was on five liters of oxygen just to be able to breathe. It greatly limited his ability for any activity. It had been years since he could tolerate going up the stairs, so he lived on the main floor of the farmhouse. He always told us he had many questions to ask God, such as things that had happened in his life of which he couldn't understand the why. After his death, I pictured Dad walking up the heaven's steps alongside God—no oxygen needed to breathe—talking and asking his many questions without any shortness of breath and mounting those steps one right after the other. I see no stress on his face as God answered all his questions. Walk tall, Dad. Walk tall as you always did.

All day long I tried to find something to get Mom involved in. All she kept wanting to do was wash dishes. I questioned making more trees...and she made a face. She didn't want to sew. She refused to play a game of solitaire with me. No interest in working a jig saw puzzle, or play a game.

Let's see, I have a story that you want to hear. It's a good read, and you don't want to miss it. I'm living through the experience...

and it's too darn good not to share. I thought maybe I could share this enticing story in a daily blog—but I've passed that goal up. This story is going to be in pieces—but you have to remember that while I recorded it...I also took care of the main actress.

August Has Arrived And Left

Hi to all my listeners—voluntary or not.

Mawmaw started with a new doctor this past week, since she was discharged from hospice after five weeks. The staff told me "it's not a bad thing to be discharged from hospice." I guess she is considered a "hospice recovery."

While in the office of her new doctor, difficulty started showing it's face with her restlessness in the waiting room. "Come on, let's go home," "this is ridiculous, let's go" "why can't we leave." Fortunately, Bri had got rained out and he was with us. When we went back into the small offices, her restlessness just escalated. I kept reassuring her that we were not leaving her, nor were we going anywhere without her. She just wanted to leave. May I remind you that she doesn't always have a "filter" on her words. If she's not looking directly at you...you may not be in her presence. As the PA worked at questions and observations, and working with her laptop, Mom would turn to me and say, "Come on, take me out of here." "Let's leave, please take me out of here."

Now the PA is my primary, so she already knew all about her new patient...so she was not surprised. Nor was she alarmed. She just continued to try and get all assessments done—and then I asked if I could take her out to the front office where my son was waiting. I walked Mom out, and told her I would be back to finish up with her plans. As I opened the waiting room door, Bri stood up. Mom almost fell into his arms—she said, "Come on, let's go," so he agreed and took her out of the building to the snowbird. The PA ordered blood work and set up a return visit for three months, so as not to work her up by coming back to soon. She started her back on half dose of her Lexapro, and stated she wasn't concerned with any other meds. She gets two Tylenol PM about 7:00 pm.

The PA thought maybe the Lexapro would help get through the obvious sundowning symptoms that seem to be a problem. Any other nerve medication, sleeping medication, or psychotic medicine would alter her improvement in memory. The PA said she could definitely help her sleep, but it would change the way her mind works. She did say that if I felt the sleeplessness and sun downing became a problem that needed addressed—that we may have to choose medication and give up some of the mental advancement that she has shown. I am to watch and see if her anxiety levels are more of a discomfort to her, than having some medication that may relax her enough to control the anxiety, then we will make other choices. Our plan is to keep her as comfortable as possible, with less anxiety.

I was thinking that we may bring her home to celebrate the holidays. I had asked the PA, and explained that she is only comfortable in my great room at home. She needs direction to go to the restroom and she will not go outside unless she is on my arm. She will not go outside and watch me work. She will go outside and sit with Bri…but only while he sits with her and holds her hand. I also told her that the hospice doctor felt that changing her environment may cause a backslide that we may—or may not regain. The PA was in total agreement.

I can't think what will happen in a month. We may not have a month. Nor can I think what could happen in a year, even if we have another year. I can only focus on the twenty-four hours in front of us. I just need to do what I can to get closer to where we want to be.

Well, move forward a week.

My roommate had on her blue pj's. She had gotten warm and removed her jacket. She went back to her bedroom and put on a purple plaid pj top and came out carrying her folded blue pj top. She said she needed to find the "one in the corner" and give it back to her. She said she had borrowed it from her and needed to give it back. There was no convincing her that it was hers, even though she had on the pj bottoms that matches it. So I guess we will wait till the "one in the corner" stops by and we can return it—right along with the kitten that no body claimed either. I'm beginning to feel I inhabit the "isle of misfit toys"—and I fit right in. Darn, I fit right in really well.

I helped her get dressed to take Millie to the beauty shop yesterday. I questioned "not" staying in town, just dropping Millie off and then going back and picking her up. I should have gone with my first gut feeling. But that's hindsight—and we all know that's twenty-twenty.

After the confusion of where we were picking Millie up at—(she walks across the street and gets in the snowbird)—and going to Walmart and pulling Mom and the cart around for one and half hours…(I felt it in my sciatic area all night). and then the confusion of where "they were" and "where are we going to pick them up at," then when we pulled into the house, she wanted to know why we were here—and she was moving up into the other seat—I explained we were home and she would be getting out of the snowbird and didn't need to move into another seat—She said she wasn't staying here, because she wasn't home…I asked her to stay in her seat until I walked Millie home and I would be right back. She got out of her seat and out of the snowbird—(which reminds me, I need to ask Bri to put the child safety lock back on the door by her seat. She kept opening it while I was driving one day—so we had to lock it with the child safety lever) and just then Bri pulled in. I was almost ready to get into his truck and just ride away.

He walked Mom into the house and she started, "How did you do this?" "This looks like my house, how did you do this?" Bri told her to come sit down at the table, because Mom brought home our supper—she said it looked like her place and, "How did we do this?" She seemed to think it looked like her house, but it wasn't her house, and how did we make it look like her house? She was quite confused and it didn't get much better as the night went on. She didn't pay any attention to the TV—she wasn't going back to bed by herself and she wasn't leaving all the kids out here by themselves. We just worked our way through the evening—and I left her refuse to go to bed because she wasn't tired—until she fell asleep in the chair. Then I went over to her, told her she was going back to bed and I would walk her back. She had moved into a different phase by then, so she went back to bed.

I drank a glass of wine, and counted my blessings, ate some semisweet chocolate and woke up early in the night. I'm pretty sure as to why she stays in the "great room" at the house. Pretty sure she gets disoriented when out of that space. I know that the confusion gets even worse if something changes in the house—electric goes off and the TV goes off—the one day she said she had to do the dishes without any hot water. As I walked to the sink, she told me she couldn't get the water to get hot. She was right. No matter how long she put the cold water spigot on, it never got hot. She was hunting for the dog food under the sink. She was looking right at it...and couldn't find it. I had to walk over and pull it out for her—she tries so hard. She comes out of her room, peaking out through the door like a kid on Christmas Eve, and asks what time it is.

She usually goes back to bed because "it is still dark out"—but she still has to inquire as to the time. I go through the days...and nights...with her—and I wonder. Why does she care what time it is? Why does she keep waiting until it's time to get up in the morning? Why does she want to get up every morning? Why is she still upset when her hair doesn't look good, or her nails are chipped? I watch her go through every day...usually just sitting and looking at whatever there is to see—with no plan or goal or purpose—and yet she goes to bed every night and gets up every morning—God bless the desire hiding behind her eyes.

So today I bought her some more narrow head bands and washed and set her hair. When it was dry, I put the headband on over her ears and her dressing—and then combed the hair around the band. She was so pleased.

As I witnessed the confusion—I realize that bringing her to another house is not a good idea for now. I can get medication to keep her more sedated...and then make the trip—but then we lose some of the mental ability that she has regained. I don't know if I want that tradeoff... at this time. At least not yet. She is usually content. She is not unhappy. She toilets and feeds herself, and hasn't fallen since May. She loves the dogs and lives to feed them and talk to them. She doesn't usually know who they are until I tell her—but she knows the "brown dog" (Lucy) and "that other one" which is Diesel. She mixes the other five up all the time…but she knows that she fixes seven bowls of food. The one night I told her she only needed to fix five bowls, and sit two bowls back empty. She counted and counted the bowls…and finally found the other two bowls and ended up with seven bowls…and then she could go forward. Now we always do seven bowls, no matter how many dogs we have.

If I tend to ramble, or repeat myself—just be patient and listen. My world is a little off axis at time—so humor me. Just know that I think about bringing our mother up north—and then I realize that you wouldn't see someone who knows you—and the price she may pay for that trip may be too costly.

I have to say this: I just polished her nails with three coats… told her to let them dry well…and we would watch the game while they dried. I walked over and sat down by my laptop to work on this email. She just came over to me…and asked, "Where is she? She told me it would take a while for these to dry—but I don't know where she went."

I checked her nails and said, "Well, they are dry."

She said—(wait for it), "Okay, but where is she? Oh, it don't matter, anyway, thank you," and she walked away.

Dear Lord, they just don't make enough chocolate for these type days. (I don't question who I am, or who I'm not, or where I went, or who took my place, or when I become "they" or when I become" she," anymore…I just imagine what it must be like inside her tangled up little mind…and know that "only by the grace of God, there go I.")

So closing off for now—and going to pour a glass of wine—and see if our mother has found me yet—love to you all—from all of me—and your mother too.

Bring on September

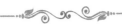

Well, it is now 1:11 AM. I am drop dead tired. As I type, she is washing the dishes. She has been walking around and through the house. In and out of her room…opening and closing her door. Her bed is made. She has been telling me she needs someone with a car so she can take her kids and go home. I just gave her anxiety medication about 12:30 AM. We go over the same conversation over and over. I have told her I am not calling anyone in the middle of the night. She's fussing and fretting about the dogs, who are laying in different places asleep. She tries to put pillows under them and cover them up—so they get up and find another place to lay. I just told her that she's going to fall, the way she is dragging her feet and moving all through the house. I told her I would then call an ambulance and she will be going to the hospital. I told her I would then have to put all the dogs in their boxes. She said she is not going to fall. That is such a relief to me—to hear her assure me that she will not fall. She is not listening—she is not receptive to any explanation. Five minutes after I explain something to her, she is back at the very same thing.

She is done with the dishes now and wandering all through the house. I don't quite understand how she moves and walks at night when her mind alters her way of thinking—the lady that waits for anyone to take over and get her home.

Try to be a rainbow in someone else's cloud

Bri has enrolled in CDL driving school for six weeks. He finishes truck school on Friday so we hope to head north that weekend. Bri has to really observe his driving record to be able to get a driving job. I'm going to pack the little trailer, because I'm thinking maybe thirty days…but it all depends on how it goes with Mom. If I have to stay longer, I want to have some stuff with me. Bri is already starting to feel lost without Mom or I here. So I'm tryin' to figure out what to bring—I'm tryin' to guess how Mom will be. I had a terrible night with her—even with Anxiety medicine in her. She is so very obsessed with the dogs…even during the night. She wanted her dogs and wanted to go home. She got upset with me because "why am I doing this to her?" I finally opened the door and told her to go ahead and take her dogs and go wherever she wants. She was trying to find all the dogs…she kept telling me they weren't here. Then she told me she had to have someone take her. I assured her I was not going out in the middle of the night when it is dark and raining…but I wouldn't keep her from going wherever she wanted to go. I told her I would call Bri and he could take her—she immediately changes her mood—cause she doesn't want to have anyone else involved.

I had tried to prepare for the hurricane before it was to arrive. I went outside and put some things in the shed. I walked back into the house as Mom looked right at me and asked me, "Where is Judy?"

The hurricane arrived with all its wind. I don't know why they always have to arrive in the dark of the night. We were without electric power for about a week but thanks to a generator—we had the comforts of home.

BACK TO PENNSYLVANIA

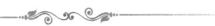

After a week without electric during a hurricane in Florida…and using a generator during that time. Bri finished his three weeks of truck driver training We felt it was the only chance we had to make the trip so I wouldn't be alone in Florida with Mom. We drove up on Wednesday a week ago. Two hundred miles into the trip, the air conditioning went out of the van. Mom wouldn't sleep and stayed restless throughout the trip. And of course, there was six dogs in the van. We hit bumper to bumper traffic in Charlotte, and heavy fog during the night. We weren't going to run straight through, but with the discomfort, Bri decided to grab a few short power naps and continue to drive. We had to have the windows down—so you couldn't talk and hear one another. The van would get very warm in the traffic jams—and heat up quickly if he didn't keep moving. Needless to say…our driver was stressed. He was concerned that Mom would be too warm or uncomfortable. It was a difficult decision, but we decided I should stay here with Mom during the time he is in orientation…since he will not be nearby. So we are staying up north.

Bri goes to the airport tomorrow morning and flies back to Orlando. His sister is taking him to the airport for a 10:35 AM flight. He needs to find a way home to Sanford, so I guess he is going to use an Uber driver. He lands about 12:55 PM. He then has to be in Jacksonville Sunday night to start orientation at a Trucking Company early Monday morning. He will have seven weeks orientation and may not be at home during that time at all. He was concerned that he wouldn't be there or available to help with Mom.

I haven't logged into my book for several days. I see deterioration in my favorite client. She doesn't jump up to keep the dishes washed in the sink. I can even draw hot water in the sink and place the dishes in the hot water. My mother watches but it's like she doesn't see. It's a household task that she has taken ownership to for quite a while now. She felt like she was being very helpful by doing the dishes—and she was. She needs help doing everything it seems. She also needs direction when listing one task…and then waiting for her to comprehend the first task, before adding another. An example would be asking her to come out to the kitchen table and sit there. She hears and recalls the last command given, which is to sit. So she sits back down on the bed.

We have completely missed the first request. She has become so dependent, so in need of help for most tasks, in total need of someone to initiate or carry out all household tasks. This is one of the things that Mom made so known before her accident. It is the one thing that she said she would never want to be—"what she calls a burden'—to her children. Bless her heart, since she doesn't know who her children are—therefore her conscious can be clear. I would never want my mother to feel that she is a burden. I don't say anything to her with that context. She thanks me every night when I tell her she will not be alone—that I will be right outside her room with all the dogs. She then told me tonight, "And I will be right here too." So I also thank her.

She doesn't request or ask for anything. She doesn't request anything to eat. She always tells us "whatever you decide." She isn't able to pick between several choices.

She sleeps more. She falls asleep after eating breakfast, and continues to fall asleep while sitting—throughout the day. This is something new…this lady has refused to take a nap during the day…ever. She still refuses to nap, even though she falls asleep so frequently. She will not consent to a nap while in the car, no matter how long the trip is. She tells me she "can't sleep in the car." She doesn't pay attention to the TV. In fact, she won't even sit in a position that makes the TV visible. She has even told me I can "change it to something else," when

I have a ball game on. I'm losing this lady slowly. I still don't know why she resists going to bed, and can't wait to get up in the morning.

Some days there wasn't a song in my heart, but I sang anyway. I have been using songs to walk Mom to bed at night. I start to sing "while strolling through the park one day—Mother would then join in with the next words—in the merry, merry month of May. She continued with, "I was taken by surprise, by a pair of pretty eyes"— and then we both ran out of words. Another song was the words to "bicycle built for two," and she joins in with the proper words. Daisy, Daisy, give me my answer true. Some nights we sing that "it won't be a stylish marriage—I can't afford a carriage"—and she completes the song. I pick some old time songs…and my mother can join me with the words. It makes the walk to her bedroom very pleasant. When we both run out of words to the songs—we had walked to our destination, so it had served its purpose.

November Is Here

She had no interest in watching me decorate for an early Christmas celebration. She'd watch me for a while, then I would look over at her seated at the kitchen table, and she would be asleep. I left her sleep.

After supper tonight, I asked her if she'd like to play cards. She declined. I ask her if she wanted to color. She declined. I told her I would like to color, so I brought out the crayons and books. She picked a picture of Santa from the one book. I asked her what color crayon she needed. She said, "Red, of course." I handed her a red crayon and proceeded to start coloring myself. She said her crayon wasn't making any color. I looked at her paper, and told her I could see that it was working, and that her page was showing the red color. She continued to color her page, but didn't look as if she was enjoying the activity. She was coloring the whole character red, with no distinction as to different parts of the character. I finished my page and started a second. She pushed her sheet across the table and said..."if you are doing this again, leave me out." She told me the crayon didn't work, and that I had given her the wrong one. She told me it didn't color very much. I take the blame—me and the crayons are at fault.

If I am already walking on thin ice, I might as well dance.

Soooo I've got Mom's home quite cluttered. I have bins of scrapbooking stuff sitting around. I have my printer set up with a box of paper supplies. I have two sewing machines set up with all the sewing supplies needed. I have several trees set up that Heath and I bought at the thrift stores. I started bringing in all the bins of Christmas Stuff from the trailer. We already had all the grandchildren and great-grandchildren's Christmas gifts sitting on every available shelf or furniture top in both bedrooms and bleeding out into the living room area. I am cleaning and putting up both Mom's and my Christmas decorations—repairing many and restringing some with working lights. I stripped the three birdhouse wooden structure that Gage gave to me. After I had all the artificial lights and flowers removed, I took it into the tub and washed and showered it. Now there are also 6 cages set up in the living room area—with a tiny kitten in one of them.

A litter of kittens was found in the shed at the farm. Apparently, something had happened to the mother, as she had moved three out of four; one was left behind. Jamey found the kitten alone in the nest. I asked her to bring it down to Mom's trailer. It was so tiny and cold that I didn't think it would survive. We fed it kitten formula with an eyedropper and positioned a heating pad in a kennel to keep it warm. A clock was put in the kennel to imitate a heartbeat. We rubbed its belly to stimulate body functions, and Mom would cuddle it and hum as she rocked back and forth. Some days, the tiny kitten would look up at her as she hummed, in total admiration. This tiny kitten survived all odds. I must say it had a whole family cheering it on and helping with its care. Mom's attention and cuddling left the kitten identifying her humming as a mother cat's purring. At the age of about five or six weeks, we had weaned it, and Jamey had found a home for it. Later, we were shown a picture of a beautiful, healthy large calico cat adopted into a home that adored it. It is such a good feeling when an abandoned, helpless kitten beats all odds.

I looked over at her and said, "I know all this clutter makes you uncomfortable, Mom. I will get it cleaned up—or put away soon. I see you looking at all the stuff piled on the counter." She quietly looked at me, while looking toward the boxes piled on the bench, then she said, "It's up to you—after all, it's not my house."

Sewing and crafts fill my days, not to mention the living room, bedroom, kitchen, and most closets.

A few of the dogs went to the door wanting to toilet outside. Mom got up, went to the door and opened it slightly. She quickly closed it, without letting any dogs out.

I said, "Mom, those dogs want out. Why didn't you let them go out?"

Innocently as she has appeared, she said, "No, it's too cold for them to go outside."

We have made yet another trip back to Florida in the snowbird van. I started to think of how Murphy travels with us and thought maybe I should see who and what "Murphy and his law" is about. I learned that, in our universe, systems naturally tend to end up in disorder and disarray. Many people see the law as a way to be pessimistic about life. It isn't true at all. It helps us think about the future and make plans for it so we can be ready for it. I understand Murphy was actually an optimist, as I feel I am. When you think about things in a way that something may go wrong, you can use practical creativity and, thus, be ready for plan B.

Now let me see how Bri may view this when I list some "happenings" during our 950-mile trips. Since Bri does all the dog walks when we stop while I stay in the van with mother, I would attach two leashes together close to the dog harnesses. In this way, he could walk more than one dog at once. The very first walk proved this as a failure. As he brought tangled dogs back to the van, he politely informed me that I shouldn't attach an older twenty-five-pound dog with a hyperactive five-pound dog. He explained how the dogs are not programmed to toilet at the same time. He also gently informed me to "not do that again," as one dog may be trying to toilet while being pulled around by the other dog. Lesson 1 learned.

We learned that we had to latch the child locks on the double door in the back of the van. When the third seat was made into a bed, it was always the way Mom tried to get off the bed to get out. Along with the darkness, her confusion, and the difficulty I had on climbing over the bed and dogs to retrieve her from the very back of the van—lesson 2 learned

On one trip, the van was overheating, so Bri pulled past the gas pumps to the back of the lot where the water was available. He got out, and I opened the side door to see if I could help him. In an instant, my little ten-pound chihuahua, Ricky, walked out the door and fell right through the large grate over the cement drainage thing.

We could see him in shallow water at the base of the culvert, swimming. Bri said, "Mom, do you think you can help me lift this grate off?" Without a thought of its size and weight, I said, "Absolutely." Together, we lifted the grate off the opening. Bri climbed down the cement sides and picked Ricky up by his harness and handed a dirty, wet, frightened dog up to me. I hugged him tightly as Bri climbed back out of the culvert.

Adrenaline does miraculously flourish when it is the only option you have. We were so fortunate that water was not running through the culvert, or he would have been washed into the tunnel. Murphy may have been with us, but plan B kicked in. Lesson learned: never park over a drainage grate again. Thank God Bri never hesitated climbing down a cement culvert to save a small life.

So when listing just a few of our travel incidents, may I take a minute to thank Bri for always being there and not throwing up his arms in defeat.

We are back in Florida. Bri didn't leave me behind in any of the truck stops or rest areas. Maybe he left Murphy behind and decided to keep me. Like I have said before, I'm always an optimist.

THANKSGIVING

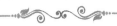

Another day set for giving thanks. Thankful for another year to share with my mother. Actually, the lady that lives with me has changed a lot in this past year. Her memory is not consistent, nor is it predictable. She talks easily when we discuss life in Rimersburg. She like to talk about her sister Fran—but does refer to her as "my daughter" at times.

I have been this lady's constant companion for three or four years now. As I drove with her to Walmart the other day, she asked, "Do you drive much?" I answered that I do, and why did she ask. She responded with another "Hallmark moment"—"because I've never seen you drive before." For years we have ridden in the car to do "shoppin' walkin'," taking Millie for her hair appointments, eating out, and all other trips. I wonder who drove us to all these places.

Her face and spirit brighten when we talk about life in Riverview or Rimersburg. Her memory seems to have stopped and stayed in that era. I tend to think the "home" she can't find is in Riverview with her parents and siblings. It's a good day when we can talk about her Uncle Oliver or Uncle Wilbur's farms, riding in a rumble seat, roller skating, Johnstown flood damage, or a childhood pet named "Troubles."

One day she was talking about Uncle Wilbur's farm and I told her I had been there, and I knew what she was talking about. She looked at me with questions all over her face and said—"I don't remember ever seeing you there." What can I say to this? I went with Mom, and had my three kids, when she visited Uncle Wilbur's farm one year. She loved going to Rimersburg for their Memorial Day

Celebrations. A distant trumpet would play the Taps…with an echo. There was a beautiful ceremony and tribute to the veterans.

We have discussed her Uncle Joe Rankin. This would be one of her father's brothers. I told her his mother's name was Ida Elvira Timblin. His father's full name was James McClelland Rankin. This was her grandparents. She said, "someone else has the name Elvira, but she couldn't remember who. Her sister Frances had the middle name of Elvira. I had joined Ancestry while she could help with some things with family history, as it doesn't come back as easily as it did. There is no pattern or depth of her memory loss that is consistent. I will keep working at it. I'm really lucky to have these other "thems" to help with the work and the cooking, laundry, cleaning etc. That way I can concentrate on researching our mother's brain… and attempt to keep her safe. She's trying to help. She wants to help, but "how to help" is causing her problems. She tells me she tries hard to remember.

No Plan B for When Plan A Gets Sick

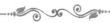

Jody has come to stay with us for the week. Mom is wearing disposable briefs, as she has had periods of incontinence. I went into my bathroom and when I came out I saw my bed. I thought it looked so good, I just stretched out across it. I don't remember anything until Bri was pulling me off the bed and said he was taking me to the emergency room. I had fell asleep across my bed and apparently Jody couldn't wake me. Bri took me to the emergency room and I was positive for the flu. Jody and Bri took care of Mom in my sleeping absence. He reported off work and we were so grateful Jody had been with us. They tell me that I slept for several days. I guess that was Influenza B.

ANOTHER REQUEST FOR HOSPICE HELP

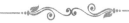

What a strange evaluation by a member of a hospice team. I'm not sure what their hiring interviews are like, but I'm thinking that a hospice member should have a little more compassion or sensitivity than what I witnessed in our home. She came in wearing a mask and sat at the dining table with her laptop. My mother was in a recliner in the living room. The nurse started reading reports on her laptop from a year ago. I brought my mother to the dining room table. The nurse never touched her, never addressed her, never did a vital sign, never ask her a question. She didn't even acknowledge that my mother was at the table…she just dealt with what she was doing on her laptop. My mother seemed confused. Why did the nurse have a mask on, was she contagious? Was my mother contagious? Whatever she did, she then went outside and talked on her phone. When she came in, I was informed that the doctor declined accepting her into the hospice program. The doctor wasn't here, so all he knew was what the nurse told him. She only spent time on her laptop. She did nothing with my mother, not even look at her head wound, which was covered with a dressing and a headband.

I can see this will not end with today's visit. This does not set well with me. I had requested the same hospice program as we had last year. I was pleased with the interaction with all members last year. This one person is a very poor representative of what is—or was—a good program. This story is not over.

ONE WEEK LATER:
A LETTER TO HOSPICE

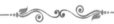

G ood morning.
It has been one week since a member of your staff was here in my home. I sent a message out to your agency the next day that my concerns couldn't be addressed in five hundred spaces—the size of the message box on your sight. I was told that Claudia or Christy would be contacting me in twenty-four to forty-eight hours. This did not happen.

Since the assessment, my mother has passed out while sitting on the toilet. My son helped me get her to her recliner, after which time she slept the entire evening and night. She is so much weaker than she had been. She has an appointment at Sanford Medical Group this afternoon—which I will give my best to get her out and to the appointment This is one of the reasons I reached out and ask for help from your agency. My mother is very difficult to transfer and ambulate—and her anxiety increases greatly when she is taken out of the home.

I sent a letter with my feelings to your agency last week, since no one has bothered to follow up on my concerns. I have nothing to gain with my opinion and correspondence. My hope is that you will follow through and do something to prevent negative attention to your agency in the future. As my letter has stated, I have forty-four years' experience working as an RN in Pennsylvania. My experience included supervisor in long term care, assistant DON, CNA instructor, and many years with home health and hospice. The assessment

I observed in my home appeared to be a joke to me. Apparently my expectations of a nursing assessment are much higher. Apparently my compassion for a patient is much higher. Apparently I have a higher understanding and more empathy of what a brain damaged and mentally altered elderly patient may feel when a stranger comes into her home. If I had given a report of having something contagious, I would have understood the use of a face mask during the entire visit. I don't see why she needed a mask, since she never addressed my mother, never touched her to do a vital sign or even show some desire to make a connection. She never got that close to my mother. In fact, my mother would have sat in a recliner in another area of my home if I hadn't brought her to the dining room table where your staff sat trying to read records and reports from a year ago on their laptop.

Your reply stated if I needed further assistance, to let you know. My mother didn't qualify for your agencies assistance. My family constantly asked, "Have you heard back from hospice yet." I have relayed your message that someone would be getting back with me. I have informed them that it didn't happen. The letter that I have sent to your agency may be destroyed, and never reach someone who might actually read it. I just thought someone should know my feelings, as the powers-that-be may want to know what happens during a home visit.

It took me quite a while to actually contact hospice, as I didn't want to accept the fact that my mother is that ill. I don't need you, but the next family that reaches out to you and receives the same type of assessment may.

I am so disappointed.

Judy Clark

(My mother, Virginia Clark, was the patient I refer to.)

(Sent from mail for Windows 10.)

ONE DAY LATER

Rather than try to repeat the day's events—I'm composing an email

I received a phone call from hospice yesterday—full of apologies. I told the caller I had an appointment with Mom's doctor in the afternoon and the caller wanted me to call her on her personal cell phone after the appointment She wanted to try and correct the experience I had with the initial assessment. I know the doctor was surprised that she was denied from hospice and remade the referral herself. Mom has lost 20# since she last saw this doctor. She wrote her up as failure to thrive, infected cranial wound, and I don't know what else. This morning I got a call from the other hospice nurse. She had my email in front of her and she was full of apologies. Everyone says that our experience is not what they are about. I left her set up a visit from a nurse for three or three thirty this afternoon. The nurse arrived. Bri had already got home from work, as they finished the job he was on. The nurse was attempting to explain to Mom what hospice is all about, and what their purpose is in the home. After a few minutes of this, while Bri sat and held her hand and Mom had the most confused look on her face, I took the nurse out to the dining room table. From then on we referred to her as a friend of mine that was visiting.

The nurse took a lot of notes and informed me of what all they offer. I explained that a few weeks ago I went down with the flu and Bri missed work because we had no back up plan. I explained that Bri actually thought they were going to admit me to the hospital. This organization has what they call a five day in house respite care for times like that. If she had been a patient, Bri could have had her admitted to their facility for five days. They also have volunteers that will come and sit with family when the end is near, so family is not left alone. I explained that I didn't need aides for personal care as she gets total personal care when she has incontinent bowel movements or diarrhea…so to schedule personal care would be double care. I also explained that when I toilet her, as I try to pull her pants down she is pulling the other side back up. I felt her vanity would be too compromised with a stranger undressing and bathing her—at least at this time. Although she has lost so much in the past few months— her vanity and bashfulness are still very much intact.

I ask for a nurse to monitor my mother's care and help me with what I am doing, and a doctor to be available without taking Mom out of the home.

This nurse called a different doctor while sitting at the table. She told the doctor that the patient had an infected head wound, with duration of about four years, told the doctor that she had three surgeries to her head and a fractured hip within the last four years. She has pain in the left knee on transfers and ambulation. She is dyspneic (short of breath on any exertion.) She only eats about four to five bites, by being fed, and then she is done. She explained that she is totally dependent on all personal activity and care. She told the doctor about her anxiety and how her memory has greatly declined. She covered the fact that she is incontinent, does not ambulate without maximum assistance…and tolerance for activity is very limited. While explaining her mental decline, Bri asked her if she had seen Brian yet today. She looked right into his face and said, "No, I don't think so."

The assessment nurse informed me that she was accepted. A staff nurse will come out within a few days and do the total assessment. Tomorrow is Millie's hair day, so Mom and I will take her and drop her off at the beauty shop, and bri will pick her up on his way home. Maybe I will take JoJo and let her hold her in her car seat.

She is on an antibiotic twice daily for ten days for her head wound. When at the doctor's office, the doctor told Mom she didn't have to come back. She remembered how badly she wanted out of there last year, but today she couldn't get up and walk out. Of course, Mom didn't understand "why" she didn't have to go back—but hearing that she didn't—made her smile.

We thought we would take her in the restaurant while we waited on the script to get filled—another experience on its own merit. After helping her walk in and getting her seated, she said, "I have to pee." Bri helped me walk her to the restroom so we could get there faster. While walking she said, "I'm already peeing." So we took her in the family restroom and bri went to the snowbird to get the bag with spare pull-ups and clothing, and also the WC. I did a change while in the restroom, then it was much easier to take her back to our table with the WC. Afterward, in a moment of weakness, I ordered a Maui margarita. Bri has a picture of Mom taking a few sips. And I wonder why I am tired.

Right now Mom is watching the pirate game and I just told her the cubs got four runs and they are winning. She said, "Are they?" End of discussion. I'm just glad she is watching the game.

I remember…not long ago…she would tell me "they are doing the same thing…they hit the ball and then they run—then they hit the ball again and they run—the same thing."

Tonight we just watch the game.

Two Days Later

It's Friday afternoon and the hospice pastor just left. He remembered me from last year—but didn't say if that was a good thing—or bad. He just said he knew my face was familiar. I must have had under eye darkness, hair up in a ponytail...and no makeup last year when he came also. Again, I went over her entire history, her decline, and the events of the last four years. It happens he also had the flu this year...and he said he actually thought he was going to die. So you can tell Jenny, we know what she dealt with.

The Pastor prayed with Mom after she gave her permission. He has told me to call him for anything.

I explained what she was like last year when she was discharged from hospice, and how she is today. She gave her usual general answers to his questions, but she doesn't cover as well as she used to. I took JoJo out of her crate...put her on Mom's lap...and showed the pastor how Mom spends her days and evenings. She broke into her smile, fussed over her little pink dress and kept holding her head and face up toward her. I told him that when I washed the "little pink dress" the other day, she didn't know who the dog was. I also told him what our mother was like the first eighty-eight years of her life.

Now yesterday the nurse and the Social Worker ended up here about the same time. Again, I reviewed the entire history of surgeries and her interests and activities for the first eighty-eight years of her life—and again—all the history since that fateful Labor Day. I told them it was a slow—stop—and start—bleed. I explained the three cranial surgeries and the broken hip—I told them about the previous denial of hospice, and when I took her to the doctor—that she ordered hospice. I told them everything that the doctor said…that I could remember—and the 20# wt loss since last year—infected head wound…anxiety disorder, etc.

So I've told Mom's story at least four or five times now. I wonder where the communication is within the staff? There are hospice volunteers who will come and sit with the patient—but do not give any care. They also have a five-day in-house respite care facility…but you need to request dates ahead of time so a bed will be available. I explained how we had no Plan B if they would have admitted me to the hospital. I said I left Bri High and Dry because he had no one to contact for help or support. As God keeps watch over this lady, my sister Jody was here visiting at the time. I honestly don't remember those days. Bri had taken me to the emergency room, they confirmed the flu, and I slept for a few days. Bri called off work and Jody and him took total care of Mom.

The social worker is going to check about some volunteers to sit with Mom at times. The nurse said she will be back next week. I think she is ordering me dressings. They have already delivered the hospice comfort box of medications. I turned down any aides coming to bathe Mom at this time. Her vanity and bashfulness is still quite intact. I explained that a stranger coming into the home to undress and bathe her—at this time—is not necessary. I explained that she gets bathed when she has an accident—so scheduling a bath would be silly.

I will send this out before I fall asleep on the keyboard again. Bri and I are both running on fumes—which is what Dad used to tell us that Mom's cars were trained to do.

Bri had a union meeting tonight, so I have all the dogs right now. Mom has the one she calls "punkin" with the little pink dress—lying on her nap. We will attempt to watch the pirate game—if I can stay awake—very questionable at this moment in time.

Love to all till the next update,

April Is Ending

Good evening everyone—and good morning (in case I fall asleep on my keyboard and wake up sometime tomorrow).

I guess to make sense of all this—if that is even possible…I need to retrace the last few months. I had a hard time making a decision to inquire about hospice again—after she was a "hospice recovery" last June and July. They held her on their service for six weeks, but her improvement didn't give them anything to justify to Medicare that she was hospice material. So after what seemed months of a downhill slide—to where she had to be fed—she had to be told when to open her mouth—totally incontinent of bowels and bladder…with episodes of incontinent diarrhea that required a bath and often a bed change. At these times, which always seemed to be early morning when she wasn't really awake, she showed no signs that she had done something that wasn't normal. She was not aware that she had hit such a level of dependence. She had to be encouraged, or tricked, to eat. She said she was "full" and didn't want anymore. She didn't really talk. She could not get out of bed or off a chair. She could walk with maximum assistance, but sometimes that was very hard. I have watched Bri pick her up and carry her as her legs wouldn't hold her up.

All the years she told us, "I will never live with any of you. I will never be a burden to my kids"—affirms that the higher power knows where we are and knows what our next chapter holds. We are truly silly if we think that our tight grip on our life would change the outcome. His eyes are on everyone, plus the sparrow. He already knows how our story ends. He knows that all the planning and worrying and fretting that we do in managing our own lives is a waste of precious energy and time. Did it matter what statements our mother made in the past? I do know now that the good Lord is not ready for her yet as he left me hold her a few weeks ago—and then he sent her back to me.

Mom's condition was so much weaker, with a 20# weight loss since last August… I was starting to figure out how and when our next trip up north would be. Bri had his boss at work updated and alerted to what seemed eminent. I was wondering how long I would stay when we came up north. I knew the changes that would take place in our lives when Mom makes that final trip. I thought I would stay and work with my sister's grandchildren—to make scrapbook albums of their childhood. I had already started purchasing an assortment of 12 × 12 albums…because I have so much scrapbooking supplies and material. I was starting to put it all together…thinking I would hold scrapbooking parties at Mom's trailer. I cleared out the pull-behind trailer and started putting crafting supplies inside. I wondered what clothes I could fit into for the events that would be taking place for our mother.

A few days later, I had Mom in the bathroom on the toilet. She started to lean against the wall and slide down. She was cold and wet and gray. Her head dropped forward on her chest and she was "out." I was getting ready to slide her onto the floor when I held her face in my hands. I then picked up her head and held it back, opening her airway. She started fluttering her eyelids slightly and then she was smiling. She couldn't, or didn't talk. She just slowly opened her eyes and continued to smile. I sat on the floor and just watched her, knowing Bri would be home in a few minutes. She just kept smiling.

I asked her, "Mom, where did you go?"

She said, "I don't know."

I asked her who she was with? Again, she smiles and says, "I don't know," and continues to smile. Her bladder had relaxed, so I cleaned up the pee. Bri came home and got her to her chair and she slept all evening. We put her to bed and she slept all night

I know her time away from us was very pleasant. I know she wasn't frightened, and she certainly wasn't sad. I truly feel she was gone and now two weeks later I am positive. The changes that have occurred in the interim from that incident are landmark moves. For example, I took her in the snowbird to Casselberry to pick up a generator today. When we left the store, she said, "Are we going to eat?" I asked her if she was hungry.

She said, "Yes, I am." So we went to McDonald's drive-thru, then parked in the shade. She ate a quarter pounder, a small shake, and an apple pie. She picked up the sandwich and ate it independently. When we came home, she then ate a kolbassi sandwich, chicken fried rice, apple sauce, and then peach/apple cobbler with cool whip. She took the kolbassi out of the bun, picked up her knife and cut it in small pieces. She is presently eating strawberry ice cream while we watch the Pirates. She is totally feeding herself.

She is walking everywhere by herself. She has "remembered" how to walk. She is toileting herself at times. When we pulled into Bri's driveway this afternoon, she said, "I was here before."

I said, "Yes, you were, we were here planting flowers yesterday."

When we pulled into our home and I walked her to the carport, she asked, "How long have you lived here?"

I said, "About five years, we have lived here."

She said, "Are you ready for it?"

"No, I mean, how long since you moved here?"

I said, "Moved from where?"

She said, "How long since you moved here from Vandergrift?"

Now we haven't said "Vandergrift" for a year. When she talked of places, it was Rimersburg or Kepple Hill. She is making complete sentences and showing some short term memory. Her appetite is back, bigger than ever. She is starting to fuss about the dogs being in crates or that they are hungry. She is back to feeding them from her plate and Annie is back to getting Oreo cookies.

I woke up on the sofa with her hand touching my face the other night. She was in her underwear with one yellow sock and one blue sock...I walked her back to her bedroom and her slacks were in the bed, along with a shop n save bag, a few other socks, another headband and a dogs Christmas neckerchief. This would be why I sleep between her and the three doors to the outside. One door is blocked with an oval table and Bri's dog's crate. The front door is blocked. The carport door is the only one she has a chance to get to. I have awakened to the dining room and kitchen lights all lite, and her sleeping with her head on the dining room table. She doesn't say a word. She moves about quietly. And yes, my house is childproofed of chemicals.

Her actions and behaviors are like those of two years ago. I can only explain that I think her brain was "rebooted" when it shut down and restarted. There is something going on within her head, because even pushing her wheelchair and being above her head—the odor from her wound is vile. And she had just finished ten days of antibiotics.

But—with these changes, I'm expecting her to get tossed off hospice again. I can understand why. Each day there seems to be more improvement. She came to the kitchen and dried the dishes a few nights ago. I am tired. Bri is holding down a full time job with a 130-mile commute daily. He fell asleep on his lunch break last week. But this is the lady we keep safe and happy. We must be doing it right, because she still doesn't want to leave us. She doesn't want to go to bed at night, and she gets up several times in the morning before the sun even comes up. She emits an incentive that inspires us both.

There is more to this story, with each breath she takes, but I want to send this before I "wake up tomorrow."

This awesome lady was knocking at death's door, decided to peek into heaven, and then rejoined us. It has to be that God knew she wanted to stay awhile yet, "rebooted" her brain, and left her return to us. There is no other explanation. People don't make that 180 turn normally. She made it easier than Bri or I. I hope she doesn't realize that Mickie is not here anymore. As long as JoJo is on her lap and in her chair...I think we will be okay. I had to have Bri's dog Lucy put down with cancer in her neck and throat. Mickie had declined so much with her blindness, diabetes, incontinence, and confusion, that I also had her put to rest. Mom no longer knew her, and the darkness of Mickie's world was sad and it frightened her. Now Mom's direction has switched paths, and her train travels down another track. God had "dropped" off JoJo and her little pick dress for Mom to love. God even left Mom change her into a "kitten" to fill the void in her world.

God understands our prayers even when we can't find the words to say them.

I have chosen not to keep repeating Mom's feeding obsession with the dogs, nor her anxiety when they are sleeping quietly. You as a reader know I have certainly addressed it enough. I as a writer have been so involved in the need to monitor her sleeplessness to keep her safe that I drop off to sleep when times are quiet. Often, I wake to pages of a single letter that my finger was on my laptop when I nodded off. Her behavior is changing. Her ability to maintain a status quo doesn't happen. Some days are drastically different from others. Some days, she has forgotten she can walk. Some days, she feeds herself without prompting, and maybe the very next meal, she has forgotten how to get the spoon of food to her mouth. Some days, she doesn't remember how to chew and swallow the food in her mouth. She often piles dishes on top of her coffee cup and then twists the dishes into the food on her plate. Behaviors have become dramatically different, and she apparently doesn't need much sleep. I'm trying to keep rested enough to survive this period of precarious activity.

Love to you all, as this awesome lady that shares our lives don't follow any rulebook or medical journal.

MIDYEAR EMAIL TO MY SISTERS AND FAMILY

This message is going to be confusing, since I haven't updated you lately. I haven't gotten an email out to family up north for so long. I send you those emails when I get them composed. Hospice has been addressing her anxiety and the fact that my mother doesn't seem to sleep—but instead has hyperactivity. They have tried several different medications—thinking it would cause her to sleep and give me some sleep also. They are wrong; medications seem to work the total opposite on my Mom—and has for almost four years now. After the last month I'm not trying any medications on Mom again. I'm not giving her anything. She's been on forty-eight-hour marathons with hyperactivity. She did a total turnabout about six weeks ago where she was acting like she did two years ago. It seems when she passed out on the toilet, while a total dependent person who needed fed and couldn't stand up on her own, she "rebooted" somehow. Then she had a bad fall a week ago. She fell against the dog crates and hit her back and head on the floor. She hit hard. She had many skin tears on her arms and legs and when I tried to sit her up, she was so dizzy. She described her head as "whuzzy, whuzzy, whuzzy" and couldn't sit up from the laying position. I called Bri over and we worked slowly to get her up to the recliner. I had been worrying about a fall that would act like the "shaken baby syndrome" to her brain. Bri sat with her while I got a cat nap, as I was totally exhausted.

Jumping ahead again, or maybe just side-winding for a few minutes, and I will return to my mother, Bri was asked to run for the executive board for his ironworker union hall as recording secretary. He then sits on the executive board. So with the campaigning and then the election on Saturday (which he won with a landslide) he has been busy with a new activity. We've been trying to get him into another psychiatrist as his had to retire quickly with bladder cancer, and have had a difficult time. After waiting for several months each time the new psychiatrist appointment has been canceled because they will not accept his insurance. We've been trying to maintain his medication routine—but running out of options. Finally he has an appointment on June 20 with a new psychiatrist. It's been a major issue to maintain his bipolar medication…and hopefully a new psychiatrist may have some new ideas—His roommate is moving out— He's staying at a place this week to watch their dogs and house while they are in Maine…so Bri almost has his house back. June 1 was his finale day. I had been going to Bri's house to clean and sort through his kitchen, etc., because Mom was standing and walking and feeding herself.

Now, I don't know where we are as far as her status. Her legs and feet are so swollen…they are like tree stumps…and it makes ambulation very difficult—even with help. I don't know whether I can get her to lift her legs to get in the van or not. She's supposed to be homebound with hospice, anyway…I was thinking of moving over with Bri for a week—after the roommate leaves—to put his house into a fresh state. It's a good therapy for me…while I spend every minute with Mom—but it would be so much easier than trying to take her back and forth—and I can get a lot more done in a shorter period of time. My heel…felt some better after the prednisone… but the discomfort is returning. I'm going to call the doctor and see if she would consider another script for prednisone for me—before I have to get the injection into my heel. Mom's lack of sleep has me so weary—she's been getting worse since the fall. She forgot how to feed herself…I left her sleep on the recliner beside the sofa last night, rather than try to keep her in bed in her room. She has a hospital bed now—but I can't duct tape her in it—there are some drastic changes in her daily—and the wound in her head has the most foul odor—I took on the job of her caretaker—and I'm going to see it through—I don't know what keeps the decay process going on inside her head from affecting a major artery—unless it's the fact that the pressure is kept off her brain by draining outside—needing frequent dressing changes.

The American heating technician came to maintain my air conditioner and heater and left me with a $1,600 estimate to get the insides cleaned of bacteria and spores—as both inside and outside unit need an ultraviolet light installed—before the units are permanently damaged—along with a new motor for it. It's only about five years old. Millie told me the same thing happened with hers—and it was about five years old then also. We have been ripped off by so many contractors and workers here—I'm afraid to believe anyone. I also haven't made it to the dentist yet, but my heel is taking front stage right now.

So that is a rough version of my life right now—I know I've missed some things…but my eyes are heavy—so I am going to close them for a little while while Mom is sitting quietly.

June Moves On

Mom was seen by the hospice doctor and the nurse yesterday. It was a very comfortable visit—but Mom couldn't answer any of the questions he asked her. She has improved so much since my initial request for them to come in—I'm wondering how they are "keeping her" with Medicare guidelines. She has two and three plus edema and has been started on some new medication for it. Sleeping medication about 9:00 PM has helped her with sleeping. I usually toilet her about 4:00 or 5:00 AM—and she will go back to bed. Her urine output has definitely increased—and per usual—I just changed her because she starts peeing before I can get her seated on the toilet. She had a mixed up day yesterday—and fretted a lot. It was difficult to even get her to eat. Everything had an issue—her surroundings, a blanket on the sofa, a pillow, the dogs—even the one that likes to sit on her chair—I can't make sense out of her fretting, so I just try to pacify her.

The doctor asked me if I tried to correct her when she is confused. I told him, "No, I just climb into her world and spend some time there."

He said that was good. I had him look at her head wound—and questioned the odor of the wound. As I thought, He said it was a necrotic odor—and antibiotics, at least oral ones, would do little to help that. He questioned when she had the last IV antibiotics, so I printed out her history of the last four years. He asked Mom her age—she said she would have to think about it—later he came back and asked her—you said you had to think about your age Virginia—can you tell me your age now? Of course she couldn't. She didn't know the year.

And then the doctor said to me, "She knows who you are, doesn't she?"

I said no—she knows that I am the one that is here—but no clue as to my relationship to her. He asked me if she uses the walker—to ambulate. I told him that she either holds onto furniture, but usually I walk her. He asked about the walker and I explained that she doesn't remember how to use it—so unless I walk with her and cue her—we don't use the walker. She's not eating as well—she always tells me she is full—she will cover her food with the napkin—or push the plate away for someone else to eat. I'm still fighting this head cold.

And Mom says, "You girls just can't get over that cold, can you?"

I told her we keep passing it back and forth—and she agreed.

I told the doctor there is always more than me here—in her world. I told him she thinks someone always brings in food—cause it just appears on the table. He told me he hoped I didn't take offense that she doesn't know me. I asked him if he saw the movie *Pay It Forward.* and he had. I just told him I think Virginia paid forward for eighty-eight years—and I'm just trying to repay her. Bri has gotten sick again. He missed work last Thursday—and spent the entire weekend in his house and usually in bed. Bri is still sick, emotionally rundown, exhausted, and weary—I guess the bad head and chest cold had an easy victim. Bri's on cold and sinus pills, several other medications, the vaporizer and cough drops. I've fixed him breakfast and lunch—and he heats up something for his supper if he is hungry—but he hasn't left the house. He showed up Thursday morning. For work—I checked his temperature because he was chilling and sweating—it was one hundred, so he went back home and to bed. his cough comes from his chest. we are lucky Mom hasn't caught any of our illnesses—she never got the flu when I had it either. so that's how run down the caregivers are of our mother—and she still doesn't want to go to bed at night—and won't stay in bed in the morning. I guess she has found a reason why she wants each new day. I'm exercising and stretching my foot and heel—I can't wait till the day it doesn't hurt at all. I think that's the basic rundown—at least for now. If I think of anything more, I will let you know.

ALMOST ANOTHER LABOR DAY

That was the beginning of the big life change.

It is the day my mother required cranial surgery, following a large subdural hematoma. When I call it a "life change," I need to define the totality of that statement. My mother had a rough summer with memory issues. I had stayed with her for almost six weeks, preceding the wedding of her granddaughter Sara. She had bruises down one side of her body. She said: "I didn't tell anyone, but I'm telling you." Apparently it wasn't the first fall she had. She had fallen on the back steps, where ice had covered the sidewalk and steps. She had fallen and hit her face or head, for her glasses were bent out of shape. Then she had the wreck with her car. I have actually lost count of the falls we have had since that day.

Mom has forgotten how to eat. She doesn't know what to do with the silverware. She doesn't know what to do with the food. She doesn't know what to do with the food that is put in her mouth. She actually asks questions while holding the food in her mouth. Verbal cues along with physical demonstrations are necessary.

Put more on your spoon. "It's not sticking on there." Yes, put it on your spoon and put it in your mouth. "And then what?" And then you chew it up and swallow it. I watch as she stirs, and stirs, and puts cereal on her spoon, and then dumps it off. I watch as she lays the spoon down, and looks confused. I sit down beside her and put cereal on her spoon, and then put it in her mouth.

She says, "Oh, thank you." She starts to stir again…frosted flakes with little tiny marshmallows, round and round in the bowl. I prompt her to put more on her spoon.

She says, "I have to let it cook or something. I can't get any more birth marks on something."

The days have been extremely interesting, but far from what would be defined as a "normal day." I have watched this modest lady pull her pantlegs up to her knees, remove her sock and slippers, and then walk in her bare feet. She never walked in bare feet. She moves chairs and lines them up in the living room. She folds, and refolds, and refolds again any dishcloth or tee towels laying on the counter in the kitchen. She moves papers about and then lays them down in the same area. Words do not match her actions. Her mind seems so very busy. Her face shows a scorn-like expression as she tries to tell me how much "has to be done."

September Has Come

Now I have to smile. I had a photo ID made for Mom in Florida when we first made a trip down after her surgery. She no longer had a driver's license, so it was advised so she could fly without problems. At that time, I didn't know where these records were shared, until Mom received a jury notice. Should I take her in a WC and see if she gets picked for a jury? No, not this time. I contacted them with her situation, her mental status and brain injury, and also the fact that she was on hospice. She received a permanent notice that she was excused from jury duty for the rest of her life. How can I not smile, knowing she received a jury notice while on hospice?

What a week it has been. Since her fall at 2:00 AM coming from the bathroom, things have changed. My son wonders how many hits her head can take. She apparently came out of her room during the night and went to the bathroom. I don't know the time element of her actions, as she doesn't ask for help. I woke to the loud noise of a fall. I found her seated in the hallway, but in a strange type of position. The back of her head had a two-inch gash, exposing the skull and bleeding well. She was alert but confused. When I moved her, I noted she was leaning against the corner of the wall where there is metal edging. It was bent in position. Later I would find a bruise on her left shoulder, and she did complain of her head hurting. I called my son from across the street, as he wants to know anytime she falls or gets an injury. I worked at getting butterfly tape to hold the wound together.

Tape would not stick to the area, and it kept bleeding. I cleaned the wound and decided to tie her hair together to approximate the wound and control the bleeding. This worked in one area, so I did it in two other parts of the wound. I put a dry gauze dressing over the sight and held it in place with the wide hair band that I use to keep the temporal dressing intact. When I checked the area of the fall, I realized that she had been in the bathroom and she did have a large bowel movement. Now I think she may have weakened as she walked from the bathroom, as she has passed out twice on the toilet during a bowel movement in the past half year. My son and I kept watch over her the rest of the night. There were no signs of lack of consciousness or escalation of neurological symptoms.

I have worried so much about falls, and the effects that happen when a baby is violently shaken. She must be a candidate for "shaken baby syndrome" when she hits her head that hard. Those are my thoughts, whether I'm right or wrong.

Each time she falls, she seems to "reboot." Behaviors that were normal related to her previous condition then change. Sometimes it seems she is more alert, and her memory does improve occasionally. Other times she regresses to where she doesn't remember how to eat. She doesn't know what to do with a spoon, or why she is to put the food into her mouth. I have had to tell her to "chew it now," only to have her open her mouth with the food on her tongue and asks, "What's this?" Somedays I must instruct her to "swallow it now." Then we sit down at another meal, and she feeds herself and eats without any hesitation or needed guidance. Just recently she couldn't seem to find the food on her plate. I just purchased white paper plates my last trip to the store. I thought maybe having no print or design on her plate would make finding her food less confusing. I will follow up on this idea and let you know how that works out in the future.

I go onto dementia web sites at times, for some guidance or direction. I saw that there are 3 main points in taking care of a dementia or Alzheimer's patient. The first of these is "patience." The second point is "patience." You guessed it, the third point is also "patience." Patience does wear very thin when you direct or give instructions in every move, for the entire day. The next day you start all over. You don't know whether she will recall anything that you guided her through the proceeding day, and then you realize that this is not a learning game. This is not a case where instruction and repetition will lead to learning a function or action. Everything depends on where the neurons of the brain decide to misfire today. Some days they connect without issue, which is always a pleasant surprise. Sadly, the next day, or the next meal, or even the next minute gives no guarantee of the behavior or ability that she is capable of.

We just open each package when it arrives, and then figure out the best way to deal with the contents. I often tease my sister about the "box of chocolates" referred to by Forrest Gump. We are never aware of what is under the chocolate until we bite into it. When caring for a dementia patient, there is no follow-through or guaranteed retention of knowledge or activity. I've learned that some days, or some nights, there just is never enough chocolate.

It's been well over four years now, and I mentioned to the hospice nurse and social worker the other day that I don't feel I will be able to carry on a normal or diversified conversation when out in the public. They laughed and said I will do just fine, but for four years now I have eaten, slept, and lived in a dementia patients world. The subject matter is limited on most days. The patient shows no interest in movies or TV, so my knowledge in these areas is very restricted. I start to watch the news and my patient may need to go to the toilet, so I miss the contents and the ending of the news story. Oh well, tomorrow is a brand new day.

October Has Slid In

I must have slept a few hours…Bri was at the door, his lunch wasn't packed, and my roommate was sitting at bedside and quite upset. Her words were confusing as I tried to transfer her to the bedside potty chair. She wouldn't let go of the bedrail, she wouldn't let me pivot her, and she was resisting any action I tried to use to sit her on the pot. She was upset and trying to tell me a story of "not finding anyone," and "where did everyone go?" It is barely 4:00 AM, and my world is up and active. My mother is agitated and wide awake. She is upset about something. Her brow is furrowed. Her voice is firm. Her resistance to any movement I try to help her make shows me her mind is on something else.

She tells me, "I'm trying to figure it out." She can't tell me what is so wrong in her world at this very early hour that has her upset.

I usually don't hit a deep sleep. I usually keep watch on the monitor most of the night. When she sits up at the side of the bed, I go to her and usually toilet her and then encourage her to "get some more sleep, which she does. I must have missed something last night. I knew I was running on empty, as far as sleep goes. She has fallen a few times in less than a week. She will not sit for any period. She is constantly getting up, pushing her wheelchair forward, sideways, and often backward. If the brakes are on, she just pushes harder. I try to watch her so closely, thinking I can prevent any more falls. In the few minutes I may look in another direction, or step outside her area of vision, seems to be the time spam that has me picking her up off the floor.

I know trying to put her back in bed this morning would only agitate her more, so I transfer her to the wheelchair and bring her to the living area. She is still trying "to figure this out." Her brow is furrowed, and her body language shows a tenseness that I have not been able to ease yet. My son is having his morning coffee, so I sit her wheelchair close to the chair he is sitting in.

He tells her, "Good morning, Mawmaw."

She looks at him and asks, "Where did you come from?"

Signs of her agitation are so evident, and it's only 4:00 AM. Thus, another day on Sunset Drive has begun. The sleep I evidently got last night felt good on first arising. I'm not sure it is worth the problems that this morning has already presented. Two hours later I have fixed my mother cereal and milk. I watch her stir the cereal nonstop. I tell her to start eating her cereal.

She tells me, "I don't know how." This is where we are this morning. One time she feeds herself without any cues. Another time I must give cues from picking up her spoon to "chew it up and then swallow it."

She has eaten most of her cereal this morning with continued cues and constant reminders when she seemed to forget what she was doing. I have sat beside her at the table during her entire breakfast. She seems very insecure this morning. That is just my opinion, but she is watching me closely. I ask her if she wants to go into her recliner chair or go back to bed. She states "I just want to sit here with you." I reassure her that we can do that, and we do.

How does her brain work? She can make a sentence that is totally understood, during other comments that have a bunch of dissociated words put together. Hand gestures often accent the disassociated group of words, making the comment even more confusing.

How do I react to her confused states? Do I correct her and reorient her to the circumstances of the day? Do I try to guess what she is saying and answer accordingly?

OCTOBER MOVES FORWARD

I must record some of the events of the past few days. She has been awake since 4:00 AM—I put magazines on a small desk and ask her to sort them and fix them She worked on the piles for hours, eyes wide open. She had breakfast about six thirty, waffles with strawberry jelly, syrup, and butter. I didn't give her ice water this morning, so it wouldn't end up in the middle of her waffles and syrup. After she had eaten most of her breakfast, I sat a cup of coffee in front of her. She loves her coffee. After the first sip, the coffee cup was "screwed" into the center of her plate, in the midst of the remaining waffle and syrup. I guess that is right where it belongs.

How can God blame me for being human—when he made me human?

She won't stay seated. She is constantly standing and trying to walk, pick things up or move things that aren't too big for her to move. She kept pushing her wheelchair away from the table while she ate. I kept pulling it back to the table. She stood again and moved her wheelchair, causing her to fall backward and land on her butt on the floor. After she hit the floor, her head went back against the wall. Fortunately, there didn't seem to be any outward injury. At least no visible injury. She had to help me get herself off the floor. She pulled herself up with the use of a kitchen chair.

After finally getting her back to bed and tucking her in, she sweetly told me: "now you go and get a good night's sleep" Almost everything this little lady says makes me smile.

The best eraser in the world is a good night's sleep.

As she finishes eating and is aware of all the food on her clothes, she tells me, "We're going to have to wash these."

I agree, my mother, we will have to wash these. If that is our biggest problem this brand-new day, we can count out blessings.

I am at the sink and she is seated at the table in her WC. It is about time for Bri to arrive from work. I turn around and see her leaning over to the side with her hand down toward the dogs. I think she is feeding them from her hands—until I realize something is wrong with her position. Her hand hasn't moved. I quickly head to the table and see that she has again "passed out." Her face is gray and unresponsive. I turn the WC away from the table and tip it backward as I lower myself and her to the floor. This put her feet and legs up in the air, and tipped her head and neck backward. I support and hold her head and face, so that her airway is open. Her body is limp. These are the longest seconds that I have ever experienced, waiting to see how far away she has gone. Again she takes a few breaths and starts to move. I don't know whether her sigh was heavy, or if it was mine. Again mother, I don't know how much I had to do with it, but together we did it—again. I can only assume you aren't ready to leave us, probably more because of the dogs and the kitten—but for whatever reason…I will take it.

Just then Bri comes to the door and is busy greeting his dog, when he sees myself under my mother's wheelchair and both his grandmother and me on the floor. By then she has started to rally. He immediately takes over finding a better position for us both. His grandmother has been somewhere peaceful again—his mother not so much.

He takes her back to her bedroom and puts her into her bed. He sits with her for quite a while, holding her hand and talking to her. She is quite tired…but again, she came back to us. How many times will she do this, before she decides not to return?

November Arrives—
Thanksgiving Email to
My Sisters and Family

How a day starts in two different worlds you ask? Let me tell you. I had a show on TV this afternoon—a very pretty lady without a hair out of place, makeup perfection, perfect slim figure in pretty nightclothes, talking about how she gets up in the morning. She rolls over in her soft sheets and fuzzy blanket, crawls out of bed, brushes her teeth, puts on her fuzzy Sherpa lined mukluk slipper socks, sits down with a cup of coffee and plans what she is going to do with her day.

Glory Be—Does a day really start like that for some people? This lady needs to step into the real world.

My days are often more like watching a squirrel attempt to cross the street.

I jump up from the sofa in the middle of the night, as I realize that my roommate and "other mother" isn't visible in the child monitor. I hurry back to her bedroom, bare feet and mismatched pj's—glasses crooked on my face—since I fell asleep with them on my head. The dogs are barking as they realize that my motion and movement is hurried. I find my other mother on the floor, as expected. She is sliding around on her behind. Apparently, nothing is broken. She pleasantly says; "Oh, Hi!" I sit down on the chair in her room to assess the mess before me. I wonder where, how, and on what body part I start to wash. I see I am going to need help for this task at hand. She is unable to help me enough to be able to get her off the floor. She needs to get onto the potty chair, although that need has already been met. In fact, the potty chair is on its side, as is the pot.

It is 2:00 AM—I call my son, and he always answers. Within a matter of minutes, he is at the door…and together we lift her onto the potty chair. I excuse him immediately, as the environment has visibly affected his gastric stability. I get two buckets of warm soapy water and start with the floor, bedrails, hands, feet and then meet the rest of the cleaning needs. I take her on the potty chair directly into the shower. My other mother isn't affected with her condition or status…only with the fact that she gets cold with a shower…and maybe this is a normal day in another's world. Finally, soaking her fingernails and now all clean clothes.

Washer is already running to fill. I transfer her to the WC, but my son helps her back into bed, since it is the middle of the night. My son returns to his home to grab a few more hours of sleep. I run the washer and change the water in the scrub bucket. I wipe up the floor in her room again. She is resting quietly, but not sleeping. I walk to the living area of my little home, lower the handle on the Keurig, and listen to the cup of coffee brew. I have changed my clothes, as I also was affected in the cleaning process. I sit down, look at the clock which is telling me 3:32 AM. I add milk to my coffee, lower myself on the sofa with a bit of a flop—take a sip of my coffee and think— hello world, my day has already started—there is no planning on my part…my day is laid out ahead of me, often with an abrupt start. So I catch the ball that's been thrown, look at the cards that's been dealt and then take another large slurp of coffee…and know that my day is already full speed ahead.

Love,
Jud

Love stretches your heart and makes you big inside.

EMAIL TO MY SISTERS AND FAMILY

Another Thanksgiving…thankful for another year to share with my mother. Actually, the lady that lives with me has changed a lot in this past year. Her maternal instincts are present. That doesn't surprise me as she was the best mother and grandmother in the world. She had a whole township of kids that called her "Mawmaw" from her time in the elementary school next to the farm. I don't know one person that doesn't speak lovingly of my mother. My mother is no longer in control of herself. The damage to her brain is more obvious.

I hold her face in my hands as I kiss her forehead and remind her that "we got this Mom. Together we got this."

Bri has drove us up to Pennsylvania while he travels to the Philippines. I have her admitted to hospice—once again.

My oldest son's birthday is two days into December. He shares the day with my younger sister Jody. I was able to celebrate his fiftieth by baking cupcakes with his two young children, Jeffrey age five and Samantha age seven. Mom sat and watched, notably enjoying the excitement and activity as they heavily decorated their dad's birthday cupcakes.

Just a few days ago, I thought we were to the end of Mom's life. It seems she has gotten another second wind.

COME ON DECEMBER, BRING ANOTHER BIRTHDAY TO OUR MOTHER

Mom has been increasingly more restless, anxious, and disturbed. She has not been sleeping at night, nor does she nap during the day. Sunday night she was so very restless, that she was sure to fall. She became mad at me and very angry—she wouldn't stay in bed and began yelling. I tried medicating her, and finally she settled down sometime early morning. I put her Broda chair next to the recliner and tried getting her to sleep so I could sleep. When the nurse came the following morning, she got the hit with the full load. I told her I couldn't do this without her sleeping at night anymore.

Sister Jane told me she never saw someone so close to exhaustion. Hospice has a "respite program" of five days in a nursing center to give the caregiver time to recharge or rest or do whatever she needs to do. She had Mom admitted into the nursing facility at 6:30 PM that same day. I didn't have to put her name on a waiting list. She admitted her on the day I became totally worn out. I spent two days just here at Mom's home napping and resting. This hospice group is so involved. Hospice delivered an electric hospital low bed this afternoon…so I can lower it at night to prevent her from falling any distance.

Thank you, gra⬛⬛⬛⬛and holding Mawmaw's ha⬛⬛⬛⬛hank you

The third day at the nursing facility, I found myself there very early in the morning. They have Mom in a geri chair sitting at the nursing station. She is heavily medicated. I got help to put her back in bed. Mom is having pain in her head now. They told me she hadn't peed, so they were going to have hospice bladder scan her. I didn't realize that when she is in the respite program, hospice comes in to do her care. I questioned if the nursing staff could do the bladder scan?

The bladder scan read 623 cc. They then catheterized her with my help and received 700 cc right away. It quickly went up to 900 cc. So now they are wondering if her behavior was related to being toxic from the urine retention. Her BP was high, and she was holding her head in pain. They have been medicating her heavily to get control of the head pain and also to find a recipe for sleep. They have had her so medicated that she had slept for like forty-eight hours…with no food or drinks. I couldn't leave.

I don't know what is causing the head pain unless something related to the head wound is increasing the pressure in her head. Hospice only treats the symptoms, keep her comfortable, so I will never know what causes the pain. The source of pain really doesn't matter at this time, as long as we can stop the pain.

It's only when we truly know and understand that we have a limited time on earth—and that we have no way of knowing when our time is up—that we will begin to live each day to the fullest, as if it was the only one we had.

I'm not feeling good about Bri leaving for Florida next week without me. But right now, I just can't take her down in the condition she is now in. Beyond that, I have no idea what is ahead. Today we had a meeting with the funeral director and made the necessary arrangements now, instead of later.

It was a difficult decision not to take Mom back to Florida in the state of health she is in now, but it is obvious I can't do that. Bri will leave th_____ay and arrive in Pittsburgh on Tuesday _____rt driving back to
Fl_____d __ back